Frontiers in Cancer Immunology

(Volume 3)

Probiotics in Anticancer Immunity

Edited by

Mitesh Kumar Dwivedi

C. G. Bhakta Institute of Biotechnology & Faculty of Science
Uka Tarsadia University
Tarsadi, Bardoli, District Surat
Gujarat, India

Alwarappan Sankaranarayanan

Department of Life Sciences
Sri Sathya Sai University for Human Excellence Kamalapur
Navanihal, Kalaburagi
Karnataka State, India

&

Sanjay Tiwari

National Institute of Pharmaceutical Education and Research
(NIPER)-Raebareli, Lucknow,
Uttar Pradesh, India

Frontiers in Cancer Immunology

(Volume 3)

Probiotics in Anticancer Immunity

Editors: Mitesh Kumar Dwivedi, A. Sankaranarayanan and Sanjay Tiwari

ISBN (Online): 978-981-5124-78-1

ISBN (Print): 978-981-5124-79-8

ISBN (Paperback): 978-981-5124-80-4

need for a court order if at any point you breach any terms of this License Agreement. In no event will any delay or failure by Bentham Science Publishers in enforcing your compliance with this License Agreement constitute a waiver of any of its rights.

3. You acknowledge that you have read this License Agreement, and agree to be bound by its terms and conditions. To the extent that any other terms and conditions presented on any website of Bentham Science Publishers conflict with, or are inconsistent with, the terms and conditions set out in this License Agreement, you acknowledge that the terms and conditions set out in this License Agreement shall prevail.

Bentham Science Publishers Pte. Ltd.
80 Robinson Road #02-00
Singapore 068898
Singapore
Email: subscriptions@benthamscience.net

**BENTHAM
SCIENCE**

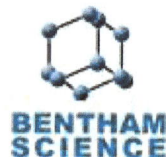

CONTENTS

FOREWORD

Nowadays, the probiotics field (a scientist that investigates; industry, production process; regulators, and protection to consumers, and consumers) is an interesting topic in the nutritional field that is constantly being discussed (medical, immunological) related to human health. Who thought that 100 years ago, when Russian immunologist Melnikoff noted that Bulgarian farmers are healthier and live longer? This Nobel Prize winner supposed that this is because the fermented milk they use contains live bacteria, which gave rise to the modern concept of probiotics, "live microorganisms which, when administered in adequate amounts, confer a health benefit on the host.

As a researcher in the probiotic field, it is always good to reinforce the knowledge and see how much we know about probiotics, and how they could help us in the prevention of children's diarrhoea, cases of allergy, or a coadjutant treatment in immunological disorders or even cancer.

Today I have the honour to introduce the volume 3 of book titled "Frontiers in Cancer Immunology [Probiotics in Anticancer Immunity]", which include a total of 11 chapters with 283 pages and edited by Dr. Mitesh Kumar Dwivedi, Dr. Alwarappan Sankaranarayanan, and Dr. Sanjay Tiwari.

The book is focused on the mechanical characteristics that probiotics generate in several human cancers, with evidence-based medicine based on human studies and its effects along with the comprehension of key molecules of cancer progression using animal studies. In my personal experience, knowing how probiotics work, we obtained a better general vision of their effects in different conditions. An expert team of researchers worked on the compilation of the book with a special final chapter related to "Future Challenges in Probiotics Based Anticancer Immunotherapy", which mention the need for more human clinical trials with a higher number of subjects that allow us to understand the correct dose/benefit of the use of probiotics as a coadjutant therapy.

I think that the present book will have an impact on the probiotics field because the topic is related to our clinical research; now, we will be investigating how microbes are present on the surface of different mucosa and how they could affect the progression of the disease or the treatment.

Hopefully, more investigation in the probiotic field will be made in the next years to understand the true mechanism of action of the probiotics in different human conditions.

All the best with the present book.

Julio Plaza-Diaz
Department of Biochemistry and Molecular Biology II
School of Pharmacy, University of Granada
Granada, Spain

PREFACE

The book 'Frontiers in Cancer Immunology (volume 3) Probiotics in Anticancer Immunity' is focused on the role of probiotics in exerting the anticancer immunity. With the diverse role of probiotics in benefitting the human health, their role in prevention and management of various human cancers cannot be denied. The book is focused on delivering the evidence of the use of probiotics in human cancers through several animal and human studies, in addition to highlighting their mechanistic role.

The book 'Probiotics in Anticancer Immunity' consists of total 11 chapters. The initial two chapters provide the basic background of the interaction of gut microbiota and host immune system in cancer and the different mechanisms by which probiotics can induce/exert the anticancer immunity.

The subsequent chapters deal with the specific cancer conditions such as cancer of skin, colon, colorectal, breast, stomach, liver, cervical, lung, and head & neck, and mechanistic role of probiotics in inducing the anticancer immunity. Moreover, the role of gut microbiota in the dysbiosis and management and/or prevention of these cancers is also put forward.

We, the editorial team, strongly believe that the contents of the individual chapters will provide recent and updated information as well as new insights into the role of probiotics in anticancer immunity. As such, the book will be useful in education and as a scientific tool for academics, clinicians, scientists, researchers, and health professionals in various disciplines including microbiology, medical microbiology, immunology, biotechnology, and medicine.

As the editors, we would like to express our sincere gratitude to all authors for their excellent contributions. We are also indebted to the publishers for their efforts to publish the book in a timely fashion.

Mitesh Kumar Dwivedi
C. G. Bhakta Institute of Biotechnology & Faculty of Science
Uka Tarsadia University
Tarsadi-394350, Bardoli, District Surat
Gujarat, India

Alwarappan Sankaranarayanan
Department of Life Sciences
Sri Sathya Sai University for Human Excellence Kamalapur
Navanihal, Kalaburagi
Karnataka State, India

&

Sanjay Tiwari
National Institute of Pharmaceutical Education and Research
(NIPER)-Raebareli Lucknow, Uttar Pradesh
India

List of Contributors

Anshul Shakya	Department of Pharmaceutical Science, Dibrugarh University, Dibrugarh, Assam, India
Amir Ghaemi	Department of Influenza and other respiratory viruses, Pasteur Institute of Iran, Tehran, Iran
Amruta Mohapatra	Institute of Life Sciences, Bhubaneswar, Odisha, India
Anderson Junger Teodoro	Universidade Federal do Estado do Rio de Janeiro, Laboratory of Functional Foods, , Rio de Janeiro, Brazil
Arul Prakash Francis	Centre of Molecular Medicine and Diagnostics (COMMAND), Saveetha Dental College and Hospitals, Saveetha Institute of Medical and Technical Sciences, Chennai, India
Archana Chaudhari	Dermatology Research Foundation, Vyara, Tapi, Gujarat, India
Alka Ahuja	College of Pharmacy, National University of Science and Technology, Muscat, Sultanate of Oman
Alwarappan Sankaranarayanan	Department of Life Sciences, Sri Sathya Sai University for Human Excellence Kamalapur, Navanihal, Kalaburagi, Karnataka State, India
Adriano Gomes da Cruz	Departamento de Alimentos, Instituto Federal de Educação, Ciência e Tecnologia do Rio de Janeiro (IFRJ), Rio de Janeiro, Brazil
Bindu Kumari	Department of Pharmacy, Central University of South Bihar, Gaya, Bihar, India
Cíntia Ramos Pereira Azara	Universidade Federal do Estado do Rio de Janeiro, Laboratory of Functional Foods, Rio de Janeiro, Brazil
Dhananjay Kumar Singh	Department of Pharmacy, Central University of South Bihar, Gaya, Bihar, India
Deog-Hwan Oh	Food Science and Biotechnology, School of Agriculture and Life Sciences, Kangwon National University, Chuncheon, Republic of Korea
Dhanalekshmi Unnikrishnan Meenakshi	College of Pharmacy, National University of Science and Technology, Muscat, Sultanate of Oman
Engkarat Kingkaew	Department of Biochemistry and Microbiology, Faculty of Pharmaceutical Sciences, Chulalongkorn University, Bangkok, Thailand
Elahe Abdolalipour	Department of Influenza and other respiratory viruses, Pasteur Institute of Iran, Tehran, Iran
Firdosh shah	C. G. Bhakta Institute of Biotechnology, Faculty of Science, Uka Tarsadia University, Tarsadi-394350, Bardoli, District Surat, Gujarat, India
Gireesh Kumar Singh	Department of Pharmacy, Central University of South Bihar, Gaya-Bihar, India
Gaurav Ranjan	Department of Pharmacy, School of Health Sciences, Central University of South Bihar-, India
Jayalaxmi Dash	Institute of Life Sciences, Bhubaneswar, Odisha, India

Kalaiselvi Selvaraj	Department of Microbiology, Goverment Arts And Science College (W), Orathanadu-, Tamil Nadu, India
Karnan Muthusamy	Grassland and Forage Division, National Institute of Animal Science, South Korea
Kaliyan Barathikannan	Food Science and Biotechnology, School of Agriculture and Life Sciences Kangwon National University, Chuncheon, Republic of Korea
Mitesh Kumar Dwivedi	C. G. Bhakta Institute of Biotechnology, Faculty of Science, Uka Tarsadia University, Tarsadi, Bardoli, District Surat, Gujarat, India
Mangala Lakshmi Ragavan	Biomedical Sciences Department, School of BioSciences and Technology, Vellore Institute of Technology, Vellore, Tamil Nadu, India
Mehran Mahooti	Department of Influenza and other respiratory viruses, Pasteur Institute of Iran, Tehran, Iran
Mahaveer Dhobi	Department of Pharmacognosy and Phytochemistry, School of Pharmaceutical Sciences, Delhi Pharmaceutical Sciences and Research University, New Delhi, India
Manisha Sethi	Institute of Life Sciences, Bhubaneswar, Odisha, India Regional Centre for Biotechnology, Faridabad, Haryana, India
Majed Abhukhader	College of Pharmacy, National University of Science and Technology, Muscat, Sultanate of Oman
Mishel Pulikondan francis	Department of Botany, Bharathidasan University, Tiruchirappalli-620 024, Tamil Nadu, India
Nathalia da Costa Pereira Soares	Universidade Federal do Estado do Rio de Janeiro, Laboratory of Functional Foods, Rio de Janeiro, Brazil
Nilanjana Das	Biomedical Sciences Department, School of BioSciences and Technology, Vellore Institute of Technology, Vellore, Tamil Nadu, India
Nosheen Masood	Department of Biotechnology, Fatima Jinnah Women University, The Mall, Rawalpindi, Pakistan
Nilanjan Ghosh	Department of Pharmaceutical Technology, Molecular Pharmacology Research Laboratory Jadavpur University, Kolkata, India
Nirupam Das	Department of Pharmaceutical Sciences, Susruta School of Medical and Paramedical Sciences, Assam University (A Central University), Silchar, Assam, India
Priyashree Sunita	Department of Health, Medical Education & Family Welfare, Bariatu, Government Pharmacy Institute, Ranchi, Jharkhand, India
Pedro Sánchez Pellicer	MiBioPath Group, Health and Science, Faculty, Catholic University of Murcia, Campus de los Jerónimos, Murcia, Spain
Pritha Bose	Institute of Nuclear Medicine and Allied Health Sciences, DRDO, Delhi, India
Panneerselvam Annamalai	P.G. and Research Department of Microbiology, A. V. V. M. Sri Pushpam College, Poondi, Tamil Nadu, India

Prashant Shankar Giri	C. G. Bhakta Institute of Biotechnology, Faculty of Science, Uka Tarsadia University, Tarsadi, Bardoli, District Surat, Gujarat, India
Rabinarayan Parhi	Department of Pharmaceutical Sciences, Susruta School of Medical and Paramedical Sciences, Assam University (A Central University), Silchar, Assam, India
Rajni Yadav	Faculty of Pharmacy, Kalinga University, Naya Raipur, Chhattisgarh, India
Ramachandran Chelliah	Food Science and Biotechnology, School of Agriculture and Life Sciences Kangwon National University, Chuncheon, Republic of Korea
Ravi Bhushan Singh	Institute of Pharmacy, HC PG College, Varanasi, Uttar Pradesh, India
Shakti Prasad Pattanayak	Department of Pharmacy, School of Health Sciences, Central University of South Bihar, India
Somboon Tanasupawat	Department of Biochemistry and Microbiology, Faculty of Pharmaceutical Sciences, Chulalongkorn University, Bangkok, Thailand
Sujitra Techo	Mahidol University, Nakhonsawan Campus, Nakhonsawan, Thailand
Saima Shakil Malik	Department of Genetics, Research Division, The University of Alabama at Birmingham, AL, USA
Shivaraju Amrutha	Department of Life Sciences, Sri Sathya Sai University for Human Excellence Kamalapur, Navanihal, Kalaburagi, Karnataka State, India
Shilpi Singh	Molecular Bioprospection Department, CSIR- Central Institute of Medicinal and Aromatic Plants, Lucknow- U.P, India
Sonal Sinha	Pragya College of Pharmaceutical Sciences, Gaya -823003, Bihar, India
Suaib Lqman	Molecular Bioprospection Department, CSIR- Central Institute of Medicinal and Aromatic Plants, Lucknow- U.P, India Department of Biotechnology, Iranian Research Organization for Science and Technology, Tehran, Iran
Seyed Mohammad Miri	Department of Influenza and other respiratory viruses, Pasteur Institute of Iran, Tehran, Iran
Suryakanta Swain	Department of Pharmaceutical Science, School of Health Sciences, Kaziranga University, Jorhat, Assam, India
Suvendu Kumar Sahoo	GITAM Institute of Pharmacy, GITAM Deemed to be University, Gandhi Nagar Campus, Visakhapatnam, Andhra Pradesh, India
Sandip Prasad Tiwari	Faculty of Pharmacy, Kalinga University, Naya Raipur, Chhattisgarh, India
Shanth Kumar Sushma	Department of Life Sciences, Sri Sathya Sai University for Human Excellence Kamalapur, Navanihal, Kalaburagi, Karnataka State, India
Swayambara Mishra	Institute of Life Sciences, Bhubaneswar, Odisha, India Regional Centre for Biotechnology, Faridabad, Haryana, India
Swati Patel	C. G. Bhakta Institute of Biotechnology, Faculty of Science, Uka Tarsadia University, Bardoli, Surat, Gujarat, India
Saikat Dewanjee	Department of Pharmaceutical Technology, Advanced Pharmacognosy Research Laboratory Jadavpur University, Kolkata, India

Selvasudha Nandakumar   Department of Biotechnology, Pondicherry University, Puducherry, India

Shantibhusan Senapati   Institute of Life Sciences, Bhubaneswar, Odisha, India

Steffi Pulikondan francis   Department of Microbiology, Cauvery College for Women, Tiruchirappalli, Tamil Nadu, India

Tamilkani Pichai   Department of Hospital Administration, Queens College of Arts and Science for Women; Punalkulam, Pudukkottai (Dt), Tamil Nadu, India

Vicente Navarro López   MiBioPath Group, Health and Science, Catholic University of Murcia, Campus de los Jerónimos, Murcia, Spain
Infectious Diseases Unit, University Hospital of Vinalopó, Carrer Tonico Sansano Mora Elche, Spain

Vijayalakshmi Selvakumar   Food Science and Biotechnology, School of Agriculture and Life Sciences, Kangwon National University, Chuncheon, Republic of Korea

CHAPTER 1

Gut Microbiota and Host Immune System in Cancer

Shakti Prasad Pattanayak[1,*], Gaurav Ranjan[1], Priyashree Sunita[2] and Pritha Bose[3]

[1] *Department of Pharmacy, School of Health Sciences, Central University of South Bihar, India*

[2] *Government Pharmacy Institute, Dept. of Health, Medical Education & Family Welfare, Bariatu, Ranchi, Jharkhand, India*

[3] *Institute of Nuclear Medicine and Allied Health Sciences, DRDO, Delhi, India*

Abstract: The mammalian gut is inhabited by more than 100 billion symbiotic microorganisms. The microbial colony residing in the host is recognised as microbiota. One of the critical functions of microbiota is to prevent the intestine against exogenous and harmful pathogen colonization mediated by various mechanistic pathways involving direct competition for limited nutrients and regulation of host immunity. Cancer accounts for one of the leading causes of mortality arising from multifactorial abnormalities. The interconnection of microbiota with various pathological conditions including cancer is recently being researched extensively for analysing tumor induction, progression, inhibition and diagnosis. The diversified microbial colony inhabiting the human gut possesses a vast and distinct metabolic repertoire complementary to the mammalian enzyme activity in the liver as well as gut mucosa which facilitates processes essential for host digestion. Gut microbiota is often considered the critical contributor to defining the biochemical profile of diet thus impacting the health and disease of the hosts. This chapter mainly focuses on understanding the complex microbial interaction with cancer either negatively or positively which may help to conceive novel precautionary and therapeutic strategies to fight cancer.

Keywords: Adenocarcinoma, Cancer, Carcinogenesis, Dysbiosis, Dysplasia, Gut microbiota, Hyperplasia, Homeostasis, Inflammatory pathways, Metaplasia, Metabolism, Metabolomics, Metagenomics, Oncogenes, Pathogens, Tumorigenesis.

[*] **Corresponding author Shakti Prasad Pattanayak:** Department of Pharmacy, School of Health Sciences, Central University of South Bihar (Gaya), Bihar India; E-mail: sppattanayak@cusb.ac.in

Mitesh Kumar Dwivedi, Alwarappan Sankaranarayanan & Sanjay Tiwari (Eds.)

1. INTRODUCTION

The gut microbiota of humans is recognized as a complex and dynamic heterogonous ecosystem which is comprised of diverse microbial communities such as bacteria, archaea, viruses, fungi, *etc.* interacting with each other and also with the host. All the genes of microorganisms taken together build a genetic repertoire representing an order of higher magnitude than that of humans. Being the most extensive micro-ecosystem existing in human body, it is considered an essential organ. Its symbiotic nature with host's body allows it to play a major role in regulating the various physiological processes. Gut microbiota is mainly categorized in four major sections namely *Firmicutes, Proteus, Bacteroides* and *actinomycetes*. The complex and cross-linked adaptive and innate immune system play a pivotal role in maintaining the homeostasis of host defence system against harmful pathogens. With the rapid advancement in molecular biology, bioinformatics, genomics, analysis technology *etc.* gut microbiota research has made immense progress. Such research has pointed out that compromised gut microbiota and their metabolites often contribute to pathological developments such as neurodegenerative problems, metabolic and gastrointestinal disorder and even cardiovascular diseases. Current evidence also reflects the involvement of microbiota in carcinogenesis and may improve the activity and efficacy of anticancer therapies or might also increase their toxicities in contrast. In this chapter we have summarized the relevance of gut microbial alteration with various cancers and also discussed the association of probable metabolic mechanisms of microbes and their derivatives with the development of cancer and also their facets of anti-tumorigenic properties. Thus, the present chapter reflects the link of gut microbiota with the host immune system and its role in the modulation of carcinogenesis.

2. HUMAN HEALTH AND DISEASE: ROLE OF GUT MICROBIOTA

More than 1000 million symbiotic microorganisms live inside human beings and exert a significant role in human health and disease. The gut microbiome has been considered a "fundamental organ" [1], containing about 150 times more genes than that of expressed in the entire human genome sequence [2]. Recent advancement in research has revealed that the microbiome is implicated in basic biological activities of human being, influencing innate immunity, regulating development of epithelium and modulation of metabolic phenotype [3 - 6]. Several chronic ailments like IBD, ulcerative colitis, obesity, metabolic disorder, atherosclerosis, ALD, NAFLD, liver cirrhosis, as well as hepatocellular cancer have been related through the human microbiome [7, 8]. In current decades, a remarkable extent of evidence has intensely recommended an important function of the gut microbiome in health and disease of humans being [9 - 23] *via* numerous mechanisms of actions. Significantly, gut microbiota has the ability to upsurge extraction of energy from nutrient, enhance nutrient production and modify signalling of appetite [9, 10]. Gut microbiota has additional multipurpose metabolic genes as compared to the genome of humans, and delivers individuals with specific and distinctive enzymes and several biological and chemical pathways [9]. Firstly, an immense quantity of the metabolic gut microbiota use that are advantageous towards the host are concerned in both acquirement of dietary or xenobiotic dispensation, comprising with the metabolic process of undigested biological compound and the vitamins production [10]. Secondly, the gut microbiota of human also delivers a bodily blockade, defending its host against external infectious agents through production of antimicrobial agents as well as competitive rejection [11 - 13]. In conclusion, gut microbiota shows a very important function in the expansion of the abdominal mucosa as well as immunity of the host [14 - 16].

2.1. The Human Microbiome in Health

The human microbiome has a significant impact on host physiology. Bacteria, viruses and trillions of other microorganisms colonize the body of human being, and the gut microbiota are directly associated with host physiology. While more than 1000 known bacterial species dwell in the body, innumerable other microbial genes have been identified in the human genome [2]. After birth, the mutualistic bacteria start colonizing in the host and subsequently evolve into a diversified ecosystem as the host body grows and develops [24]. Symbiotic bacteria assist in metabolism of indigestible food, supplement with requisite nutrients, extend protection against other pathogenic colonization and also play pivotal role in forming intestinal architecture [25]. Thus host-bacteria interrelation has evolved to be beneficial. The intestinal microbiota is involved in maintaining energy homeostasis and often facilitates the digestion of indigestible dietary fibres present in vegetables. While specific *Bacteroides* species help in digestion of xyloglucans present in vegetables, beneficial microorganisms like *Lactobacillus* and *Bifidobacterium* utilize fructo-oligosaccharides and oligosaccharides which are difficult for digestion by host [26, 27]. Moreover, earlier reports indicate that gut microbiota essentially participate in maintaining lipid and protein homeostasis and are involved in synthesis of microbial nutrients like vitamins [28]. Each day, 50 to 100 mmol/L of SCFAs produced by gut microbiota, including acetic acid, butyric and propionic acids, supply energy to the host intestine [29]. These easily absorbable SCFAs in the colon perform diversified roles and regulate motility of gut, inflammatory response, and metabolism of glucose and energy management [30, 31]. Additionally, the gut microbiota is also associated with the supply of essential vitamins to the host, like riboflavin, folates, cobalamine, biotin, *etc*. Gut-bacteria also regulate the gut immune system (humoral as well as cellular) [32]. The microbial metabolites, once recognized by hematopoietic and/or non-hematopoietic cells, trigger innate immunity that translates into physiological responses [33]. Tolerogenic response generated by gut colonizing bacteria restricts Th17 induced anti-inflammatory pathway in dendritic cells of gut [34].

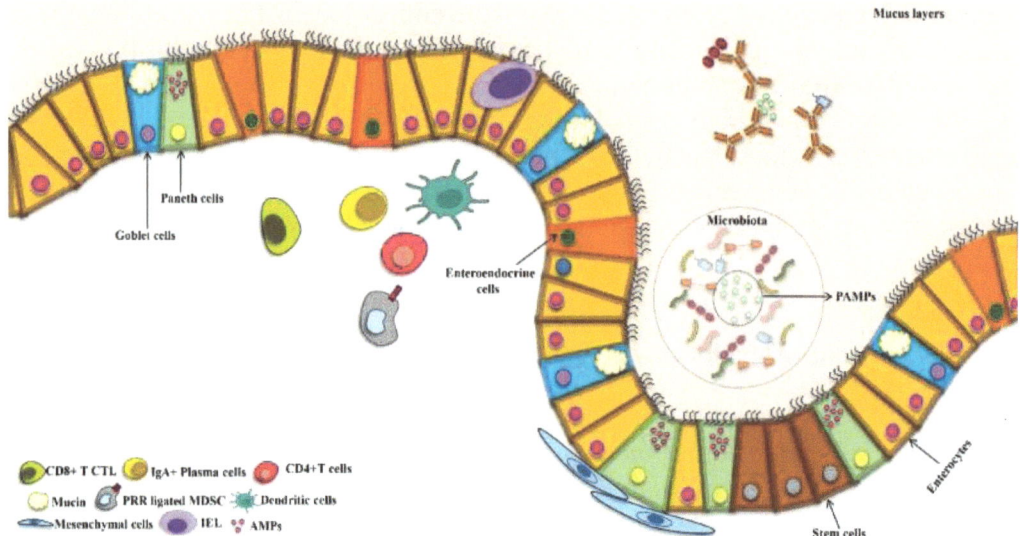

Fig. (1). The gut-immune axis. The GI lumen embodies the interface between the Gut Microbiota and the immune system. Intestinal cells consist of microvilli and embrace Goblet cells, Paneth cells, enterocytes, enteroendocrine cells and stem cells. IELs may exist within the epithelial cells. Goblet cells secrete mucin protein which enhances the intraluminal mucus layer. Paneth cells secrete AMPs. GM and GM-derived molecules form PAMPs, which are recognized by PRRs expressed on immune cells and gut epithelial cells. IgA molecules are secreted in the lumen, and they help to bind microbes and microbial-derived molecules. Immune cells are crucial in the initiation of immune-tolerance versus commensals and immune-reactivity against pathogens. Both innate immunity and adaptive immunity are involved in it. The immune cells are comprised of DCs, CD8$^+$ CTLs, MDSCs, IgA-producing plasma cells, and CD4$^+$ T-cells. The latter can be distinguished into different phenotypes which are involved in immune reactivity or tolerance (*i.e.*, Th1, Th2, Th17 and Tregs). [**Abbreviations:** CD, cluster of differentiation; CTL, cytotoxic T lymphocytes; PRR, pattern recognition receptors; MDSC, myeloid-derived suppressor cells; IEL, Intraepithelial lymphocytes; AMPs, Antimicrobial peptides; GI, gastro-intestinal; GM, gut microbiota; PAMPs, pathogen-associated molecular patterns; DCs, dendritic cells]

3. THE ROLE OF THE HUMAN MICROBIOME IN CANCER INDUCTION

3.1. Human Microbiome and Gastrointestinal Malignancy

Globally, gastrointestinal cancer is one of the main causes of death. In addition to the well-known genetic factors, non-genetic factors often accentuate the risk of

GIT cancer which the residential GIT microorganisms contribute majorly (Fig. 1). Progress in research related to microbial-induced GIT malignancies, like gastric, colorectal and esophageal cancer, has revealed novel roles of human gut microbiota in tumor development (Table 1).

Table 1. Composition of gut microbiota associated with various cancers.

Bacterial Strains and Virulence Factors (if known)	Types of Cancers	Deciphered Mechanisms and Signalling Pathways	Experimental Models	Reference
Helicobacter pylori (VacA)	Gastric cancer	Stimulates autophagic and Wnt/β-catenin pathway, upregulates expression of Kinases (MAPK, ERK1/2)	Mouse Epithelial cells	[35]
Porphyromonas gingivalis	Pancreatic cancer	Induces apoptosis, triggers STAT3 and NF-KB mechanistic pathways, interacts with toll-like receptors TLR2/4	Mouse Macrophages	[36]
Helicobacter hepaticus (Cytolethal distending toxin)	Hepatocellular cancer	Facilitates endoreplication and upregulates proliferation markers like p21 and Ki67	Mouse	[37]
Fusobacterium nucleatum (FadA and Fap2)	Colorectal cancer	Tiggers cellular proliferation, modulates E-cadherin and Wnt/B-catenin molecular signallings, increases cyclin D, NF-kB expressions. Modulation of TLR4 interactions, stimulation of β-catenin and NF-kB pathways, induces microRNA21 expression	Mice	[38]
Escherichia coli (Colibactin)		Accelerates formation of p-H2AX foci	Mice	[39]
Peptostreptococcus anaerobius		Aggravates cellular proliferation with simultaneous oxidative degeneration and also activates SREBP2/AMPK signalling nexus. Modulates interaction sod TLR2/4	Mice	[40]
Enterotoxigenic Bacteroides fragilis (Fragilysin)		Increases IL-1 expression and response of Th-17. Promotes cleavage of E-cadherin and activates B-catenin-STAT3 signalling	Stool sample	[41]

3.1.1. Gastric Cancer

Chronic inflammation induced by *H. pylori* is considered one of the distinctive causes of gastric cancer and is classified by World Health Organization (WHO) as a class I carcinogen. Almost 6,60,000 new gastric cancer cases reported each year are related to *H. pylori* infection that causes degeneration of parietal cells instigating gastric tissue deterioration, metaplasia and dysplasia, which lead to carcinogenesis [42]. Studies reported that *H. pylori* elimination prior to the initiation of degenerative gastritis limits the risk of gastric cancer [43]. However, the predisposition to gastric tumorigenesis is often dependent on various factors such as genetic variation in the *H. pylori* strain, diversities in retaliation of the host, and also on the distinct interactions between host and microbe [44]. The risk of gastric cancer development is often found to be essentially related to the phylogenetic origin of *H. pylori* [45]. Among the various *H. pylori* determinants, the two which primarily aggravated the carcinogenic risks are CagA (cytotoxin-associated antigen-A) and VacA (vacuolating cytotoxin) [46]. In response to specific *H. pylori* infection in the host, VacA stimulates gastric cell apoptosis and induces mitochondrial dysfunction leading to carcinogenesis [47]. Moreover, host immunity is also documented to be suppressed by VacA *via* dendritic cells' expression and release of anti-inflammatory cytokines (IL-10/ IL-8). Such a disrupted host immune system facilitates the evasion of *H. pylori* and potentiates tumor survival [48]. In contrast to VaCA, the risk of developing gastric adenocarcinoma is exponentiated by PAI (cag pathogenicity island) existing in certain *H. pylori* strains [49]. The cag PAI houses specific genes encoding the proteins that are responsible for forming bacterial secretion system- type IV (T4SS). CagA and other peptidoglycans exported into the host system from *H. pylori via* activation of PI3K signalling nexus, stimulate cell migration and contribute to tumorigenesis [50]. Moreover, phosphorylated CagA, through interaction and activation of different cellular proteins within the host, alters morphological characteristics such as cell scattering along with elongation [51]. Lertpiriyapong *et al.* [52] also documented that insulin-gastrin mice develop worse gastric pathology due to the synergetic establishment of ASF (Altered Schaedler's flora) that caused inflammation of gastric corpus, hyperplasia and dysplasia of gastric epithelial cells.

3.2. Colorectal Cancer

Recent research also focuses on deciphering the interlink between colonizing gut microbes and colon cancer incidence. Microbial dysbiosis often contributes to the complex etiology of adenomas and colorectal cancer. The adenomas exhibit a pathological lack of diversity and imbalance in the microbial community [53, 54]. Various studies revealed that both adenomas and colorectal cancer result due to a lack of "good" bacteria colonization, such as butyrate-producing bacteria, and infestation of of high proportion of pathogenic bacterial strains like *Pseudomonas, Acinetobacter, Helicobacter, etc* [53]. The gut microbiota from neoplasmic-generating mice has been shown to stimulate tumor formation and inflammation in selected animals, thus explicitly contributing to colorectal cancer [54]. The relationship between the gut microbiome and colorectal cancer progression is studied *via* mechanistic insight. Though, this fact remains still uncertain from clinical trials whether any alteration or change in the gut microbiota is a reason or repercussion of colorectal cancer or adenomas. Furthermore, the role of certain bacterial agents in cancer risk has yet to be clearly elucidated. *Fusobacterium nucleatum*, one of the periodontal infectious agents, was proposed to be excessive in the course of the progression of infection from adenomas to cancer [55]. A noteworthy upsurge in many bacteria, including *Bacteroides* species like *Bacteroides ovatus, Bacteroides fragilis, Bacteroides vulgatus, Bacteroides massiliensis* and *Escherichia coli,* has been witnessed from high-grade adenoma to carcinoma [56]. The progression of infection or inflammation, as well as the growth of tumors, are the most likely mechanisms that cause this growth [57, 58]. Fragilysin, a toxin produced by the Entero-toxigenic bacterium *Bacteroides fragilis*, stimulates the NF-κB pathway as well as the Wnt signalling pathway. This can escalate the proliferation of cells and the generation of several inflammatory mediators like TNF-α, IL-8, GRO-alpha, IL-1β, and IL-5 [59 - 61]. The protagonist by *Enterotoxigenic Bacteroides fragilis* (ETBF) in CRC was additionally exemplified in the study of Wu *et al.* [62]. The study revealed that ETBF colonized mice showed a noticeable proliferation in colon carcinomas and tumorigenesis as compared to normal control. Moreover, *Enterococcus faecalis* and *Escherichia coli* may possibly cause DNA impairment by stimulating the discharge of O_2^- in host cells extracellularly and encrypting the enzymatic mechanism of action that produces a genotoxic metabolite called colibactin by means of complex enzymes, namely polyketide synthases (PKSs) [63, 64]. Though these reports illustrate a causative involvement by gut microbiota in the colorectal neoplastic process, further detailed studies are required to conclude their effectiveness as colorectal carcinoma biomarkers, and also their efficacy as theranostic targets. Furthermore, many metabolites isolated from bacteria have been associated with the subdual of CRC progression, which includes short-chain fatty acids (SCFAs) that are formed *via* microbial enzymatic decomposition of complex carbohydrates, including a salt of acetic acid, salt of propionate and salt of butyrate, which acts as source of energy for colonic columnar epithelium. Ester of butyric acid, which is predominantly produced by several species within the obligate anaerobic bacterium family, mainly *Oscillospiraceae* and

Lachnospiraceae, has shown its potential to be defensive against colonic neoplastic process. A fibre-rich diet has apparently shown a decrease in the possibility of causing colon maliciousness due to the secretion of ester of butyric acid [65, 66]. *In vitro* cancer cell line study revealed that ester of butyric acid has the potential to suppress tumorigenesis by inducing apoptosis, hindering proliferation, causing epigenetic variations in transcription, modifying inflammatory mediators and production of cytokines [67]. Therefore, modification of the intestinal microbiome *via* nutritional regulation as well as microbicidal therapy can propose an abundant theranostic prospective. The synthesis of SCFAs occurs due to manipulation of intestinal microbiota and can be attained with the use of non-nutritious food or prebiotic ingredients and might be a promising method to sequence host metabolic rate, which ultimately influences risk against cancer.

3.3. Oesophageal Cancer

Current research revealed that gastro-oesophageal reflux causes oesophageal chronic inflammation and is very closely associated with esophageal adeno-carcinoma. The complete pathophysiology of the progression method could be referred to as "gastro-esophageal reflux disease-Barrett's esophagus esophageal adeno-carcinoma" (GERD–BE–EA) [68 - 70]. Local alterations in its occurrence seem to be interrelated with fiscal expansion. As a result, scientists have recommended that the disease from esophageal adenocarcinoma can be associated with the practice of microbicidal globally. Continuing alterations in the esophageal microenvironment after repeated microbicidal experiences may cause a greater incidence of gastro-esophageal reflux disease, consequently leading to an upsurging disease from esophageal adenocarcinoma [71]. A number of detailed researches have described noticeable esophageal micro-environmental changes in subjects with gastro-esophageal-reflux disease [72]. However, the regional microbiome does not differentiate between adenocarcinoma and epidermoid carcinoma [73]. Furthermore, the action of *Helicobacter pylori* in the pathophysiology of GERD and esophageal adenocarcinoma still remains indistinct and contentious. *H. pylori* bacterium was primarily recognized by the World health Organization as a cancer-causing agent related to adenocarcinoma of the stomach before the 2000s. Moreover, scientists have discovered that, with the drop in *H. pylori* infection, gastro-esophageal reflux disease frequency has augmented [74]. A sequence of case-referent studies also recommended that *H. pylori* may cause the development of gastro-esophageal reflux disease and associated esophageal adenocarcinoma. Nevertheless, the elimination of *H. pylori* therapy may not exacerbate gastro-esophageal reflux disease or surge new GERD [75].

4. FUNCTION OF GUT MICROBIOTA IN HOST PHYSIOLOGY AND METABOLISM OF NUTRIENTS

The fact that the gut microbiota plays such an important role in the host's metabolic process and health, has prompted research into the microbial population and their activity in related metabolic processes, especially those involving nutritional component metabolism. For survival, most intestinal bacteria depend on undigested dietary in the upper digestive tract. While useful metabolites are generally produced by Saccharolytic bacteria, in case of limited carbohydrate sources, the bacteria rely on alternative sources for energy leading to detrimental metabolite production for the host body [76], thereby affecting the health also. The SCFAs are the key substances produced by bacteria through the fermentation of dietary carbohydrates. Among them, acetate, propionate, and butyrate are the three most abundantly found SCFAs in faeces (ratio ranging from 3:1:1 to 10:2:1) [77]. These major SCFAs regulate diversified and critical roles in human physiology. Butyrate is mostly recognized as the essential SCFA for human well-being, as it produces a key energy source necessary for host colonocytes and also possesses anticarcinogenic properties. Butyrate also exerts an apoptotic effect on colon cancer cells and also leads to histone deacetylase inhibition, thereby regulating the gene regulation [78]. Evidence also supports the ability of butyrate to activate the intestinal gluconeogenesis (IGN) mediated by the CAMP-dependent pathway, which facilitates glucose along with energy homeostasis [79]. Propionate, on the other hand, also acts as a source of energy for epithelial cells, and when transferred to the liver, it participates in hepatic gluconeogenesis. Its role in satiety signalling is also becoming increasingly prominent because of its interaction with gut receptors like GPR41 (G-protein coupled receptor) and GPR43 (also recognised as FFAR2 (fatty acid receptors FFAR2/3) which consequently may lead to IGN activation [79 - 81]. The IGN-mediated formation of glucose from propionate directly stimulates energy homeostasis *via* reduction of hepatic glucose production, subsequently reducing obesity [79]. Acetate is not only the furthermost abundantly found SCFAs but it is also an important metabolite or cofactor that promotes the growth of bacteria such as *Faecalibacterium prausnitzii* [82]. In humans, acetate is found to accentuate cholesterol metabolism as well as lipogenesis whereas; studies in rodents indicate its pivotal role in regulating appetite [83]. Lactate, fumarate, succinate and other fermentation products synthesized intermediately by bacteria are usually detectable in faeces of healthy individual in lower levels due to their maximum utilization by other bacteria. For example, other bacteria have been observed to convert lactate into propionate or butyrate, which results in trace amount of lactate in adult faeces. However, a significant rise in lactate levels is often detected in patients suffering from ulcerative colitis which in turn serve as a disease indicator also [84]. Moreover, the effect of interactions between different bacteria on final detection of SCFA has also been discussed in different co-culture cross feeding studies. *Bifidobacterium longum* grown on fructo-oligosaccharides (FOS) produced lactate; however, the lactate completely disappeared when co-cultured with *Eubacterium hallii*. Moreover, significant high levels of butyrate replaced the lactate, though *Eubacterium hallii* solely failed to grow on carbohydrate-rich substrate [85]. On the other hand, acetate is known to stimulate growth of *Roseburia intestinalis,* and when it was co-cultured with *B. longum,* a delay in *the* growth of *R. intestinalis* was observed on fructo-oligosaccharides till enough acetate was formed in the growth medium by *B. longum* [86].

SCFA production specificity by intestinal bacterial species: While most bacteria are reported to produce acetate, only a few bacterial species produce butyrate and propionate [87, 88]. *Firmicutes* are major butyrate producers in gastrointestinal environment and include *Lachnospiraceae* and *Faecalibacterium prausnitzii,* and *Negativicutes.*Certain *Clostridium* species are predominant producers of propionate. Also, different organisms possessing butyrate synthesis pathways have also been identified by metagenomic studies [89]. Since bacterial phylogeny does not define SCFA production, different approaches targeting typical genes are necessary for enumerating bacteria with specific metabolic processes. Two major butyrate production routes and three propionate synthesis pathways have been identified by Louis and co-workers in a colonic microbial colony [90]. The primers intended against the critical metabolic genes involved in these signalling pathways may assist in revealing bacterial functional groups in different cohorts. This technique may also be more beneficial than the recently studied *16S rRNA* gene sequencing, which indicates bacterial composition but provides no information about fluctuations in metabolic activities.

5.   ISOLATION   OF   INTESTINAL   MICROBES   IN   DIETARY METABOLIZATION

Various studies, including those reporting gut microbiota-mediated daidzein (soy isoflavone) metabolism to equol, indicate the specific role of certain gut microorganisms in metabolizing dietary components. Matthies *et al.* [91] reported the isolation of a new microbial strain from an equol-producing participant by serially diluting faecal homogenate and successively incubating in daidzein and tetracycline-containing broth which potentially prevented the growth of different faecal microorganisms without affecting the daidzein metabolism. A novel species was thus identified after characterizing the pure culture both phenotypically and phylogenetically and was named *Slackia isoflavoniconvertans.* Environmental microbiology includes methods like enrichment techniques for the isolation of organisms mediating contaminants and xenobiotic degradation in the environment. Usually, suspension batch or continuous batch culture enrichment techniques are employed in which mixed microbial culture is subjected to incubation with xenobiotics, behaving as a selection factor and a sole source of carbon [92]. Although these methods promote organism's isolation or sometimes consortia which facilitate dietary substance metabolism, such techniques have not been extensively employed in the field of gut microbiota of human. In one study [93], carbon sources like xylan and pectin or cellulose-containing nutrient medium were inoculated with faeces from cattle for 8-weeks in continuous culture fermenters under conditions mimicking the environment of cattle colon and caecum. Subsequently, serial dilutions of samples were followed with carbohydrate-specific agar plating for isolation of colonies which were successively identified with the help of 16S rRNA gene sequencing. This enrichment procedure led to the growth of communities that represented a wide microbial spectrum demonstrating six main phyla, namely *Actinobacteria, Bacteroidetes, Fusobacteria, Synergistetes, Firmicutes* and *Proteobacteria*. Among the isolated strains, *Bacteroidetes* and *Firmicutes* were associated with species known for possessing enzymes required for the fermentation of components of plant cell walls. However, they did not identically match sequences of cultured bacteria in the ribosomal database project, signifying a new genera or species. Thus, this technique may propel newer opportunities for characterizing metabolic capabilities of different members belonging to gut microbiota. Even though the isolation methods of strain with the potential to metabolize dietary compounds reflect potential microbes complicated in *in vivo* processes, they have a few drawbacks. Particularly, such techniques only focus on the bacteria that have been cultured in *in vitro* [94]. Currently, microbiota research focuses on sequencing techniques for describing either the composition or probable abundance of the microbial colony. However, the evaluation of specific functions performed by the diversified microorganism still remains to be widely explored, which will be beneficial for the elucidation of mechanisms linking gut microbiota and metabolism [95].

5.1. Omics Approaches

The incorporation of top-down methods for researching the functionality and composition of microbiota, known as 'omics' approaches, is being extensively explored. While, metagenomics gives the perception of the genes which might be articulated, meta-transcriptomics exposes evidences regarding regulatory systems as well as the expression of gene. Metabolomics, on the other hand, notifies the functionality of the microbiome and consequently gives a lot of information on the intestinal microbial community. Because each 'omic' technology enables a distinct perspective on the microbiota and its effect on the host, numerous 'omic' techniques can be used concurrently and the results are merged, usually from the same samples, to completely harness their potential. This enables to understand the impact of the microbial community on the entire biological process at the molecular scale with the use of computer modelling [96].

5.2. Metagenomics

Metagenomics has been widely utilised to look at variations in microbiota composition in illness states like diabetes, obesity and inflammatory bowel disease related to healthy people; however, it has also found new modifications in microbiome activity in specific disorders [97]. In contrast to control participants, the faecal microbiome of 20-patients using hepatitis-B cirrhosis of the liver showed elevation of branched-chain AA (amino-acids), glutathione, nitrogen, gluconeogenesis and lipids, as well as a reduction in AAA and bile acid linked metabolism, according to Wei *et al* [98]. The functional genes of intestinal microbiota are progressively being studied using metagenomic analysis. This methodology was used by Jones *et al.* to investigate the location of *BSH* genes [99]. They discovered the functioning BSH in each of the major bacterial groups and Archaea within the gut using metagenomic analysis, demonstrating that bioidentical synthetic hormone is a persistent response to the quantity of combined bile-acids inside the intestine with a greater level of duplication. The technique employed in a recent study by Mohammed & Guda is particularly related to the current review [100]. The approach was subsequently used to examine the effect of microbe-derived enzymes responsible for metabolism and anticipate enzymes transcribed by human gut microbiome using the gut metagenomic data. They found 48 pathways with at least one enzyme encoded by bacteria. Vitamins, amino acids, lipids and co-factors were all metabolised by these pathways. The approaches were then used to show variations in the profile of gut microbiota-derived enzymes in obese and lean participants, as well as in IBD patients. Polygalactouronase, which is produced by *Prevotella* and *Bacteroides* species, was found to be abundant in obese persons' gut microbiota. However, in obese versus thin people, the urease-encoding bacteria were identified in lower numbers.

5.3. Meta Transcriptomics

Meta transcriptomics is the process of extracting and sequencing mRNAs from the microbial environment in order to determine which genes are articulated in those ecosystems. It generally begins with reverse transcription to create c-DNA, which is subsequently sequenced by using metagenomics-related methods. Meta transcriptomics enables the discovery of new non-coding RNAs that are hypothesised to be involved in biochemical functions, including quorum detection as well as stress outcomes [101, 102]. In a clinical meta-transcriptomic investigation of faecal microbiota [103], the microbial c-DNAs of every sample were decoded using 454 methodologies. Moreover, evaluation of the 16S ribosomal RNA transcription demonstrated that *Bacteroidetes*, as well as *Firmicutes*, caused most of the transcription (31 and 49%), with fewer amounts from *Actinobacteria* (0.4%), *Lentisphaerae* (0.2%) and *Proteobacteria* (3.7%). Meta transcriptomics, like all 'omics' techniques, has limits, and investigations are technically and bioinformatically demanding. Because of the small half-life of mRNA, detecting short-term reactions to changes in the environment is challenging [104].

5.4. Meta-proteomic

Meta-proteomic tries to define the entire profile of translation of gene outcomes and can provide extra information regarding posttranslational alterations and localization than meta-transcriptomics data [105]. One benefit of meta-proteomic is the ability to relate proteins to particular taxonomic groupings, giving insight into microbiota at the species and subspecies levels complicated in certain catalytic activities and signalling pathways, for example, phenotype-genotype correlations [106]. Meta-proteomic approaches are still in progress; however, they typically entail heat treatment of a faeces sample and intensive beads battering to extract as well as deform the peptides, which are then enzymatically degraded to peptides. The most common method of peptide testing is nano-2D-LC-MS-MS, with COG designations obtained using BLAST against the NCBI COG dataset for every peptide sequence. The functions of microbial communities are studied by categorising proteins into Children's Oncology Group groups. The meta-proteomic investigations on the intestine microbes have been conducted in a limited number of participants (typically n=1 to 3), limiting the inferences which can be taken; however, the outcomes have exposed consistency. Verberkmoes *et al.* performed a faecal meta-proteomic investigation on a group of mature female twins of monozygotic [107]. The proteins found by selected databases were categorised into COG categories after being analysed using nano-2D-LC-MS-MS. Nucleotide metabolism, amino acid metabolism, energy production, glucose metabolism, protein folding and translation were the COG activities with the highest frequency in both patients. The authors have compared the meta-proteomic profiles to a previously released meta-genomic status of two participants, which disclosed, in comparison to, the greatest plentiful roles recognised in the meta-proteome. The metagenome has been controlled *via* proteins related to the metabolism of inorganic ion, cellular biogenesis, cell proliferation, and bioactive compound bio-synthesis. Meta-proteomic was also used on faecal samples from an obese and lean person, as well as assessments of CDP (Crohn's Disease Patients) and normal participants by Xiong *et al.* [105]. Young *et al.* employed acoustic proteomics to investigate modifications in the faecal bacteria of a premature new-born (72 to 21 days of delivery) [106]. According to the findings, the growing bacterial population emphasizes its energies on cellular division, creation of protein, and metabolism of lipids before shifting to more complicated metabolic roles like metabolism of glucose and protein secretion and proteins trafficking. It is worth noting that the operational distribution observed after three weeks, matched that of the adolescent human intestine [107].

5.5. Metabolic Summarizing (metabolomics/ Metabonomics)

The metabolic profile has been developed by means of a potent systems biology tool for obtaining the metabolic activity or phenotype by simultaneously detecting the low-molecular-weight molecules within the biological fluid. These metabolic profiles inside the host consist of thousands of biological macromolecules derived endogenous and external metabolic signalling pathways, ecological stimuli, and host-environment metabolic collaborations. Dietary ingredients and by-products of gut microbes' activity might be considered environmental factors. The capacity to quantify metabolites in host specimens that are directly derived from the microbiota, such as SCFAs, is a significant advantage of employing metabonomic to examine the intestinal flora. This shows the detail of gut microbes action and changes because of food. Moreover, after absorption from intestine, bacterial substances can infiltrate the metabolic systems of host, causing down-stream metabolic disruptions and the formation of microbial host co-metabolites, which can then be detected by metabolic sequencing.

6. THE CROSSTALK BETWEEN IMMUNE SYSTEM AND MICRO-BIOTA

Because the microbiota flora is formed during the prenatal stage together with immunological formation, and the gut, as that of the major immunological organ, seems to be the main microbiota host, it is apparent that the microbiome could play a role in immune system response regulation [108]. Research on germ-free (GF) mice revealed that a loss of microbiome is associated with a significant impairment in the intestine's lymphoid tissue development and immunological activities [109]. At different levels, the gut microbiome has a wide range of impacts on adaptive and innate immune systems. Similarly, these microorganisms have the ability to influence both systemic and local immune responses in their hosts [110 - 113]. Several body cells, especially immune cells, carry pattern recognition receptors as pathogenic component detectors. TLRs are mostly expressed on macrophages and B-cell among PRRs. Microbes interact with this category of receptor to induce local immunogenicity [114, 115]. Furthermore, interactions with pattern recognition receptors trigger local dendritic cells by microorganisms or their metabolites and by-products [111 - 116]. The locally activated dendritic cells (DCs) can subsequently move to regional lymph nodes, causing novice T-cells to differentiate into Th17 as well as regulatory T-cells (Tregs) [117]. A subset of such effector T-cells returns to their initial place and governs local immune function once more. However, a subpopulation of T-cells relocates to the circulatory system, where they generate systemic immunity. Th17 cells, by secreting cytokines like IL-17 or stimulating neutrophils, can cause inflammatory immune reactions [118]. In contrast, Tregs, which are considered important gatekeepers in immunological regulation, orchestrate inflammation reduction to inhibit unwanted immune reactions *via* engaging dendritic cells and secreting TGF-β and IL-10 [119]. The Th17 cells are typically found in the small intestine's basal lamina. During intriguing research, GF mice lacking Th17 cells were identified and colonised by the particular subgroup of bacteria known as segmental filamentous bacteria. Such commensal bacteria may cause Th17 cells to accumulate in the intestinal lumen. This intriguing link endorses the important function of commensal bacteria in Th17 cell stimulation and promotes human defence against microbial diseases [120]. During the 1st year of life, the microbial population in the new-born gut influences Treg population formation [121]. The number of Treg cells in the basal lamina was reduced considerably in antibiotic-treated or GF mice, implying that the microbiome plays a role in Treg development or maintenance. The colonisations of GF mice with numerous *Clostridium* strains are sufficient to generate Treg in the gastrointestinal system [122]. Transfection of *Bacteroides fragilis*, a common human intestinal bacterium, also resulted in the production of Tregs in mice [123]. B-lymphocytes, which are the key mediators of gastrointestinal mucosal homeostasis, by generating immunoglobulin-A (IgA), are also affected by the composition of human microbes. Several investigations have shown that the concentration of this secreted antibody is notably reduced in GF as well as new-born mice, but that this is reversible after the microbiota colonises the animals [124].

7. MECHANISM OF GUT MICROBIOTA IN ANTICANCER IMMUNITY

Several studies have highlighted the microbiota's dual function in maintaining the host's health. Commercial microorganisms can safeguard the host's homeostasis in a number of different ways, including by producing a variety of metabolites and by-products [125, 126]. The microbiome often helps in lowering cancer rates and inflammatory response. The host microbiome has a number of roles that can help to prevent tumour growth and progression.

7.1. Improvement of Antitumor Immunity

Microbiota may be able to reduce tumour cell power by modifying anti-tumor immunity. In the tumour microenvironment (TME), for example, beneficial microbiota activates the NK cell-DC axis by regulating monocytes [127, 128]. In comparison to control mice, *Lactobacillus acidophilus*, *Bifidobacterium lactis* and *Lactobacillus rhamnosus*, fed mice showed improved immune systems as it increased the phagocytic activity of peritoneal macrophages as well as peripheral blood leucocytes. Furthermore, compared to untreated cells, spleen cells of mice nourished with these probiotics showed increased cytotoxic effects of NK cells. As a result, lactic acid bacteria alter both innate and acquired immune responses [129]. Mice colonised with 11 strains of bacteria taken from healthy human faeces and accomplished of IFN-γ producing CD8$^+$ T-cells demonstrated significant resistance to tumour formation, according to the study. Human microbiota and their anti-tumor immunity effects were ascribed with this ability [130].

7.2. Inflammation Reduction

Inflammation is now widely recognised as a key factor in cancer development. Anti-inflammatory mechanisms in certain commensal microorganisms can help them modulate tumour formation. For example, *E. coli,* such as KUB-36, which has the ability to generate 7 SCFAs, triggered anti-inflammatory action resulting in slowed tumour growth. The inflammatory cytokines such as IL-1β, IL-6, IL-8 and TNF-α were all suppressed by SCFAs as well as additional metabolites of *E. coli* like KUB-36 [131]. *Faecalibacterium prausnitzii* is yet another common bacterium that has anti-inflammatory properties. *F. prausnitzii* has been revealed to exert anti-inflammatory action in Caco2 colorectal cells by inhibiting NF-kB stimulation and IL-8 release. This microbiome's activation of peripheral blood mononuclear cells led to a rise in the IL-10/IL-12 ratio [132]. These findings support the argument that existing in gluten-free environs makes people more prone to infections and illness growth [133].

7.3. Systemic Genotoxicity Reduction

Gluten-free diet mice transfected with wild microbiota from related animals reported enhanced resistance to certain mutagen factors, as well as a higher chance of survival [113]. As observed in the oral injection of *L. johnsonii* into B-cell lymphoma-sensitive animals, the positive effect of certain bacteria against cancer could be due to a decrease in systemic genotoxicity [134]. Inflammatory mediators are the primary cause of systemic genotoxicity [135], and *L. johnsonii* drastically decreases the number of immune cells like T-cells and NK, along with pro-inflammatory factors, while increasing anti-inflammatory cytokines. As a result, it contributed to the removal of intra-cellular and systemic genotoxic substances [134].

7.4. Stimulation Of Anti-tumor Signalling Pathways

According to new data, anticancer benefits of healthy microbiota are thought to be mediated *via* anti-tumor signalling stimulation. For example, P8, a probiotic-derived protein, has been shown to be a novel therapeutic for colorectal carcinoma [136]. The entangled mechanism in P8's anti-proliferative effects was cell-cycle apprehension in G2-phase through p53-p21 pathway. Surprisingly, endogenous P8 articulation had a two-fold anti-proliferative effect when compared to exogenous cure. Oral administration of *L. acidophilus* to mice with colorectal cancer could control tumour growth by enhancing apoptosis [137]. Another study found that this probiotic hindered cancer cell growth and pushed them toward apoptosis by down-regulating MAPK and NF-kB signalling. *Lactobacillus reuteri* inhibited cell growth proteins like cyclin D1 and Cox-2 and antiapoptotic proteins like Bcl-xL and Bcl-2 [138]. Secondary substance bile acids inhibited mammary cancer cell growth and repressed the primary tumour aggressive nature by provoking the mesenchymal to epithelial transition [139]. Disruption to the cell surface of HT29 colon carcinoma cells was prevented by cell-free *Lactobacillus* supernatants [140]. Another study found that isolated lactic-acid bacteria cell-free supernatant exhibits anticancer effects in two colorectal cancerous cells [141].

8. INTERLINK OF CANCER RISK WITH MICROBIOME

Although it is widely established that the existence of the host microbiota causes mutagen resistance in contrast to viral resistance, increasing evidence suggests that specific microbiomes are linked to the progression and development of particular cancers [142]. Microbes and associated metabolites are thought to be responsible for approximately 20% of all cancer cases globally [143]. *Helicobacter pylori* have been recognized as a significant microorganism in the growth of gastric cancer [144, 145]. Numerous modes of action (MOA) are recommended which demonstrate that gut microbiota adds to the development of cancer, which includes the occurrence of inflammation [146], relocation of observable traits of vulnerable tumor [147], suppression of immune system, induction of promotion of generation of tumor environment, and mutagenic growth [148].

8.1. Induction of Inflammation

Carcinogenesis is frequently thought to be subsequent to localised long-term inflammation, which is one of cancer's hallmarks [149]. For example, carcinogenesis can occur as a result of the production of pro-inflammatory toxins generated by bacteria such as *Bacteroides fragilis* [150, 151]. The microbiome influences inflammatory actions mainly by increasing the synthesis of IL-1, IL-23 and IL-17 *via* myeloid cells and T-cells in dysbiotic conditions [152]. In the host, some *Streptococcus* species, including *Streptococcus parasanguinis* and *Streptococcus australis,* were associated with elevated IFN-γ, a pro-inflammatory cytokine. Various inflammatory cytokines produced by specific microbiomes can cause DNA damage in a variety of ways, including abnormal methylation of DNA. Over time, these DNA alterations may result in tumorigenesis [153]. TLR5 stimulates the production of IL-6 in the existence of commensal microbes, resulting in inflammation and increased tumour growth [154]. Long-term inflammation can also cause dysbiosis by modifying the composition of typical flora and raising the possibility of particular bacteria with genotoxic abilities, thereby providing an environment conducive to tumour development [155, 156] (Fig. **2**). However, some bacteria, like *Helicobacter pylori*, have significant genotoxic actions on the cell growth signalling pathway [145].

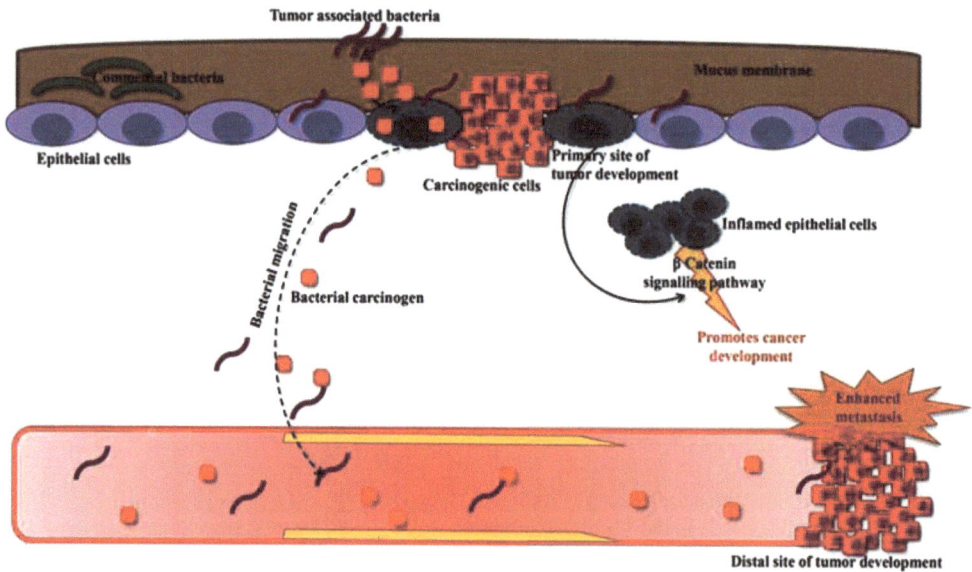

Fig. (2). **Role of microbes and their metabolites in the tumor environment.** Many bacteria secrete metabolites and carcinogens that initiate oncogenic and inflammatory responses which influence the gut microbiota constitution, thereby enhancing the development of cancer. Lastly, tumor-associated bacteria move from their primary site to the distal tumor site *via* systemic circulation to initiate metastasis.

8.2. Immunosuppression

Fusobacterium nucleatum, a periodontal microorganism found in the micro-environment of a variety of malignancies [156], suppresses the immune system by inhibiting NK cells. These immune cells were inhibited in the presence of *F. nucleatum* due to the interaction of the *F. nucleatum* Fap2 protein with the inhibitory NK-cell receptor TIGIT. Because CD4+ memory T- cells also prompt T cell immune-globulin and domain of ITIM, their behaviour in the presence of *Fusobacterium nucleatum* was investigated, and IFN-γ-secretion was found to be inhibited. As a result, this bacterium evades the immune system by interacting with inhibitory receptors on immune cells [157]. According to research, patients with pancreatic cancer have more microbiomes than individuals who have a healthy pancreas. Due to immune response reprogramming after the removal of this microbial population from the pancreas, the tumour invasion was slowed. This depletion resulted in an enhanced CD4+ T-cell Th-1 differentiation, stimulation of CD8+ T cells, M1 macrophage differentiation, and a decrease in myeloid-derived repressor cell penetration [158].

8.3. Protumorigenic Environment Development and Genotoxin Aggregation

The generation of cytolethal toxin *via Campylobacter jejuni* [159], as well as colibactin by *E. coli* [160], appear to have a function in malignancy and tumour growth by microbial populations dwelling in our bodies [161]. The research findings on *Enterotoxigenic Bacteroides fragilis* in colon cancer demonstrated that this pathogen could break E-cadherin, such as a tumour suppressor, leading to the stimulation of the Wnt signalling, that enhances the MYC expression as a proto-oncogene, cell growth, and tumorigenesis by generating *Bacteroides fragilis* toxin [162]. Tumor angiogenesis, which allows tumours to develop quickly, may potentially be influenced by human microbiome. Unmethylated CpG and LPS, two bacterial ligands, can stimulate the host Toll-like receptors at the tumorigenic region. In this circumstance, activated TLRs can synthesise and produce VEGF, which promotes angiogenesis [163]. By quorum sensing peptides, the human microbiome potentially stimulates angiogenesis and cancer development [164]. In addition, quorum peptide-induced metastasis is triggered by interactions between these peptides as well as EGF receptors, which promote the Ras STAT signalling pathways. An elevation in NF-kB, a protein that can stimulate angiogenesis as well as invasion, was also considered as a possible mechanism through which microbiota led to metastasis [164].

9. GUT MICROBIOME AND ALLEVIATION OF IMMUNE CHECK-POINT INHIBITION RESISTANCE IN CARCINOMA IMMUNO-THERAPY

9.1. Cancer Immunotherapy

Nowadays, cancer immunotherapy has improved the treatment of cancer by targeting PD-1, PD-L1 and CTLA-4. It is greatly associated with the blockade of an immune checkpoint. Normalization of tumor immune response is done by immune checkpoint inhibitors (ICIs) [165]. Nobel Prize in the field of Physiology or Medicine in the year 2018 was awarded for cytotoxic T-lymphocyte associated protein-4 (CTLA-4), as well as apoptotic protein-1 checkpoint immunotherapy. The US-FDA 2011 approved the first anti-CTLA-4 blockade, such as, ipilimumab and then, for therapy of ten different types of cancers, seven ICIs were released into the marketplace. However, response to ICI was low, as it was less than 30% in cancer by august 2018, which revealed primary or acquired resistance [166]. Several factors, including environmental conditions, host-related factors, and also tumor-intrinsic factors, mainly contribute to the resistance mechanistic insights. For example, the presence of T cells in the tumor microenvironment (TME) is determined by intrinsic factors of tumour cells such as low levels of mutations, mutations in an antigen-presenting pathway, the signalling pathway dedicated to interferon or cancer signalling pathways, thereby attributing to escape from the immune system [167] (Fig. **3**). The age of an individual, diet, hormones levels, HLA type, genetic variation or polymorphisms, the habit of smoking, and some ongoing secondary diseases or infections play important roles in specifying characteristics of individual host-bearing tumour [168]. Studies are being conducted for agents that are cytotoxic and therapy given in combination with ICIs with radiation, as they are seen as some of the relevant approaches to overcome primary resistance by increasing the immunogenicity of tumor cells.

Recent studies showed that there is an impact of microbiota in the gut for melanoma resistance and the response of ICIs [169 - 171] towards NSCLC, urothelial cancer and kidney cancer [172]. Gut microbiota is diverse and helps to determine the responsiveness to ICIs. Greater sensitivity to anti-programmed cell death protein-1 immunotherapy was shown in patients who had more diversity of *Ruminococcaceae/Faecalibacterium,* and these patients showed longer and overall survival [170]. Baruch *et al.* transferred microbiota from faeces from a responder to a non-responder (Computed tomography or PET was used to measure the response of the treatment and progression of the disease RECIST version 1.1.) and again, treatment was provided with the anti-programmed cell death protein-1 blockade. The microbiota in the gut of recipients was seen to be gaining shape again and enhanced the infiltration T cells in tumor [173]. Thus, these studies suggest that microbes can be used as biomarkers and for therapeutic intervention strategies involving ICIs.

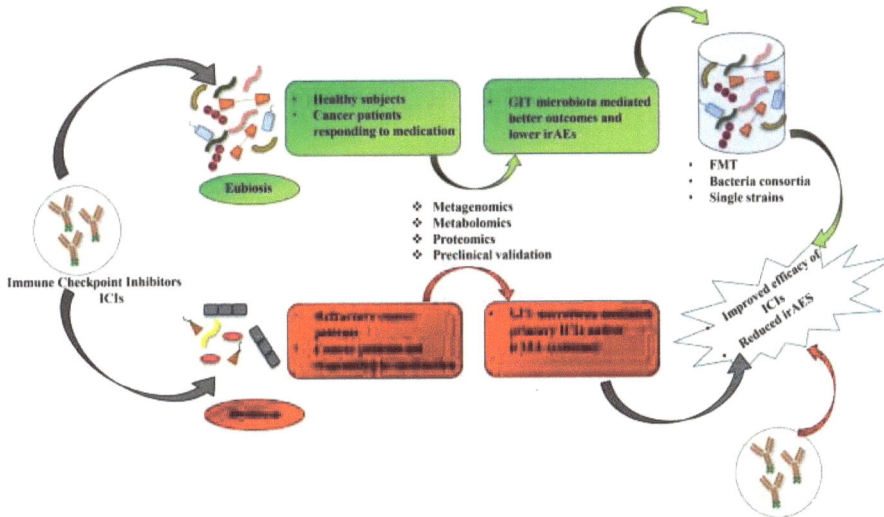

Fig. (3). Effect of Gut microbiota (GM) on immune checkpoint inhibition. ICIs mark the gut microbiota. Microbiota composition varies in the case of responders (eubiotic microbiota) and non-responders (dysbiotic and depauperated microbiota). GM from responders or from healthy individuals is analysed *via* metagenomics, metabolomics, metatranscriptomics, metaproteomic and preclinical studies. This description permits identifying whole stools to accomplish a faecal microbiota transplant (FMT), otherwise microbial consortia that can be administered to non-responder cancer patients or cancer patients who (after an initial response) became refractory to ICIs. The therapeutic modulation of gut microbiota can be associated with ICIs to obtain an improved efficacy and/or a reduction in irAEs in refractory cancer patients. [**Abbreviations**: GM, gut microbiota; ICIs, immune checkpoint inhibitors; FMT, faecal microbiota transplantation; irAEs, immune-related adverse events].

9.2. The Gut Microbiota is Linked to ICI Treatment Sensitivity

Important functions in the stimulation of the immune system and the effect of cytotoxic T-lymphocyte related protein-4, and apoptosis protein-1 obstruction, for *Bacteroides* species and *Bifidobacterium,* was reported in 2015, by two Science reports [174, 175]. Mice were transplanted with patient's microbiomes who were suffering from melanoma. CTLA-4 blockade was seen to be provided by *Bacteroides fragilis* [175]. In melanoma, mice that had tumors were fed *Bifidobacterium,* and it was seen that it helped against tumor when treated together with apoptosis protein-1 obstruction [174]. Patients with melanoma who were given ipilimumab, and patients who had an overexpression of *Bacteroides* were seen to be resistant to ipilimumab-induced colitis, whereas the patients with rich *Faecalibacterium* showed longer and overall survival [176]. *Akkermanasia muciniphila* and *Alistipes indistinctus* over-representation was shown by Routy *et al.* in a study. The response was reversed by *A. muciniphila* for apoptosis protein-1 obstruction in mice with tumors who received microbiota of gut from donors, specifically non-responders, by the method of transplanting microbial from faeces. A study by Gopalakrishnan *et al.* revealed a greater relative abundance of *Ruminococcaceae,* which showed a lot better response, whereas the microorganism *Bacteroidales* showed a lot of resistance in patients suffering from melanoma [177]. Another cohort of patients suffering from melanoma who received a combination of ICIs showed an increase of *Bacteroides stercoris* and *Parabacteroides distasonis* which were attributed to an increased response to ICIs. A study provided by Matson *et al.* revealed that *Bifidobacterium longum,* *Enterococcus faecium* and *Collinsellaaero faciens* enrichment was associated with increased response to anti-programmed cell death protein 1 therapy (Fig. **4**). Some research explored the possibility of whether the effect of microbiota in gut sensitization can be used in the treatment of patients suffering from cancer worldwide. A total of eleven strains were isolated by Tanoue *et al.*, including IFN-γ^+ CD8$^+$ T cells inducing bacteria from the gut microbiota of healthy humans in Japan. It was seen that mice with tumor had enhanced efficacy. Among 11 bacteria identified are *Alistipes senegalensis*, *Parabacteroides* spp., five *Eubacterium limosum*, *Phascolarctobacterium faecium*, *Ruminococcaceae bacterium* cv2, *Fusobacterium ulcerans*, and *Bacteroides* spp. Patients who were suffering from liver cancer were studied by Zheng *et al.*, and they revealed a greater presence of *Ruminococcus* spp. and *A. muciniphila* with greater sensitivity to anti-programmed cell death protein-1 immunotherapy [178]. Another research by Jin *et al.* revealed that patients suffering from advanced lung cancer of non-small cells had an abundance of *Alistipes putredinis* and were more prone to apoptosis protein-1 blockade, whereas the patient with *Ruminococcus* unclassified was less sensitive to apoptosis protein-1 blockade [179]. Therefore, gut microbiota can be used as an important biomarker to check the efficacy of checkpoints in immune therapy.

10. CHALLENGES OF MICROBIOME RESEARCH IN CANCER IMMUNOTHERAPY

The relationship between cancer, the immune system and gut microbiota are complicated. Hence, there is a need for standardized microbiome analysis, network analysis, a good approach to research and preclinical model optimization [180].

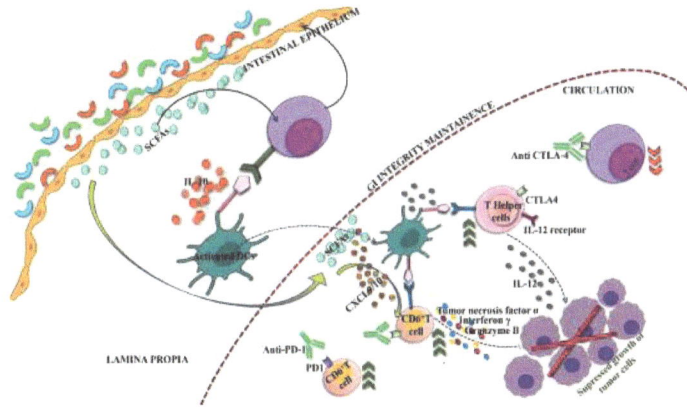

Fig. (4). Potential mechanisms of gut microbiota to overcome resistance to immune checkpoint inhibitors (ICI's). Gut microbes are recognized by dendritic cells (DCs) to instruct local as well as systemic immune responses. In lamina propria, activated DCs can bring Treg and IL-10 to sustain gut integrity. On the other hand, activated DCs may translocate into mesenteric lymph nodes to prime adaptive immune response, which can circulate systemically and suppress the growth of tumor cells by the expansion of Th1 and CD8$^+$ T cells and upregulation of IFN-γ, TNF-α in anti-CTLA4 and anti-PD-1/PD-L1 therapies. Microbial metabolites such as SCFAs induce Treg cells or IL-10 to protect the gut integrity from the invasion of foreign microorganisms in the colon. In the circulation system, SCFAs, such as an ester of butyric acid, directly interact with CD8$^+$ T cells and augment their antitumor effect.

10.1. Preclinical Model

Animal models that are free of germs are referred to as germ-free (GF), and animal models treated with antibiotics are mainly used to establish a relationship between gut microbiota and ICIs. Animal models linked with human microbiota provide good proof of its role in therapy by transplantation of faecal microbiota into GF mice from patients [181, 182]. However, specialized isolators are needed for GF mice breeding in order to prevent bacterial virus and fungus contamination, which requires a lot of labour, care and optimization of study design; however, these result in less commercially available GF mouse strains. Mice required in *in vivo* test of checkpoints in the immune system of humans are humanized programmed cell death protein-1 knock-in mouse models, to help *in vivo* experiment of human-immune checkpoints including humanized programmed cell death protein-1 receptor. Pembrolizumab, using the abovementioned model, can obstruct MC38 colorectal cancer and GL261 glioblastoma tumorigenesis [183, 184]. Moreover, there is another similar mouse model that is very similar to the immune system of humans, *i.e.*, humanized NSGTM-SGM3 and NSGTM evaluation of the effectiveness of Keytruda in PS4050 and hu-NSG-SGM3 mice with tumor was done to validate this study [185]. Thus, further optimization of HMA models is needed for researches which are immunologically and metabolically humanized. Nowadays, microfluidic organ chip technologies are used to overawe the restrictions of animal models, and it can be used to mimic cellular collaborations and physiological activities *in vivo,* such as TME. In both, tumor fragments of mice and biopsy of human tumor methods like EVIDENT, microfluidic devices, and *ex vivo* systems, were used to show the effect of programmed cell death protein-1 inhibitor. Quantification of death of tumor and tumor-infiltrating lymphocytes is done by this system, and it also provides a way to examine either the individual effect of immunotherapies or the effect of immunotherapies in different combinations [186]. Tailored-made organ chips are used to establish living microbiomes' culture of human intestinal cells, like an anaerobic intestine-on a chip, which gives an association between interactions between microbiome and host. A micro physiological system (MPS) was created by Trapecar *et al.*, which helps in connecting the liver circulating immune system and gut with the help of a liver chip. Induction or exacerbation of inflammation in UC by SCFAs depends on the function of T cells and CD4$^+$ cells [187]. Thus, *ex vivo* platform establishes a complex relationship between the microbiota of gut and different diseases and establishes a way to screen and evaluate therapeutics that target the gut.

11. NEW INSIGHTS ON THE MODULATION OF THE GUT MICROBIOTA AND THE SUPPRESSION OF IMMUNOLOGICAL CHECKPOINTS IN CANCER

The relationship between the efficacy and safety of ICI-related immunotherapy and GM-CSF characteristics in patients suffering from cancer has been shown by different studies. The first time observation in GF mice treated with antibodies was done by Vétizou *et al.* [188] in 2015. The study revealed that the mice did not show any effect to anti-CTLA4 immunotherapy. *Bacteroides fragilis* specifically was responsible for the antitumor action of anti-CTLA4. Apart from it, *Bacteroides* spp. was also responsible for the action. Oral gavage of *Bacteroides fragilis*, immunization with *Bacteroides* T-cells, transfer of *Bacteroides fragilis*-specific *in vitro* and fragilis-derived polysaccharides showed high antitumor response [188]. FMT in tumor-bearing mice was done and then treated with anti-CTLA4 antibody. Melanoma Patient's stool sample was taken and enriched with *Bacteroides* spp. Faeces derived from mice were tested and were found to be rich in *Bacteroides fragilis*. Negative association was established with the size of the tumor followed by CTLA-4 blockade in mice. Modification of *Bacteroides* spp. in the gut that is immunogenic in nature can be done by anti-CTLA4 antibody treatment. This affected the anti-cancer efficacy of ICI [188]. A comparison of the development of melanoma in mice suggested dissimilar breeding abilities [189]. Major differences in the growth of melanoma were seen, which revealed the various T-cell responses that were cancer-specific. Oral administration of faeces to *Bifidobacterium* in non-responder mice with anti-PD-L1 increased their action to anti-PD-L1 therapy [189]. Moreover, major changes in tumor growth were seen, such as the reduced tumor, along with an increased DC response led to enhanced CD8$^+$ T-cell activity and accumulation of T-cells within the TME [189]. Therefore, these studies suggest that by changing the GM, we could increase the effectiveness of ICIs and their antitumor action [188, 189]. Another study published in 2016 by Dubin *et al*. suggested that in cancer patients, anti-CTLA4 antibody led to inflammatory colitis and dysbiosis [190]. An association between *Bacteroidetes* and increased resistance to colitis induced by the ICI was established. Patients who did not have genetic pathways for the synthesis of vitamin-B and transport of polyamine were subjected to microbiome analysis, which confirmed that there is more risk of colitis development [190]. Frankel *et al*., in the year 2017, studied the association of GM and its efficacy in ICIs in patients with multiple myeloma (MM) [191]. The study used a meta-genomic shotgun with sequencing profiling of metabolomics. It was observed that among 39 patients with MM, there was a group that showed ICI response (equivalent to 67% of nivolumab and ipilimumab, and 23% of pembrolizumab-treated participants). Faeces from ICI-responders were evaluated and were found to be rich in *Bacteroides caccae* [191]. A combination of anti-CTLA4 and anti-PD-L1 showed GM rich in *Bacteroides thetaiotamicron, Holdemania filiformis* and *Faecalibacterium prausnitzii*. The responders treated with anti-PD1 antibody had rich GM with more *Dorea formicogenerans*. Anacardic acid was the metabolite present in the GM obtained from the responders [191]. It was found that before infusion of anti-CTLA4 antibody, patients who exhibited *Faecalibacterium* genus and other *Firmicutes* showed a lesser PFS than patients who exhibited *Bacteroides*. The presence of *Firmicutes* was associated with baseline colitis-associated phylotypes [192]. The patients who exhibited *Faecalibacterium* with MM after the development of colitis, induced by anti-CTLA4 showed greater CD4$^+$ T-cells and the T-cell promoted T-cell co-stimulator indicator on the surface upon ICI treatment. The following observation revealed that an essential contributing factor of the immune outcome may be represented in carcinoma patients by the baseline GM composition, and by anti-CTLA-4 colitis [192]. Furthermore, metagenomics and metabolomics were combined together to study the GM in patients suffering from cancer. The study revealed that ICIs treatments affect GM. Thus, a better prognosis can include a certain composition of GM along with enriched metabolite. The relationship of effectiveness of ICI-related therapy and the composition of GM was established in 2018 [193, 194]. The effects of FMT from the RCC and NSCLC were studied and evaluated by Routy *et al*. in ICI-responder as well as ICI-non responder donors, together with recipient mice with epithelial tumor that were antibiotic-treated or germ-free. The study revealed that the efficacy of FMT from patients who were non-responder did not show any effect, while there was a reduction in tumor growth in ICIs responders [195].

CONCLUSION

Numerous conclusive confirmations prove that gut microbiota is a significant factor in immunotherapy against cancer. Though defined and precise mechanisms as well as the clinical translation from preclinical studies, are still the most important challenges to be disclosed. For example, the selection of donor, its preparation, route of administration, colonization resistance and possible adverse reactions; any of these may obstruct the application of FMT [196]. In contrast, the gut microbiota appears to play an essential part in the development of the immune system of the host and immunity against tumor. Furthermore, the commensal bacteria-derived metabolites such as an ester of butyric acid and propionic acid can limit the progression of Treg cells by stimulating the nuclear factor kappa-B, overexpressing the Toll-like receptors, liberating interleukins including IL-5, IL-6 and TNF-α and lastly causing continuous inflammation in the TME.

Hereafter, an integrative methodology must be developed to authenticate the interpretations and enhance the achievability of FMT to aid patients suffering from cancer. Moreover, it fetches several novel opportunities to relate prebiotics as well as probiotics in modulating microbiota and augment its anti-tumor therapeutic activity against cancer. Although the link between gut microbiota and different cancers has been confirmed, a further advanced investigation is required to completely solve this multifaceted network. For instance, it is important to understand by what means numerous infectious agents impact the microbiota environment, and the precise molecular mechanism of actions by which the gut microbiota influences cancerous tumor cells and anti-oncogenes. The significant capability of gut microbiota to either modulate or hinder with cancer treatment can be an alternative field of research.

In conclusion, cancer patients can be precisely medicated and treated with the aid of gut-tumor axis microbiota. In the future, more theranostic approaches should be dedicated to microbiota environment modulation to overcome the resistance against cancer immunotherapy.

CONSENT OF PUBLICATION

Not applicable.

CONFLICT OF INTEREST

The authors declare no conflict of interest, financial or otherwise.

ACKNOWLEDGEMENT

This work was supported by the Central University of South Bihar, providing research support.

REFERENCES

[1]   O'Hara AM, Shanahan F. The gut flora as a forgotten organ. EMBO Rep 2006; 7(7): 688-93.
      [http://dx.doi.org/10.1038/sj.embor.7400731] [PMID: 16819463]

[2]   Ursell LK, Haiser HJ, Van Treuren W, *et al.* The intestinal metabolome: an intersection between microbiota and host. Gastroenterology 2014; 146(6): 1470-6.
      [http://dx.doi.org/10.1053/j.gastro.2014.03.001] [PMID: 24631493]

[3]   Whitman WB, Coleman DC, Wiebe WJ. Prokaryotes: The unseen majority. Proc Natl Acad Sci USA 1998; 95(12): 6578-83.
      [http://dx.doi.org/10.1073/pnas.95.12.6578] [PMID: 9618454]

[4]   Savage DC. Microbial ecology of the gastrointestinal tract. Annu Rev Microbiol 1977; 31(1): 107-33.
      [http://dx.doi.org/10.1146/annurev.mi.31.100177.000543] [PMID: 334036]

[5]   Ley RE, Peterson DA, Gordon JI. Ecological and evolutionary forces shaping microbial diversity in the human intestine. Cell 2006; 124(4): 837-48.
      [http://dx.doi.org/10.1016/j.cell.2006.02.017] [PMID: 16497592]

[6]   Wang B, Li L. Who determines the outcomes of HBV exposure? Trends Microbiol 2015; 23(6): 328-9.
      [http://dx.doi.org/10.1016/j.tim.2015.04.001] [PMID: 25864882]

[7]   Ley RE, Turnbaugh PJ, Klein S, *et al.* Human gut microbes associated with obesity. Nature 2006; 444(7122): 1022-3.
      [http://dx.doi.org/10.1038/4441022a] [PMID: 17183309]

[8]   Wang B, Jiang X, Cao M, *et al.* Altered fecal microbiota correlates with liver biochemistry in nonobese patients with non-alcoholic fatty liver disease. Sci Rep 2016; 6(1): 32002.
      [http://dx.doi.org/10.1038/srep32002] [PMID: 27550547]

[9]   Gill SR, Pop M, DeBoy RT, *et al.* Metagenomic analysis of the human distal gut microbiome. Science 2006; 312(5778): 1355-9.
      [http://dx.doi.org/10.1126/science.1124234] [PMID: 16741115]

[10] Roberfroid MB, Bornet F, Bouley C, Cummings JH. Colonic microflora: nutrition and health. Summary and conclusions of an International Life Sciences Institute (ILSI) [Europe] workshop held in Barcelona, Spain. Nutr Rev 1995; 53(5): 127-30.
      [http://dx.doi.org/10.1111/j.1753-4887.1995.tb01535.x] [PMID: 7666984]

[11] Cash HL, Whitham CV, Behrendt CL, Hooper LV. Symbiotic bacteria direct expression of an intestinal bactericidal lectin. Science 2006; 313(5790): 1126-30.
      [http://dx.doi.org/10.1126/science.1127119] [PMID: 16931762]

[12] Hooper LV, Stappenbeck TS, Hong CV, Gordon JI. Angiogenins: a new class of microbicidal proteins involved in innate immunity. Nat Immunol 2003; 4(3): 269-73.
      [http://dx.doi.org/10.1038/ni888] [PMID: 12548285]

[13] Schauber J, Svanholm C, Termén S, *et al.* Expression of the cathelicidin LL-37 is modulated by short chain fatty acids in colonocytes: relevance of signalling pathways. Gut 2003; 52(5): 735-41.
      [http://dx.doi.org/10.1136/gut.52.5.735] [PMID: 12692061]

[14] Bouskra D, Brézillon C, Bérard M, *et al.* Lymphoid tissue genesis induced by commensals through NOD1 regulates intestinal homeostasis. Nature 2008; 456(7221): 507-10.
      [http://dx.doi.org/10.1038/nature07450] [PMID: 18987631]

[15]   Rakoff-Nahoum S, Medzhitov R. Innate immune recognition of the indigenous microbial flora. Mucosal Immunol 2008; 1 (Suppl. 1): S10-4.
[http://dx.doi.org/10.1038/mi.2008.49] [PMID: 19079220]

[16]   Macpherson AJ, Harris NL. Interactions between commensal intestinal bacteria and the immune system. Nat Rev Immunol 2004; 4(6): 478-85.
[http://dx.doi.org/10.1038/nri1373] [PMID: 15173836]

[17]   Sekirov I, Russell SL, Antunes LCM, Finlay BB. Gut microbiota in health and disease. Physiol Rev 2010; 90(3): 859-904.
[http://dx.doi.org/10.1152/physrev.00045.2009] [PMID: 20664075]

[18]   Sartor RB. Microbial influences in inflammatory bowel diseases. Gastroenterology 2008; 134(2): 577-94.
[http://dx.doi.org/10.1053/j.gastro.2007.11.059] [PMID: 18242222]

[19]   Liu Q, Duan ZP, Ha DK, Bengmark S, Kurtovic J, Riordan SM. Synbiotic modulation of gut flora: Effect on minimal hepatic encephalopathy in patients with cirrhosis. Hepatology 2004; 39(5): 1441-9.
[http://dx.doi.org/10.1002/hep.20194] [PMID: 15122774]

[20]   Scanlan PD, Shanahan F, Clune Y, *et al.* Culture-independent analysis of the gut microbiota in colorectal cancer and polyposis. Environ Microbiol 2008; 10(3): 789-98.
[http://dx.doi.org/10.1111/j.1462-2920.2007.01503.x] [PMID: 18237311]

[21]   Verhulst SL, Vael C, Beunckens C, Nelen V, Goossens H, Desager K. A longitudinal analysis on the association between antibiotic use, intestinal microflora, and wheezing during the first year of life. J Asthma 2008; 45(9): 828-32.
[http://dx.doi.org/10.1080/02770900802339734] [PMID: 18972304]

[22]   Finegold SM, Molitoris D, Song Y, *et al.* Gastrointestinal microflora studies in late-onset autism. Clin Infect Dis 2002; 35(s1) (Suppl. 1): S6-S16.
[http://dx.doi.org/10.1086/341914] [PMID: 12173102]

[23]   Wen L, Ley RE, Volchkov PY, *et al.* Innate immunity and intestinal microbiota in the development of Type 1 diabetes. Nature 2008; 455(7216): 1109-13.
[http://dx.doi.org/10.1038/nature07336] [PMID: 18806780]

[24]   Rogier EW, Frantz AL, Bruno MEC, *et al.* Lessons from mother: Long-term impact of antibodies in breast milk on the gut microbiota and intestinal immune system of breastfed offspring. Gut Microbes 2014; 5(5): 663-8.
[http://dx.doi.org/10.4161/19490976.2014.969984] [PMID: 25483336]

[25]   Round JL, Mazmanian SK. The gut microbiota shapes intestinal immune responses during health and disease. Nat Rev Immunol 2009; 9(5): 313-23.
[http://dx.doi.org/10.1038/nri2515] [PMID: 19343057]

[26]   Larsbrink J, Rogers TE, Hemsworth GR, *et al.* A discrete genetic locus confers xyloglucan metabolism in select human gut *Bacteroidetes.* Nature 2014; 506(7489): 498-502.
[http://dx.doi.org/10.1038/nature12907] [PMID: 24463512]

[27]   Goh YJ, Klaenhammer TR. Genetic mechanisms of prebiotic oligosaccharide metabolism in probiotic microbes. Annu Rev Food Sci Technol 2015; 6(1): 137-56.
[http://dx.doi.org/10.1146/annurev-food-022814-015706] [PMID: 25532597]

[28]   Morowitz MJ, Carlisle EM, Alverdy JC. Contributions of intestinal bacteria to nutrition and metabolism in the critically ill. Surg Clin North Am 2011; 91(4): 771-85.
[http://dx.doi.org/10.1016/j.suc.2011.05.001] [PMID: 21787967]

[29]   Duncan SH, Louis P, Thomson JM, Flint HJ. The role of pH in determining the species composition of the human colonic microbiota. Environ Microbiol 2009; 11(8): 2112-22.
[http://dx.doi.org/10.1111/j.1462-2920.2009.01931.x] [PMID: 19397676]

[30]   Cani PD, Everard A, Duparc T. Gut microbiota, enteroendocrine functions and metabolism. Curr Opin Pharmacol 2013; 13(6): 935-40.
[http://dx.doi.org/10.1016/j.coph.2013.09.008] [PMID: 24075718]

[31]   Flint HJ, Scott KP, Louis P, Duncan SH. The role of the gut microbiota in nutrition and health. Nat Rev Gastroenterol Hepatol 2012; 9(10): 577-89.
[http://dx.doi.org/10.1038/nrgastro.2012.156] [PMID: 22945443]

[32]   Cebra JJ. Influences of microbiota on intestinal immune system development. Am J Clin Nutr 1999; 69(5): 1046-51.
[http://dx.doi.org/10.1093/ajcn/69.5.1046s] [PMID: 10232647]

[33]   Thaiss CA, Zmora N, Levy M, Elinav E. The microbiome and innate immunity. Nature 2016; 535(7610): 65-74.
[http://dx.doi.org/10.1038/nature18847] [PMID: 27383981]

[34]   Magrone T, Jirillo E. The interplay between the gut immune system and microbiota in health and disease: nutraceutical intervention for restoring intestinal homeostasis. Curr Pharm Des 2013; 19(7): 1329-42.
[PMID: 23151182]

[35]   Ki MR, Lee HR, Goo MJ, *et al.* Differential regulation of ERK1/2 and p38 MAP kinases in VacA-induced apoptosis of gastric epithelial cells. Am J Physiol Gastrointest Liver Physiol 2008; 294(3): G635-47.
[http://dx.doi.org/10.1152/ajpgi.00281.2007] [PMID: 18096609]

[36]   Huck O, Al-Hashemi J, Poidevin L, *et al.* Identification and characterization of microRNA differentially expressed in macrophages exposed to *Porphyromonas gingivalis* infection. Infect Immun 2017; 85(3): e00771-16.
[http://dx.doi.org/10.1128/IAI.00771-16] [PMID: 28069815]

[37]   Péré-Védrenne C, Prochazkova-Carlotti M, Rousseau B, *et al.* The cytolethal distending toxin subunit CdtB of *Helicobacter hepaticus* promotes senescence and endoreplication in xenograft mouse models of hepatic and intestinal cell lines. Front Cell Infect Microbiol 2017; 7: 268.
[http://dx.doi.org/10.3389/fcimb.2017.00268] [PMID: 28713773]

[38]   Rubinstein MR, Wang X, Liu W, Hao Y, Cai G, Han YW. *Fusobacterium nucleatum* promotes colorectal carcinogenesis by modulating E-cadherin/β-catenin signaling *via* its FadA adhesin. Cell Host Microbe 2013; 14(2): 195-206.
[http://dx.doi.org/10.1016/j.chom.2013.07.012] [PMID: 23954158]

[39]   Cuevas-Ramos G, Petit CR, Marcq I, Boury M, Oswald E, Nougayrède JP. *Escherichia coli* induces DNA damage *in vivo* and triggers genomic instability in mammalian cells. Proc Natl Acad Sci USA 2010; 107(25): 11537-42.
[http://dx.doi.org/10.1073/pnas.1001261107] [PMID: 20534522]

[40]   Tsoi H, Chu ESH, Zhang X, *et al. peptostreptococcus anaerobius* induces intracellular cholesterol biosynthesis in colon cells to induce proliferation and causes dysplasia in mice. Gastroenterology 2017; 152(6): 1419-1433.e5.
[http://dx.doi.org/10.1053/j.gastro.2017.01.009] [PMID: 28126350]

[41]   Ulger Toprak N, Yagci A, Gulluoglu BM, *et al.* A possible role of *Bacteroides fragilis* enterotoxin in the aetiology of colorectal cancer. Clin Microbiol Infect 2006; 12(8): 782-6.
[http://dx.doi.org/10.1111/j.1469-0691.2006.01494.x] [PMID: 16842574]

[42]   De Martel C, Ferlay J, Franceschi S, *et al.* Global burden of cancers attributable to infections in 2008: a review and synthetic analysis. Lancet Oncol 2012; 13(6): 607-15.
[http://dx.doi.org/10.1016/S1470-2045(12)70137-7] [PMID: 22575588]

[43]   Wong BCY, Lam SK, Wong WM, *et al. Helicobacter pylori* eradication to prevent gastric cancer in a high-risk region of China: a randomized controlled trial. JAMA 2004; 291(2): 187-94.

[http://dx.doi.org/10.1001/jama.291.2.187] [PMID: 14722144]

[44]   El-Omar EM, Carrington M, Chow WH, *et al.* Interleukin-1 polymorphisms associated with increased risk of gastric cancer. Nature 2000; 404(6776): 398-402.
        [http://dx.doi.org/10.1038/35006081] [PMID: 10746728]

[45]   De Sablet T, Piazuelo MB, Shaffer CL, *et al.* Phylogeographic origin of *Helicobacter pylori* is a determinant of gastric cancer risk. Gut 2011; 60(9): 1189-95.
        [http://dx.doi.org/10.1136/gut.2010.234468] [PMID: 21357593]

[46]   Rhead JL, Letley DP, Mohammadi M, *et al.* A new *Helicobacter pylori* vacuolating cytotoxin determinant, the intermediate region, is associated with gastric cancer. Gastroenterology 2007; 133(3): 926-36.
        [http://dx.doi.org/10.1053/j.gastro.2007.06.056] [PMID: 17854597]

[47]   Cover TL, Krishna US, Israel DA, Peek RM Jr. Induction of gastric epithelial cell apoptosis by *Helicobacter pylori* vacuolating cytotoxin. Cancer Res 2003; 63(5): 951-7.
        [PMID: 12615708]

[48]   Oertli M, Sundquist M, Hitzler I, *et al.* DC-derived IL-18 drives Treg differentiation, murine *Helicobacter pylori*-specific immune tolerance, and asthma protection. J Clin Invest 2012; 122(3): 1082-96.
        [http://dx.doi.org/10.1172/JCI61029] [PMID: 22307326]

[49]   Blaser MJ, Perez-Perez GI, Kleanthous H, *et al.* Infection with *Helicobacter pylori* strains possessing CagA is associated with an increased risk of developing adenocarcinoma of the stomach. Cancer Res 1995; 55(10): 2111-5.
        [PMID: 7743510]

[50]   Kaparakis M, Turnbull L, Carneiro L, *et al.* Bacterial membrane vesicles deliver peptidoglycan to NOD1 in epithelial cells. Cell Microbiol 2010; 12(3): 372-85.
        [http://dx.doi.org/10.1111/j.1462-5822.2009.01404.x] [PMID: 19888989]

[51]   Odenbreit S, Püls J, Sedlmaier B, Gerland E, Fischer W, Haas R. Translocation of *Helicobacter pylori* CagA into gastric epithelial cells by type IV secretion. Science 2000; 287(5457): 1497-500.
        [http://dx.doi.org/10.1126/science.287.5457.1497] [PMID: 10688800]

[52]   Lertpiriyapong K, Whary MT, Muthupalani S, *et al.* Gastric colonisation with a restricted commensal microbiota replicates the promotion of neoplastic lesions by diverse intestinal microbiota in the *Helicobacter pylori* INS-GAS mouse model of gastric carcinogenesis. Gut 2014; 63(1): 54-63.
        [http://dx.doi.org/10.1136/gutjnl-2013-305178] [PMID: 23812323]

[53]   Sanapareddy N, Legge RM, Jovov B, *et al.* Increased rectal microbial richness is associated with the presence of colorectal adenomas in humans. ISME J 2012; 6(10): 1858-68.
        [http://dx.doi.org/10.1038/ismej.2012.43] [PMID: 22622349]

[54]   Zackular JP, Baxter NT, Iverson KD, *et al.* The gut microbiome modulates colon tumorigenesis. MBio 2013; 4(6): e00692-13.
        [http://dx.doi.org/10.1128/mBio.00692-13] [PMID: 24194538]

[55]   Keku TO, McCoy AN, Azcarate-Peril AM. *Fusobacterium* spp. and colorectal cancer: cause or consequence? Trends Microbiol 2013; 21(10): 506-8.
        [http://dx.doi.org/10.1016/j.tim.2013.08.004] [PMID: 24029382]

[56]   Feng Q, Liang S, Jia H, *et al.* Gut microbiome development along the colorectal adenoma–carcinoma sequence. Nat Commun 2015; 6(1): 6528.
        [http://dx.doi.org/10.1038/ncomms7528] [PMID: 25758642]

[57]   Rubinstein MR, Wang X, Liu W, Hao Y, Cai G, Han YW. *Fusobacterium nucleatum* promotes colorectal carcinogenesis by modulating E-cadherin/β-catenin signaling *via* its FadA adhesin. Cell Host Microbe 2013; 14(2): 195-206.
        [http://dx.doi.org/10.1016/j.chom.2013.07.012] [PMID: 23954158]

[58]   Kostic AD, Chun E, Robertson L, *et al. Fusobacterium nucleatum* potentiates intestinal tumorigenesis and modulates the tumor-immune microenvironment. Cell Host Microbe 2013; 14(2): 207-15.
[http://dx.doi.org/10.1016/j.chom.2013.07.007] [PMID: 23954159]

[59]   Sokol SY. Wnt signaling and dorso-ventral axis specification in vertebrates. Curr Opin Genet Dev 1999; 9(4): 405-10.
[http://dx.doi.org/10.1016/S0959-437X(99)80061-6] [PMID: 10449345]

[60]   Sears CL. *Enterotoxigenic Bacteroides fragilis*: a rogue among symbiotes. Clin Microbiol Rev 2009; 22(2): 349-69.
[http://dx.doi.org/10.1128/CMR.00053-08] [PMID: 19366918]

[61]   Shiryaev SA, Remacle AG, Chernov AV, *et al.* Substrate cleavage profiling suggests a distinct function of *Bacteroides fragilis* metalloproteinases (fragilysin and metalloproteinase II) at the microbiome-inflammation-cancer interface. J Biol Chem 2013; 288(48): 34956-67.
[http://dx.doi.org/10.1074/jbc.M113.516153] [PMID: 24145028]

[62]   Wu S, Rhee KJ, Albesiano E, *et al.* A human colonic commensal promotes colon tumorigenesis *via* activation of T helper type 17 T cell responses. Nat Med 2009; 15(9): 1016-22.
[http://dx.doi.org/10.1038/nm.2015] [PMID: 19701202]

[63]   Huycke MM, Abrams V, Moore DR. *Enterococcus faecalis* produces extracellular superoxide and hydrogen peroxide that damages colonic epithelial cell DNA. Carcinogenesis 2002; 23(3): 529-36.
[http://dx.doi.org/10.1093/carcin/23.3.529] [PMID: 11895869]

[64]   Cuevas-Ramos G, Petit CR, Marcq I, Boury M, Oswald E, Nougayrède JP. *Escherichia coli* induces DNA damage *in vivo* and triggers genomic instability in mammalian cells. Proc Natl Acad Sci USA 2010; 107(25): 11537-42.
[http://dx.doi.org/10.1073/pnas.1001261107] [PMID: 20534522]

[65]   Howe GR, Benito E, Castelleto R, *et al.* Dietary intake of fiber and decreased risk of cancers of the colon and rectum: evidence from the combined analysis of 13 case-control studies. J Natl Cancer Inst 1992; 84(24): 1887-96.
[http://dx.doi.org/10.1093/jnci/84.24.1887] [PMID: 1334153]

[66]   Clausen MR, Bonnén H, Mortensen PB. Colonic fermentation of dietary fibre to short chain fatty acids in patients with adenomatous polyps and colonic cancer. Gut 1991; 32(8): 923-8.
[http://dx.doi.org/10.1136/gut.32.8.923] [PMID: 1653178]

[67]   Singh N, Gurav A, Sivaprakasam S, *et al.* Activation of Gpr109a, receptor for niacin and the commensal metabolite butyrate, suppresses colonic inflammation and carcinogenesis. Immunity 2014; 40(1): 128-39.
[http://dx.doi.org/10.1016/j.immuni.2013.12.007] [PMID: 24412617]

[68]   Lagergren J, Bergström R, Lindgren A, Nyrén O. Symptomatic gastroesophageal reflux as a risk factor for esophageal adenocarcinoma. N Engl J Med 1999; 340(11): 825-31.
[http://dx.doi.org/10.1056/NEJM199903183401101] [PMID: 10080844]

[69]   Lagergren J. Adenocarcinoma of oesophagus: what exactly is the size of the problem and who is at risk? Gut 2005; 54(Suppl 1) (Suppl. 1): i1-5.
[http://dx.doi.org/10.1136/gut.2004.041517] [PMID: 15711002]

[70]   Anderson LA, Murphy SJ, Johnston BT, *et al.* Relationship between *Helicobacter pylori* infection and gastric atrophy and the stages of the oesophageal inflammation, metaplasia, adenocarcinoma sequence: results from the FINBAR case-control study. Gut 2008; 57(6): 734-9.
[http://dx.doi.org/10.1136/gut.2007.132662] [PMID: 18025067]

[71]   Pei Z, Bini EJ, Yang L, Zhou M, Francois F, Blaser MJ. Bacterial biota in the human distal esophagus. Proc Natl Acad Sci USA 2004; 101(12): 4250-5.
[http://dx.doi.org/10.1073/pnas.0306398101] [PMID: 15016918]

[72]   Yang L, Lu X, Nossa CW, Francois F, Peek RM, Pei Z. Inflammation and intestinal metaplasia of the

distal esophagus are associated with alterations in the microbiome. Gastroenterology 2009; 137(2): 588-97.
[http://dx.doi.org/10.1053/j.gastro.2009.04.046] [PMID: 19394334]

[73]   Finlay IG, Wright PA, Menzies T, McArdle CS. Microbial flora in carcinoma of oesophagus. Thorax 1982; 37(3): 181-4.
[http://dx.doi.org/10.1136/thx.37.3.181] [PMID: 7101222]

[74]   El-Serag HB, Sonnenberg A. Opposing time trends of peptic ulcer and reflux disease. Gut 1998; 43(3): 327-33.
[http://dx.doi.org/10.1136/gut.43.3.327] [PMID: 9863476]

[75]   Hamada H, Haruma K, Mihara M, *et al.* High incidence of reflux oesophagitis after eradication therapy for *Helicobacter pylori* : impacts of hiatal hernia and corpus gastritis. Aliment Pharmacol Ther 2000; 14(6): 729-35.
[http://dx.doi.org/10.1046/j.1365-2036.2000.00758.x] [PMID: 10848656]

[76]   Boyd SD, Liu Y, Wang C, Martin V, Dunn-Walters DK. Human lymphocyte repertoires in ageing. Curr Opin Immunol 2013; 25(4): 511-5.
[http://dx.doi.org/10.1016/j.coi.2013.07.007] [PMID: 23992996]

[77]   Macfarlane GT, Gibson GR, Cummings JH. Comparison of fermentation reactions in different regions of the human colon. J Appl Bacteriol 1992; 72(1): 57-64.
[http://dx.doi.org/10.1111/j.1365-2672.1992.tb04882.x] [PMID: 1541601]

[78]   Steliou K, Boosalis MS, Perrine SP, Sangerman J, Faller DV. Butyrate histone deacetylase inhibitors. Biores Open Access 2012; 1(4): 192-8.
[http://dx.doi.org/10.1089/biores.2012.0223] [PMID: 23514803]

[79]   De Vadder F, Kovatcheva-Datchary P, Goncalves D, *et al.* Microbiota-generated metabolites promote metabolic benefits *via* gut-brain neural circuits. Cell 2014; 156(1-2): 84-96.
[http://dx.doi.org/10.1016/j.cell.2013.12.016] [PMID: 24412651]

[80]   Brown AJ, Goldsworthy SM, Barnes AA, *et al.* The Orphan G protein-coupled receptors GPR41 and GPR43 are activated by propionate and other short chain carboxylic acids. J Biol Chem 2003; 278(13): 11312-9.
[http://dx.doi.org/10.1074/jbc.M211609200] [PMID: 12496283]

[81]   Tazoe H, Otomo Y, Kaji I, Tanaka R, Karaki SI, Kuwahara A. Roles of short-chain fatty acids receptors, GPR41 and GPR43 on colonic functions. J Physiol Pharmacol 2008; 59 (Suppl. 2): 251-62.
[PMID: 18812643]

[82]   Duncan SH, Holtrop G, Lobley GE, Calder AG, Stewart CS, Flint HJ. Contribution of acetate to butyrate formation by human faecal bacteria. Br J Nutr 2004; 91(6): 915-23.
[http://dx.doi.org/10.1079/BJN20041150] [PMID: 15182395]

[83]   Frost G, Sleeth ML, Sahuri-Arisoylu M, *et al.* The short-chain fatty acid acetate reduces appetite *via* a central homeostatic mechanism. Nat Commun 2014; 5(1): 3611.
[http://dx.doi.org/10.1038/ncomms4611] [PMID: 24781306]

[84]   Bjerrum JT, Wang Y, Hao F, *et al.* Metabonomics of human fecal extracts characterize ulcerative colitis, Crohn's disease and healthy individuals. Metabolomics 2015; 11(1): 122-33.
[http://dx.doi.org/10.1007/s11306-014-0677-3] [PMID: 25598765]

[85]   Belenguer A, Duncan SH, Calder AG, *et al.* Two routes of metabolic cross-feeding between *Bifidobacterium adolescentis* and butyrate-producing anaerobes from the human gut. Appl Environ Microbiol 2006; 72(5): 3593-9.
[http://dx.doi.org/10.1128/AEM.72.5.3593-3599.2006] [PMID: 16672507]

[86]   Falony G, Vlachou A, Verbrugghe K, Vuyst LD. Cross-feeding between *Bifidobacterium longum* BB536 and acetate-converting, butyrate-producing colon bacteria during growth on oligofructose. Appl Environ Microbiol 2006; 72(12): 7835-41.

[http://dx.doi.org/10.1128/AEM.01296-06] [PMID: 17056678]

[87]   Louis P, Young P, Holtrop G, Flint HJ. Diversity of human colonic butyrate-producing bacteria revealed by analysis of the butyryl-CoA:acetate CoA-transferase gene. Environ Microbiol 2010; 12(2): 304-14.
        [http://dx.doi.org/10.1111/j.1462-2920.2009.02066.x] [PMID: 19807780]

[88]   Reichardt N, Duncan SH, Young P, *et al.* Phylogenetic distribution of three pathways for propionate production within the human gut microbiota. ISME J 2014; 8(6): 1323-35.
        [http://dx.doi.org/10.1038/ismej.2014.14] [PMID: 24553467]

[89]   Vital M, Howe AC, Tiedje JM (2014) Revealing the bacterial butyrate synthesis pathways by analyzing (meta)genomic data. MBio 5:e00889

[90]   Louis P, Duncan SH, McCrae SI *et al.* Restricted distribution of the butyrate kinase pathway among butyrateproducing bacteria from the human colon. J Bacteriol 2004; 186:2099–2106.

[91]   Matthies A, Blaut M, Braune A. Isolation of a human intestinal bacterium capable of daidzein and genistein conversion. Appl Environ Microbiol. 2009; 75: 1740-4.

[92]   Bastos F, Bessa J, Pacheco CC *et al.* Enrichment of microbial cultures able to degrade 1,3-dichloro-2-propanol: a comparison between batch and continuous methods. Biodegradation. 2002; 13: 211-20.

[93]   Ziemer CJ. Newly cultured bacteria with broad diversity isolated from eight-week continuous culture enrichments of cow feces on complex polysaccharides. Appl Environ Microbiol 2014; 80(2): 574-85.
        [http://dx.doi.org/10.1128/AEM.03016-13] [PMID: 24212576]

[94]   Cole CB, Fuller R, Mallet AK, Rowland IR. The influence of the host on expression of intestinal microbial enzyme activities involved in metabolism of foreign compounds. J Appl Bacteriol 1985; 59(6): 549-53.
        [http://dx.doi.org/10.1111/j.1365-2672.1985.tb03359.x] [PMID: 3938453]

[95]   Mallett AK, Rowland IR. Bacterial enzymes: their role in the formation of mutagens and carcinogens in the intestine. Dig Dis 1990; 8(2): 71-9.
        [http://dx.doi.org/10.1159/000171241] [PMID: 2178815]

[96]   Roume H, EL Muller E, Cordes T, Renaut J, Hiller K, Wilmes P. A biomolecular isolation framework for eco-systems biology. ISME J 2013; 7(1): 110-21.
        [http://dx.doi.org/10.1038/ismej.2012.72] [PMID: 22763648]

[97]   Wang WL, Xu SY, Ren ZG, Tao L, Jiang JW, Zheng SS. Application of metagenomics in the human gut microbiome. World J Gastroenterol 2015; 21(3): 803-14.
        [http://dx.doi.org/10.3748/wjg.v21.i3.803] [PMID: 25624713]

[98]   Wei X, Yan X, Zou D, *et al.* Abnormal fecal microbiota community and functions in patients with hepatitis B liver cirrhosis as revealed by a metagenomic approach. BMC Gastroenterol 2013; 13(1): 175.
        [http://dx.doi.org/10.1186/1471-230X-13-175] [PMID: 24369878]

[99]   Jones BV, Begley M, Hill C, Gahan CGM, Marchesi JR. Functional and comparative metagenomic analysis of bile salt hydrolase activity in the human gut microbiome. Proc Natl Acad Sci USA 2008; 105(36): 13580-5.
        [http://dx.doi.org/10.1073/pnas.0804437105] [PMID: 18757757]

[100]   Mohammed A, Guda C. Application of a hierarchical enzyme classification method reveals the role of gut microbiome in human metabolism. BMC Genomics 2015; 16(S7) (Suppl. 7): S16.
        [http://dx.doi.org/10.1186/1471-2164-16-S7-S16] [PMID: 26099921]

[101]   Abram F. Systems-based approaches to unravel multi-species microbial community functioning. Comput Struct Biotechnol J 2015; 13: 24-32.
        [http://dx.doi.org/10.1016/j.csbj.2014.11.009] [PMID: 25750697]

[102]   Turnbaugh PJ, Hamady M, Yatsunenko T, *et al.* A core gut microbiome in obese and lean twins.

Nature 2009; 457(7228): 480-4.
[http://dx.doi.org/10.1038/nature07540] [PMID: 19043404]

[103] Gosalbes MJ, Durbán A, Pignatelli M, *et al.* Metatranscriptomic approach to analyze the functional human gut microbiota. PLoS One 2011; 6(3): e17447.
[http://dx.doi.org/10.1371/journal.pone.0017447] [PMID: 21408168]

[104] Walker AW, Duncan SH, Louis P, Flint HJ. Phylogeny, culturing, and metagenomics of the approaches to unravel multi-species microbial community functioning. Comput Struct Biotechnol J 2014; 13: 24-32.
[PMID: 25750697]

[105] Xiong W, Abraham PE, Li Z, Pan C, Hettich RL. Microbial metaproteomics for characterizing the range of metabolic functions and activities of human gut microbiota. Proteomics 2015; 15(20): 3424-38.
[http://dx.doi.org/10.1002/pmic.201400571] [PMID: 25914197]

[106] Young JC, Pan C, Adams RM, *et al.* Metaproteomics reveals functional shifts in microbial and human proteins during a preterm infant gut colonization case. Proteomics 2015; 15(20): 3463-73.
[http://dx.doi.org/10.1002/pmic.201400563] [PMID: 26077811]

[107] Verberkmoes NC, Russell AL, Shah M, *et al.* Shotgun metaproteomics of the human distal gut microbiota. ISME J 2009; 3(2): 179-89.
[http://dx.doi.org/10.1038/ismej.2008.108] [PMID: 18971961]

[108] Schirmer M, Smeekens SP, Vlamakis H, *et al.* Linking the human gut microbiome to inflammatory cytokine production capacity. Cell 2016; 167(4): 1125-1136.e8.
[http://dx.doi.org/10.1016/j.cell.2016.10.020] [PMID: 27814509]

[109] Bauer H, Horowitz RE, Levenson SM, Popper H. The response of the lymphatic tissue to the microbial flora. Studies on germfree mice. Am J Pathol 1963; 42(4): 471-83.
[PMID: 13966929]

[110] Mazmanian SK, Liu CH, Tzianabos AO, Kasper DL. An immunomodulatory molecule of symbiotic bacteria directs maturation of the host immune system. Cell 2005; 122(1): 107-18.
[http://dx.doi.org/10.1016/j.cell.2005.05.007] [PMID: 16009137]

[111] Hooper LV, Littman DR, Macpherson AJ. Interactions between the microbiota and the immune system. Science 2012; 336(6086): 1268-73.
[http://dx.doi.org/10.1126/science.1223490] [PMID: 22674334]

[112] Cerf-Bensussan N, Gaboriau-Routhiau V. The immune system and the gut microbiota: friends or foes? Nat Rev Immunol 2010; 10(10): 735-44.
[http://dx.doi.org/10.1038/nri2850] [PMID: 20865020]

[113] Kamada N, Seo SU, Chen GY, Núñez G. Role of the gut microbiota in immunity and inflammatory disease. Nat Rev Immunol 2013; 13(5): 321-35.
[http://dx.doi.org/10.1038/nri3430] [PMID: 23618829]

[114] Takeda K, Kaisho T, Akira S. Toll-Like Receptors. Annu Rev Immunol 2003; 21(1): 335-76.
[http://dx.doi.org/10.1146/annurev.immunol.21.120601.141126] [PMID: 12524386]

[115] Kawai T, Akira S. The role of pattern-recognition receptors in innate immunity: update on Toll-like receptors. Nat Immunol 2010; 11(5): 373-84.
[http://dx.doi.org/10.1038/ni.1863] [PMID: 20404851]

[116] Iwasaki A, Medzhitov R. Control of adaptive immunity by the innate immune system. Nat Immunol 2015; 16(4): 343-53.
[http://dx.doi.org/10.1038/ni.3123] [PMID: 25789684]

[117] Lathrop SK, Bloom SM, Rao SM, *et al.* Peripheral education of the immune system by colonic commensal microbiota. Nature 2011; 478(7368): 250-4.
[http://dx.doi.org/10.1038/nature10434] [PMID: 21937990]

[118] Weaver CT, Elson CO, Fouser LA, Kolls JK. The Th17 pathway and inflammatory diseases of the intestines, lungs, and skin. Annu Rev Pathol 2013; 8(1): 477-512.
[http://dx.doi.org/10.1146/annurev-pathol-011110-130318] [PMID: 23157335]

[119] Lindau D, Gielen P, Kroesen M, Wesseling P, Adema GJ. The immunosuppressive tumour network: myeloid-derived suppressor cells, regulatory T cells and natural killer T cells. Immunology 2013; 138(2): 105-15.
[http://dx.doi.org/10.1111/imm.12036] [PMID: 23216602]

[120] Ivanov II, Atarashi K, Manel N, *et al.* Induction of intestinal Th17 cells by segmented filamentous bacteria. Cell 2009; 139(3): 485-98.
[http://dx.doi.org/10.1016/j.cell.2009.09.033] [PMID: 19836068]

[121] Ruohtula T, de Goffau MC, Nieminen JK, *et al.* Maturation of gut microbiota and circulating regulatory T cells and development of IgE sensitization in early life. Front Immunol 2019; 10: 2494.
[http://dx.doi.org/10.3389/fimmu.2019.02494] [PMID: 31749800]

[122] Atarashi K, Tanoue T, Shima T, *et al.* Induction of colonic regulatory T cells by indigenous *Clostridium* species. Science 2011; 331(6015): 337-41.
[http://dx.doi.org/10.1126/science.1198469] [PMID: 21205640]

[123] Round JL, Lee SM, Li J, *et al.* The Toll-like receptor 2 pathway establishes colonization by a commensal of the human microbiota. Science 2011; 332(6032): 974-7.
[http://dx.doi.org/10.1126/science.1206095] [PMID: 21512004]

[124] Hapfelmeier S, Lawson MAE, Slack E, *et al.* Reversible microbial colonization of germ-free mice reveals the dynamics of IgA immune responses. Science 2010; 328(5986): 1705-9.
[http://dx.doi.org/10.1126/science.1188454] [PMID: 20576892]

[125] Johansson MEV, Hansson GC. Immunological aspects of intestinal mucus and mucins. Nat Rev Immunol 2016; 16(10): 639-49.
[http://dx.doi.org/10.1038/nri.2016.88] [PMID: 27498766]

[126] Deplancke B, Gaskins HR. Microbial modulation of innate defense: goblet cells and the intestinal mucus layer. Am J Clin Nutr 2001; 73(6): S1131-41.
[http://dx.doi.org/10.1093/ajcn/73.6.1131S] [PMID: 11393191]

[127] McCoy KD, Geuking MB. Microbiota regulates intratumoral monocytes to promote anti-tumor immune responses. Cell 2021; 184(21): 5301-3.
[http://dx.doi.org/10.1016/j.cell.2021.09.024] [PMID: 34624223]

[128] Lam KC, Araya RE, Huang A, *et al.* Microbiota triggers STING-type I IFN-dependent monocyte reprogramming of the tumor microenvironment. Cell 2021; 184(21): 5338-5356.e21.
[http://dx.doi.org/10.1016/j.cell.2021.09.019] [PMID: 34624222]

[129] Gill HS, Rutherfurd KJ, Prasad J, Gopal PK. Enhancement of natural and acquired immunity by *Lactobacillus rhamnosus* (HN001), *Lactobacillus acidophilus* (HN017) and *Bifidobacterium lactis* (HN019). Br J Nutr 2000; 83(2): 167-76.
[http://dx.doi.org/10.1017/S0007114500000210] [PMID: 10743496]

[130] Tanoue T, Morita S, Plichta DR, *et al.* A defined commensal consortium elicits CD8 T cells and anti-cancer immunity. Nature 2019; 565(7741): 600-5.
[http://dx.doi.org/10.1038/s41586-019-0878-z] [PMID: 30675064]

[131] Nakkarach A, Foo HL, Song AAL, Mutalib NEA, Nitisinprasert S, Withayagiat U. Anti-cancer and anti-inflammatory effects elicited by short chain fatty acids produced by *Escherichia coli* isolated from healthy human gut microbiota. Microb Cell Fact 2021; 20(1): 36.
[http://dx.doi.org/10.1186/s12934-020-01477-z] [PMID: 33546705]

[132] Sokol H, Pigneur B, Watterlot L, *et al. Faecalibacterium prausnitzii* is an anti-inflammatory commensal bacterium identified by gut microbiota analysis of Crohn disease patients. Proc Natl Acad Sci USA 2008; 105(43): 16731-6.

[http://dx.doi.org/10.1073/pnas.0804812105] [PMID: 18936492]

[133]   Rosshart SP, Vassallo BG, Angeletti D, *et al.* Wild mouse gut microbiota promotes host fitness and improves disease resistance. Cell 2017; 171(5): 1015-1028.e13.
[http://dx.doi.org/10.1016/j.cell.2017.09.016] [PMID: 29056339]

[134]   Yamamoto ML, Maier I, Dang AT, *et al.* Intestinal bacteria modify lymphoma incidence and latency by affecting systemic inflammatory state, oxidative stress, and leukocyte genotoxicity. Cancer Res 2013; 73(14): 4222-32.
[http://dx.doi.org/10.1158/0008-5472.CAN-13-0022] [PMID: 23860718]

[135]   Westbrook AM, Wei B, Braun J, Schiestl RH. Intestinal mucosal inflammation leads to systemic genotoxicity in mice. Cancer Res 2009; 69(11): 4827-34.
[http://dx.doi.org/10.1158/0008-5472.CAN-08-4416] [PMID: 19487293]

[136]   An BC, Hong S, Park HJ, *et al.* Anti-colorectal cancer effects of probiotic-derived p8 protein. Genes (Basel) 2019; 10(8): 624.
[http://dx.doi.org/10.3390/genes10080624] [PMID: 31430963]

[137]   Chen CC, Lin WC, Kong MS, *et al.* Oral inoculation of probiotics *Lactobacillus acidophilus* NCFM suppresses tumour growth both in segmental orthotopic colon cancer and extra-intestinal tissue. Br J Nutr 2012; 107(11): 1623-34.
[http://dx.doi.org/10.1017/S0007114511004934] [PMID: 21992995]

[138]   Iyer C, Kosters A, Sethi G, Kunnumakkara AB, Aggarwal BB, Versalovic J. Probiotic *Lactobacillus reuteri* promotes TNF-induced apoptosis in human myeloid leukemia-derived cells by modulation of NF-κB and MAPK signalling. Cell Microbiol 2008; 10(7): 1442-52.
[http://dx.doi.org/10.1111/j.1462-5822.2008.01137.x] [PMID: 18331465]

[139]   Mikó E, Vida A, Kovács T, *et al.* Lithocholic acid, a bacterial metabolite reduces breast cancer cell proliferation and aggressiveness. Biochim Biophys Acta Bioenerg 2018; 1859(9): 958-74.
[http://dx.doi.org/10.1016/j.bbabio.2018.04.002] [PMID: 29655782]

[140]   Sadeghi-Aliabadi H, Mohammadi F, Fazeli H, Mirlohi M. Effects of *Lactobacillus plantarum* A7 with probiotic potential on colon cancer and normal cells proliferation in comparison with a commercial strain. Iran J Basic Med Sci 2014; 17(10): 815-9.
[PMID: 25729553]

[141]   Chandel D, Sharma M, Chawla V, Sachdeva N, Shukla G. Isolation, characterization and identification of antigenotoxic and anticancerous indigenous probiotics and their prophylactic potential in experimental colon carcinogenesis. Sci Rep 2019; 9(1): 14769.
[http://dx.doi.org/10.1038/s41598-019-51361-z] [PMID: 31611620]

[142]   Meurman JH. Oral microbiota and cancer. J Oral Microbiol 2010; 2(1): 5195.
[http://dx.doi.org/10.3402/jom.v2i0.5195] [PMID: 21523227]

[143]   Pevsner-Fischer M, Tuganbaev T, Meijer M, *et al.* Role of the microbiome in non-gastrointestinal cancers. World J Clin Oncol 2016; 7(2): 200-13.
[http://dx.doi.org/10.5306/wjco.v7.i2.200] [PMID: 27081642]

[144]   Wang F, Meng W, Wang B, Qiao L. *Helicobacter pylori*-induced gastric inflammation and gastric cancer. Cancer Lett 2014; 345(2): 196-202.
[http://dx.doi.org/10.1016/j.canlet.2013.08.016] [PMID: 23981572]

[145]   Ishaq S, Nunn L. *Helicobacter pylori* and gastric cancer: a state of the art review. Gastroenterol Hepatol Bed Bench 2015; 8 (Suppl. 1): S6-S14.
[PMID: 26171139]

[146]   Vergara D, Simeone P, Damato M, Maffia M, Lanuti P, Trerotola M. The cancer microbiota: EMT and inflammation as shared molecular mechanisms associated with plasticity and progression Journal of Oncology, vol. 2019, Article ID 1253727, 16 pages, 2019.

[147]   Dzutsev A, Badger JH, Perez-Chanona E, *et al.* Microbes and Cancer. Annu Rev Immunol 2017;

35(1): 199-228.
[http://dx.doi.org/10.1146/annurev-immunol-051116-052133] [PMID: 28142322]

[148] Nešić D, Hsu Y, Stebbins CE. Assembly and function of a bacterial genotoxin. Nature 2004; 429(6990): 429-33.
[http://dx.doi.org/10.1038/nature02532] [PMID: 15164065]

[149] Hanahan D, Weinberg RA. Hallmarks of cancer: the next generation. Cell 2011; 144(5): 646-74.
[http://dx.doi.org/10.1016/j.cell.2011.02.013] [PMID: 21376230]

[150] Wu S, Rhee KJ, Albesiano E, *et al.* A human colonic commensal promotes colon tumorigenesis *via* activation of T helper type 17 T cell responses. Nat Med 2009; 15(9): 1016-22.
[http://dx.doi.org/10.1038/nm.2015] [PMID: 19701202]

[151] Boleij A, Hechenbleikner EM, Goodwin AC, *et al.* The *Bacteroides fragilis* toxin gene is prevalent in the colon mucosa of colorectal cancer patients. Clin Infect Dis 2015; 60(2): 208-15.
[http://dx.doi.org/10.1093/cid/ciu787] [PMID: 25305284]

[152] Jin C, Lagoudas GK, Zhao C, *et al.* Commensal microbiota promote lung cancer development *via* γδ T cells. Cell 2019; 176(5): 998-1013.e16.
[http://dx.doi.org/10.1016/j.cell.2018.12.040] [PMID: 30712876]

[153] Hattori N, Ushijima T. Epigenetic impact of infection on carcinogenesis: mechanisms and applications. Genome Med 2016; 8(1): 10.
[http://dx.doi.org/10.1186/s13073-016-0267-2] [PMID: 26823082]

[154] Rutkowski MR, Stephen TL, Svoronos N, *et al.* Microbially driven TLR5-dependent signaling governs distal malignant progression through tumor-promoting inflammation. Cancer Cell 2015; 27(1): 27-40.
[http://dx.doi.org/10.1016/j.ccell.2014.11.009] [PMID: 25533336]

[155] Arthur JC, Perez-Chanona E, Mühlbauer M, *et al.* Intestinal inflammation targets cancer-inducing activity of the microbiota. Science 2012; 338(6103): 120-3.
[http://dx.doi.org/10.1126/science.1224820] [PMID: 22903521]

[156] Arthur JC, Gharaibeh RZ, Mühlbauer M, *et al.* Microbial genomic analysis reveals the essential role of inflammation in bacteria-induced colorectal cancer. Nat Commun 2014; 5(1): 4724.
[http://dx.doi.org/10.1038/ncomms5724] [PMID: 25182170]

[157] Sobhani I, Tap J, Roudot-Thoraval F, *et al.* Microbial dysbiosis in colorectal cancer (CRC) patients. PLoS One 2011; 6(1): e16393.
[http://dx.doi.org/10.1371/journal.pone.0016393] [PMID: 21297998]

[158] Gur C, Ibrahim Y, Isaacson B, *et al.* Binding of the Fap2 protein of *Fusobacterium nucleatum* to human inhibitory receptor TIGIT protects tumors from immune cell attack. Immunity 2015; 42(2): 344-55.
[http://dx.doi.org/10.1016/j.immuni.2015.01.010] [PMID: 25680274]

[159] Pushalkar S, Hundeyin M, Daley D, *et al.* The pancreatic cancer microbiome promotes oncogenesis by induction of innate and adaptive immune suppression. Cancer Discov 2018; 8(4): 403-16.
[http://dx.doi.org/10.1158/2159-8290.CD-17-1134] [PMID: 29567829]

[160] He Z, Gharaibeh RZ, Newsome RC, *et al. Campylobacter jejuni* promotes colorectal tumorigenesis through the action of cytolethal distending toxin. Gut 2019; 68(2): 289-300.
[http://dx.doi.org/10.1136/gutjnl-2018-317200] [PMID: 30377189]

[161] Dalmasso G, Cougnoux A, Delmas J. A. DarfeuilleMichaud, and R. Bonnet, "The bacterial genotoxincolibactin promotes colon tumor growth by modifying the tumor microenvironment,". Gut Microbes 2014; 5(5): 675-80.
[http://dx.doi.org/10.4161/19490976.2014.969989] [PMID: 25483338]

[162] Sears CL, Garrett WS. Microbes, microbiota, and colon cancer. Cell Host Microbe 2014; 15(3): 317-28.
[http://dx.doi.org/10.1016/j.chom.2014.02.007] [PMID: 24629338]

[163]   Osherov N, Ben-Ami R. Modulation of host angiogenesis as a microbial survival strategy and therapeutic target. PLoS Pathog 2016; 12(4): e1005479.
[http://dx.doi.org/10.1371/journal.ppat.1005479] [PMID: 27078259]

[164]   Wynendaele E, Verbeke F, D'Hondt M, *et al.* Crosstalk between the microbiome and cancer cells by quorum sensing peptides. Peptides 2015; 64: 40-8.
[http://dx.doi.org/10.1016/j.peptides.2014.12.009] [PMID: 25559405]

[165]   Sanmamed MF, Chen L. A paradigm shift in cancer immunotherapy: from enhancement to normalization. Cell 2019; 176(3): 677.
[http://dx.doi.org/10.1016/j.cell.2019.01.008] [PMID: 30682374]

[166]   Haslam A, Prasad V. Estimation of the percentage of US patients with cancer who are eligible for and respond to checkpoint inhibitor immunotherapy drugs. JAMA Netw Open 2019; 2(5): e192535-5.
[http://dx.doi.org/10.1001/jamanetworkopen.2019.2535] [PMID: 31050774]

[167]   Kalbasi A, Ribas A. Tumour-intrinsic resistance to immune checkpoint blockade. Nat Rev Immunol 2020; 20(1): 25-39.
[http://dx.doi.org/10.1038/s41577-019-0218-4] [PMID: 31570880]

[168]   Pitt JM, Vétizou M, Daillère R, *et al.* Resistance mechanisms to immune-checkpoint blockade in cancer: tumor-intrinsic and -extrinsic factors. Immunity 2016; 44(6): 1255-69.
[http://dx.doi.org/10.1016/j.immuni.2016.06.001] [PMID: 27332730]

[169]   Matson V, Fessler J, Bao R, *et al.* The commensal microbiome is associated with anti–PD-1 efficacy in metastatic melanoma patients. Science 2018; 359(6371): 104-8.
[http://dx.doi.org/10.1126/science.aao3290] [PMID: 29302014]

[170]   Gopalakrishnan V, Spencer CN, Nezi L, *et al.* Gut microbiome modulates response to anti–PD-1 immunotherapy in melanoma patients. Science 2018; 359(6371): 97-103.
[http://dx.doi.org/10.1126/science.aan4236] [PMID: 29097493]

[171]   Chaput N, Lepage P, Coutzac C, *et al.* Baseline gut microbiota predicts clinical response and colitis in metastatic melanoma patients treated with ipilimumab. Ann Oncol 2017; 28(6): 1368-79.
[http://dx.doi.org/10.1093/annonc/mdx108] [PMID: 28368458]

[172]   Routy B, Le Chatelier E, Derosa L, *et al.* Gut microbiome influences efficacy of PD-1–based immunotherapy against epithelial tumors. Science 2018; 359(6371): 91-7.
[http://dx.doi.org/10.1126/science.aan3706] [PMID: 29097494]

[173]   Baruch EN, Youngster I, Ortenberg R, *et al.* Abstract CT042: Fecal microbiota transplantation (FMT) and re-induction of anti-PD-1 therapy in refractory metastatic melanoma patients - preliminary results from a phase I clinical trial (NCT03353402). Cancer Res 2019; 79(13_Supplement): CT042-2.
[http://dx.doi.org/10.1158/1538-7445.AM2019-CT042]

[174]   Sivan A, Corrales L, Hubert N, *et al.* Commensal *Bifidobacterium* promotes antitumor immunity and facilitates anti–PD-L1 efficacy. Science 2015; 350(6264): 1084-9.
[http://dx.doi.org/10.1126/science.aac4255] [PMID: 26541606]

[175]   Vétizou M, Pitt JM, Daillère R, *et al.* Anticancer immunotherapy by CTLA-4 blockade relies on the gut microbiota. Science 2015; 350(6264): 1079-84.
[http://dx.doi.org/10.1126/science.aad1329] [PMID: 26541610]

[176]   Dubin K, Callahan MK, Ren B, *et al.* Intestinal microbiome analyses identify melanoma patients at risk for checkpoint-blockade-induced colitis. Nat Commun 2016; 7(1): 10391.
[http://dx.doi.org/10.1038/ncomms10391] [PMID: 26837003]

[177]   Yoo JY, Hurwitz BS, Bolyard C, *et al.* Bortezomib-induced unfolded protein response increases oncolytic HSV-1 replication resulting in synergistic antitumor effects. Clin Cancer Res 2014; 20(14): 3787-98.
[http://dx.doi.org/10.1158/1078-0432.CCR-14-0553] [PMID: 24815720]

[178] Zheng Y, Wang T, Tu X, *et al.* Gut microbiome affects the response to anti-PD-1 immunotherapy in patients with hepatocellular carcinoma. J Immunother Cancer 2019; 7(1): 193.
[http://dx.doi.org/10.1186/s40425-019-0650-9] [PMID: 31337439]

[179] Jin Y, Dong H, Xia L, *et al.* The diversity of gut microbiome is associated with favorable responses to anti-programmed death 1 immunotherapy in chinese patients with NSCLC. J Thorac Oncol 2019; 14(8): 1378-89.
[http://dx.doi.org/10.1016/j.jtho.2019.04.007] [PMID: 31026576]

[180] Elinav E, Garrett WS, Trinchieri G, Wargo J. The cancer microbiome. Nat Rev Cancer 2019; 19(7): 371-6.
[http://dx.doi.org/10.1038/s41568-019-0155-3] [PMID: 31186547]

[181] De Groot PF, Frissen MN, de Clercq NC, Nieuwdorp M. Fecal microbiota transplantation in metabolic syndrome: History, present and future. Gut Microbes 2017; 8(3): 253-67.
[http://dx.doi.org/10.1080/19490976.2017.1293224] [PMID: 28609252]

[182] Walter J, Armet AM, Finlay BB, Shanahan F. Establishing or exaggerating causality for the gut microbiome: lessons from human microbiota-associated rodents. Cell 2020; 180(2): 221-32.
[http://dx.doi.org/10.1016/j.cell.2019.12.025] [PMID: 31978342]

[183] Barham WJ, Harrington SM, Liu X, Dong H. Humanized PD-1/PDL1 (HuPD) mice facilitate the direct functional comparison of immune checkpoint inhibitors *in vivo.* J Immunol 2019; 202(195): 191-5. 191

[184] Lin Q, Ma H, Zhang X, *et al.* Abstract 1495: Alternative humanized PD-1 mouse models provide more options for PD-1 antibody efficacy study *in vivo.* Cancer Res 2019; 79(13_Supplement): 1495-5.
[http://dx.doi.org/10.1158/1538-7445.AM2019-1495]

[185] Yao LC, Cheng M, Aryee KE, *et al.* Abstract 5676: Patient-derived tumor xenografts in humanized NSG-SGM3 mice: An improved immuno-oncology platform. Cancer Res 2018; 78(13_Supplement): 5676-6.
[http://dx.doi.org/10.1158/1538-7445.AM2018-5676]

[186] Moore N, Doty D, Zielstorff M, *et al.* A multiplexed microfluidic system for evaluation of dynamics of immune–tumor interactions. Lab Chip 2018; 18(13): 1844-58.
[http://dx.doi.org/10.1039/C8LC00256H] [PMID: 29796561]

[187] Trapecar M, Communal C, Velazquez J, *et al.* Gut-liver physiomimetics reveal paradoxical modulation of IBD-related inflammation by short-chain fatty acids. Cell Syst 2020; 10(3): 223-239.e9.
[http://dx.doi.org/10.1016/j.cels.2020.02.008] [PMID: 32191873]

[188] Vétizou M, Pitt JM, Daillère R, *et al.* Anticancer immunotherapy by CTLA-4 blockade relies on the gut microbiota. Science 2015; 350(6264): 1079-84.
[http://dx.doi.org/10.1126/science.aad1329] [PMID: 26541610]

[189] Sivan A, Corrales L, Hubert N, *et al.* Commensal *Bifidobacterium* promotes antitumor immunity and facilitates anti–PD-L1 efficacy. Science 2015; 350(6264): 1084-9.
[http://dx.doi.org/10.1126/science.aac4255] [PMID: 26541606]

[190] Dubin K, Callahan MK, Ren B, *et al.* Intestinal microbiome analyses identify melanoma patients at risk for checkpoint-blockade-induced colitis. Nat Commun 2016; 7(1): 10391.
[http://dx.doi.org/10.1038/ncomms10391] [PMID: 26837003]

[191] Frankel AE, Coughlin LA, Kim J, *et al.* Metagenomic shotgun sequencing and unbiased metabolomic profiling identify specific human gut microbiota and metabolites associated with immune checkpoint therapy efficacy in melanoma patients. Neoplasia 2017; 19(10): 848-55.
[http://dx.doi.org/10.1016/j.neo.2017.08.004] [PMID: 28923537]

[192] Chaput N, Lepage P, Coutzac C, *et al.* Baseline gut microbiota predicts clinical response and colitis in metastatic melanoma patie 2017; 1; 28(6): 1368-1379.

[193] Matson V, Fessler J, Bao R, *et al.* The commensal microbiome is associated with anti–PD-1 efficacy in metastatic melanoma patients. Science 2018; 359(6371): 104-8.
[http://dx.doi.org/10.1126/science.aao3290] [PMID: 29302014]

[194] Gopalakrishnan V, Spencer CN, Nezi L, *et al.* Gut microbiome modulates response to anti–PD-1 immunotherapy in melanoma patients. Science 2018; 359(6371): 97-103.
[http://dx.doi.org/10.1126/science.aan4236] [PMID: 29097493]

[195] Routy B, Le Chatelier E, Derosa L, *et al.* Gut microbiome influences efficacy of PD-1–based immunotherapy against epithelial tumors. Science 2018; 359(6371): 91-7.
[http://dx.doi.org/10.1126/science.aan3706] [PMID: 29097494]

[196] Leshem A, Horesh N, Elinav E. Fecal microbial transplantation and its potential application in cardiometabolic syndrome. Front Immunol 2019; 10: 1341.
[http://dx.doi.org/10.3389/fimmu.2019.01341] [PMID: 31258528]

CHAPTER 2

Mechanism of Probiotic Action in Anticancer Immunity

Mangala Lakshmi Ragavan[1] and **Nilanjana Das**[1,*]

[1] *Biomedical Sciences Department, School of BioSciences and Technology, Vellore Institute of Technology, Vellore, Tamil Nadu, India*

Abstract: Gut microbiota plays a significant role in human physiology which includes metabolism, nutrition uptake and immune responses. The imbalance of gut microbiota leads to various disorders or diseases like inflammatory bowel disease, infectious diseases, cancer and obesity. Cancer is one of the major health problems worldwide. Moreover, colorectal cancer (CRC) is the most common cancer in humans which is considered the fourth leading health problem worldwide. The role of probiotics in the regulation of CRC includes enhancement of immune barrier function, intestinal immune state, inhibition of enzymatic activity, cell proliferation and apoptosis, redox homeostasis, and modifying the composition of intestinal microbiota. It can be treated using chemotherapy, radiotherapy, or surgical eradication. However, these treatments may cause the demolition of the intestinal mucosal barrier system as well as dysfunction of the immune system in cancer patients. Hence, biotherapeutic drugs are used along with probiotics and their metabolites *viz.* polysaccharides, short-chain fatty acids, and inhibitory compounds like proteins and other substances to treat cancer. *Lactobacillus rhamnosus* GG (LGG) is a widely used probiotic strain in oncology. Also, it has been proven to exert beneficial effects on cancer patients after anticancer therapy. Therapeutic potential of the gut microbiome in cancer treatment *via* the administration of probiotic supplementations is being investigated using several clinical studies. Probiotic-incorporated biotheraupetic drugs are considered an alternative medicine for various types of cancer. The effectiveness of biotheraupetic drugs mainly depends on the dosage of probiotic strain and their exposure time. However, the mechanism behind the role of probiotics in cancer immunity is unclear so far. The present work summarizes the action of probiotics in anticancer immunity.

Keywords: Biotheraupetics, Cancer, Chemotherapy, Gut microbiome, Immunity, Probiotics.

---

* **Corresponding author Nilanjana Das:** Biomedical Sciences Department, School of BioSciences and Technology, Vellore Institute of Technology, Vellore, Tamil Nadu, India; E-mails: nilanjanadasvit@gmail.com and nilanjanamitra@vit.ac.in

Mitesh Kumar Dwivedi, Alwarappan Sankaranarayanan & Sanjay Tiwari (Eds.)

1. INTRODUCTION

The gut microbiota is considered one of the most significant factors in maintaining homeostasis. Bacterial strains are involved in the detection and degradation of possible carcinogens,the production of immune system signalling molecules like short-chain fatty acids (SCFAs), which influence cell death and proliferation during carcinogenesis [1]. Due to their capacity to affect cancer cell proliferation and death, probiotics have gotten a lot of attention from consumers. These potential properties are helpful to treat cancer through innovative therapies, which are considered an alternative method to more invasive treatments like chemotherapy or radiotherapy [2]. Several studies have indicated that dysbiosis of the intestinal microbiota contributes to the development of metabolic and intestinal diseases, including obesity, diabetes, and cancer [3]. The microbiota can be tumorigenic or tumor-suppressive, and its regulation and maintenance are critical for the host's overall health. Consumption of probiotics modulates the microbiota, maintains a symbiotic relationship with the host, and ensures the optimal development of the immune system and the efficacy of cancer treatment [4 - 6]. In this chapter, the cancer immunity achieved by probiotic strains is discussed with their mechanism of action.

1.1. Gut Microbiome

The human microbiome is made up of a range of microorganisms that live on the surface of our body's epithelial barrier, including bacteria, fungi, archaea, protozoa, and viruses. The gut microbiome can modulate the host's immune system to maintain the host's health. Probiotic bacteria have been proven to have an important function in immunomodulation and have antitumor effects in humans. Also, probiotics have the potential to boost and reduce the production of cytokines which are anti-inflammatory molecules and play a vital role in carcinogenesis prevention. Lactic acid bacteria in the gut have been demonstrated to play a role in carcinogenesis regression by producing metabolites that interact with immunological and epithelial cells due to their influence on immunomodulation [1]. Multiple physiological functions can be affected by the microbiota, especially metabolism, inflammation and immunity. The gut microbiota collaborates with epithelial and stromal cells to perform a variety of important regulatory activities. It maintains mucosal immunological homeostasis and host-microbial symbiosis, as well as prevents pathogen infection [7]. Microbial components in the intestine have a significant impact on the peripheral immune system, especially in the case of cancer [8].

An effect of the microbiota on host bile acids was reported as a carcinogenic driver in some of the studies. Primary bile acids are created in the liver and released into the small intestine, where bacteria convert them to deconjugated, secondary and tertiary bile acid moieties, which are then reabsorbed by the intestine and transported to the liver *via* portal circulation. Deoxycholic acid (DCA), a secondary bile acid product, is particularly carcinogenic and leads to DNA damage in hepatocytes [9].

1.2. Current Status of Cancer and Treatments

Cancer is the world's second-largest cause of death. In the United States alone, around 18,98,160 persons were diagnosed with cancer in 2021, with 6,08,570 of them dying due to the disease [10]. In India, 13,24,413 people were affected, and 8,51,678 people died of cancer [11]. Thus, cancer is a major issue that has an impact on the health of all human communities. Colorectal cancer (CRC) is the third most commonly diagnosed malignancy and the fourth leading cause of cancer-related death in the world. The treatment for colon cancer is illustrated in Fig. (**1**).

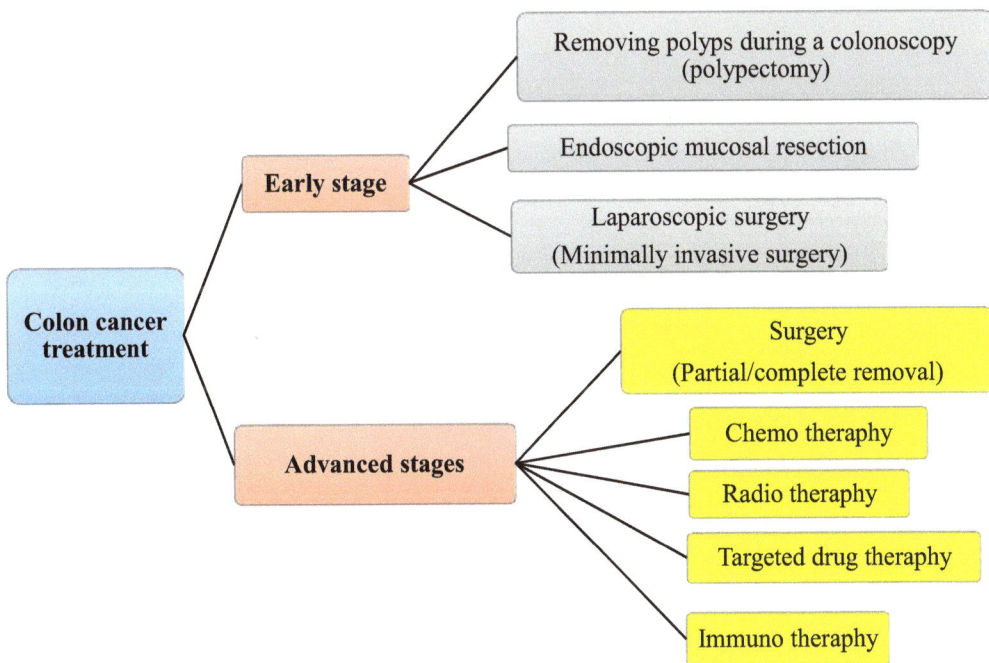

Fig. (1). Treatment strategies for Colon cancer.

Cancer immunotherapy is becoming more popular as a treatment option for cancer patients. It acts as an anti-tumor agent by utilising the immune system. As innovative immunotherapeutic drugs, immune checkpoint inhibitors (ICIs) showed encouraging clinical results for advanced hematologic malignancies. Recent research has shown that the gut microbiota influences the therapeutic efficacy of ICIs against cancer [12]. *Lactobacilli* strains are widely used probiotics for cancer treatment due to their anti-inflammatory properties, which modulate cytokine production in human dendritic cells [13, 14].

2. PROBIOTIC STRAINS USED FOR CANCER TREATMENT

Probiotics have a strong rebalancing effect on the gut microbiota with possible favourable effects on gastrointestinal immune regulation to maintain the host's health. Also, recent studies support the concept that taking certain probiotics on a daily basis can be a viable way to successfully prevent patients from the risk of serious side effects from radiation therapy or chemotherapy [15]. *Lactobacillus acidophilus* and *Lactobacillus salivarius* were found to have preventive effects on the development of precancerous growths and colorectal carcinogenesis in the rat model, respectively [16]. Probiotic strains reported for their anticancer activity are tabulated in Table **1**.

Table 1. Probiotic strains used for cancer treatment.

Probiotic bacteria	*Lactobacillus sp.*	*Bifidobacterium sp.*	Otder strains
	L. acidophilus	B. infantis	Enterococcus faecium
	L. casei	B. breve	Streptococcus tdermophilus
	L. plantarum	B. longum	Propionibacterium freudenreichii
	L. delbrueckii		
	L. rhamnosus		
	L. fermentum		
	L. reuteri		
Probiotic yeasts	*Saccharomyces sp.*	*Kluyveromyces sp.*	Other strains
	S. cerevisiae	K. marxianus	Debaryomyces hansenii
	S. boulardii	K. lactis	Pichia kudriavzevii

3. MECHANISM OF PROBIOTICS ON CANCER IMMUNITY

The gut mucosal immune system relies on a complex network of signals involving many interactions between commensal and foreign antigens as well as eukaryotic cells, to maintain host health. These include non-specific barrier cells like epithelial cells, macrophages, dendritic cells (DCs), and other mucus-producing cells such as goblet cells, as well as Paneth cells which exude antimicrobial peptides and make defensins to prevent the pathogens [17]. The mechanism of probiotic's action is illustrated in Fig. (**2**).

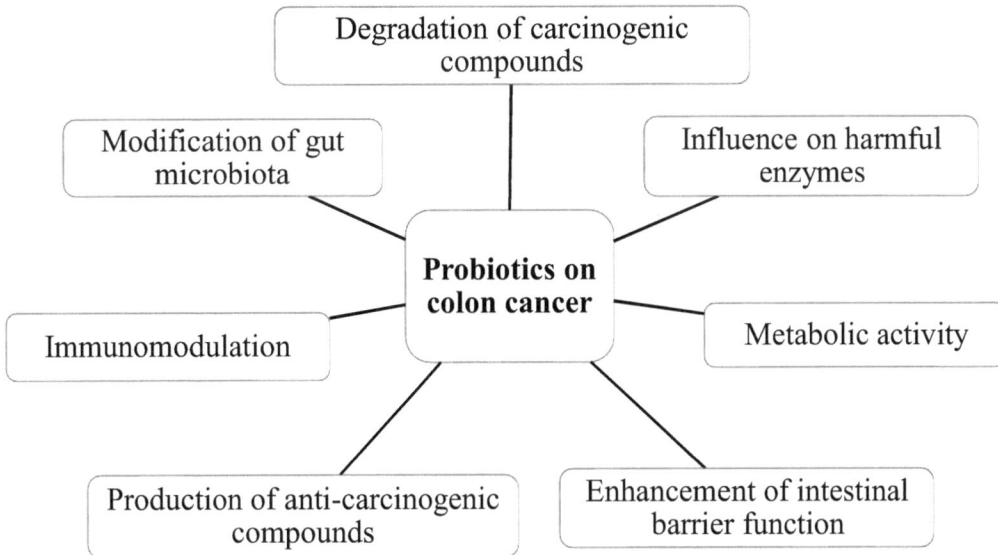

Fig. (2). Mode of actions of probiotics on colon cancer.

3.1. Modifications of Gut Microbiota

To maintain homeostasis, the healthy gut microbiota must be well-balanced and diverse (eubiosis). A disruption in the gut microbiota balance can lead to a lack of helpful bacteria and an overabundance of pathogens (dysbiosis). Dysbiosis can also lead to persistent inflammation and increased synthesis of carcinogenic chemicals, thereby raising the risk of colorectal cancer (CRC) [18, 19]. The production of toxic and genotoxic bacterial metabolites, which can cause mutations by binding to specific cell surface receptors and affecting intracellular signal transduction, has been linked to the development of gastrointestinal cancers [20]. Thus, the use of probiotic bacteria during the early stages of carcinogenesis significantly reduced the risk of colon cancer.

3.2. Immunomodulation

The composition of the gut microflora has been linked to the onset and progression of cancer, as well as therapeutic efficiency. These effects are mediated by anti-tumour immune responses and have been found in a range of tumours, not just in the stomach but also in other organs [21, 22]. The gut microbiota cancer immunity is usually divided into three categories: (i) T cell responses induced by microorganisms cross-react with tumour antigens, (ii) pattern recognition receptors (PRRs) generated by microbes regulate immunological and anti-inflammatory responses, and (iii) metabolite secretion influences systemic effects [23, 24]. Probiotic bacteria change the composition of the gut microbiota, which plays a key role in CRC carcinogenesis. Immunity to cancer is a cyclic, self-replicating process that results in an accumulation of immune-stimulatory substances that should amplify and expand T-cell responses. Inhibitory factors also play a role in the cycle, leading to immune regulatory feedback mechanisms that can prevent or limit immunity development [25]. This cycle has seven stages starting from the release of antigens from the cancer cell to the death of cancer cells (Fig. 3).

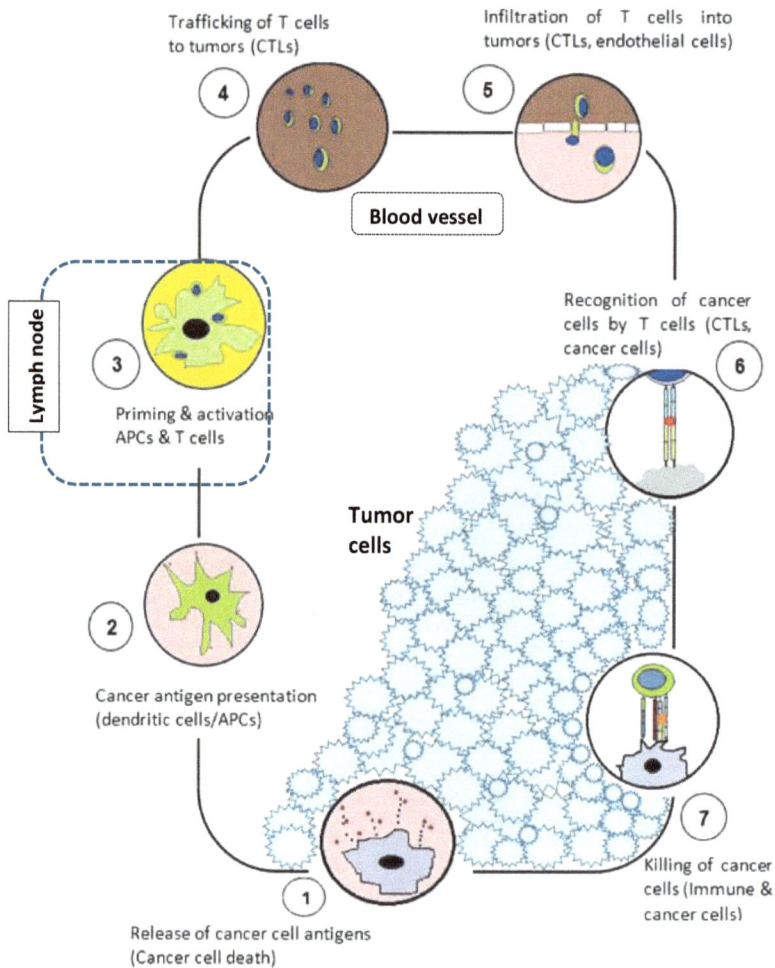

Fig. (3). Cancer immunity cycle.

The cancer immunity cycle requires the synchronization of a variety of stimulatory and inhibitory factors. The inhibitors include cytokines like IL-4 &

IL-13 (which play a key role in the inflammatory process), Programmed death ligands like PD-L1, PD-L1/B7.1 (proteins that inhibit T cell proliferation & cytokine production) and the immunosuppressive cytokines (*e.g.*, IL-10 & TGF-β) which have a pleiotropic effect on the following immune cells *viz*. DCs, natural killer (NK) cells, macrophages, CD4$^+$, CD8$^+$ T cells and stimulates the differentiation of immune-suppressive regulatory T cells (Tregs) [26, 27]. The stimulatory factors like cytokines include IL-1, IL-2, IL-12 (interleukins), IFN-α, IFN-γ, CD28, CD40, CD27, CD137 (proteins that activate antigen-presenting cells during the downstream process), TLRs (Toll-like receptors), inflammatory chemokines (CXCL-5, CXCL-10, CCL-5, & CX3CL-1) and T cell receptors (TCR plays an essential role as a regulator in the immune system) [28].

Several studies suggest that probiotics can stimulate the inhibition of cancer cell proliferation as well as maintain host cell immunity. IFN-cytokine promotes cellular proliferation in the intestine and is required for the maturation of immune cells such as DCs, IL-4, IL-5, and IL-10. By activating NK cells and macrophages, IFN-γ protects against viruses, intracellular infections, and carcinogens [29]. IL-8 is a chemokine frequently produced in the tumour microenvironment (TME) by human malignant cells. IL-8 is involved in the immune biology of human cancers as well as therapy resistance. Moreover, the change in serum IL-8 is a biomarker to follow the treatment with checkpoint inhibitors [30]. *L. casei* BL23 has immunomodulatory properties mediated by IL-22 cytokine's downregulation and anti-proliferative properties mediated by Bik, caspase-7 and caspase-9 upregulation [31]. Anticancer efficacy of *Lactobacilli* combinations in a colon cancer mouse model was demonstrated by combining multiple anti-inflammatory pathways and IL-10 activation [32]. *Lactobacilli* and *Bifidobacteria* have been widely studied for their potential activity against cancer and the anti-inflammatory effect in modifying cytokine production in human DCs. *E. faecium* CRL 183 possesses antitumor properties by provoking the immune system. *Lactobacillus* supplementation in mice modulated the expression of Toll-like receptor 2 (TLR2), TLR4, and TLR9, and notably, TLR2 lowered the tumour incidence [33]. Probiotics have been linked with better immunological functions in CRC patients, according to the research. The supplementation of *B. longum* and *L. johnsonii* resulted in increased expression of T helper (CD4) and cytotoxic T (CD8) cell markers in a double-blind, randomised controlled study by Gianotti *et al.* [34].

Probiotic bacteria also engage with PRRs on innate immune cells and trigger the powerful anti-tumour Th1 and CD8$^+$ T cell responses in DCs. *Lactobacillus* strains increased the expression of activation and maturation markers like MHC-II, CD83, CD40, CD80, and CD86 on the surface of human myeloid dendritic cells [35]. The expression of co-stimulation and maturation markers on DCs, as well as the production of cytokines such as IFN-γ and the efficacy of CD8$^+$ T cell activation, were improved by a *Lactobacillus kefiri* formulation [36]. Similar effects were noted for *Lactobacilli* species with co-culture in priming human DCs for IL-12-mediated Th1 polarisation and IFN-γ production. The combination of IL-12 and IL-18-induced production of IFN-γ was also observed in murine DCs activated by *Lactococcus lactis* subsp. *cremoris* FC [37, 38]. *Lactobacilli* can stimulate the host's immune cells, such as DCs or NK cells, and the T helper type 1 (TH1) response, which plays a role in precancerous or anti-cancerous cells. In an *in vivo* breast cancer murine model (8–10-week old *Balboa*), oral administration of probiotic *Lactobacillus acidophilus* isolated from traditional home-made yoghurt and neonatal stool reduced the tumour growth by modulating immune response or changing the cytokine milieu, reducing the tumour growth rate, increasing lymphocyte proliferation, protecting TH cells, and activating anti-tumor cell [39].

3.3. Metabolic Activity

Some bacteria in the human intestines are capable of creating carcinogenic chemicals from both the food and endogenously produced bile salts. Some enzymes, such as azoreductase, β-glucuronidase, β-glucosidase, and nitrate reductase, *etc.*, are capable of converting heterocyclic aromatic amines, polycyclic aromatic hydrocarbons, and primary bile acids into active carcinogens and synthetizing aglycones, ammonia, cresols, phenols, and N-nitroso compounds [40]. These compounds have genotoxic and cytotoxic properties leading to aberrant cell proliferation and activation of anti-apoptotic pathways in colonocytes, which then lead to colorectal cancer (CRC) development in humans. The risk of CRC can be reduced by changing the microbial metabolism through regulating these enzymes by probiotics and this can be considered as an efficient strategy to prevent the colon cancer [19]. *L. acidophilus* NCFM had a positive effect on the activity of azoreductase, nitroreductase, and β-glucuronidase in 21 healthy volunteers, according to Goldin and Gorbach [41]. The procarcinogens can be converted to proximal carcinogens by these faecal enzymes. Administration of *L. rhamnosus* GG or *L.acidophilus* to DMH-mediated CRC-induced rats resulted in the reduction of β-glucuronidase activity. In another trial, *L. plantarum* or *L. casei* reduced the nitroreductase activity, whereas *B. bifidum* exhibited inhibition of glucosidase activity [42].

3.4. Enhancement of Intestinal Barrier Function

The intestinal environment deteriorated in CRC patients compared to healthy controls, and the intestinal environment was improved upon probiotics' administration, suggesting that probiotics could be used to prevent CRC. Also, probiotic formulations considerably reduce the risk of postoperative complications, like mechanical ventilation, infections and anastomotic leakage for colon cancer [43]. The immune system and mucosal barrier homeostasis can be disrupted by dysbiosis in the gastrointestinal tract (GIT), resulting in increased mucosal barrier permeability and a persistent state of inflammation. This disruption can activate cytokines and growth factors such as transforming growth factor-beta (TGF-β), tumour necrosis factor-α (TNF-α), interleukin-6 (IL-6) and vascular endothelial growth factor (VEGF), which can promote the growth of dysplastic cell growth [44]. Increased bile acid metabolism, cell proliferation *via* Toll-like receptors, and other pathways can also contribute to malignant transformation in dysbiosis with bacterial biofilm development [7]. Goblet cells create a protective coating of mucin made up of gel-forming glycoproteins that act as lubricants and a barrier between the body and the environment. *MUC1, MUC2, MUC3, MUC4,* and *MUC5AC genes* are expressed, and at least nine human mucins (*MUC*) genes have been found in the human colon. *MUC2* is the main structural component of the mucus gel and is the principal gel-forming mucin of the small and large intestines. Mucin synthesis is reduced, and their composition is less glycosylated, as a result of the carcinogenic process. Some probiotics have been shown to boost mucin synthesis by goblet cells by upregulating *MUC* genes, particularly *MUC2* [45]. Inflammatory and cancerous processes enhance intestinal permeability by altering the structure and expression of cellular junction proteins, which induce colonocytes to stick together. Probiotics can lower intestinal permeability by altering the distribution of cell junction proteins and improving their distribution throughout the colonic epithelium resulting in a more continuous distribution. Administration of *Lactobacillus plantarum* WCFS1 to healthy subjects led to alterations in epithelial tight junctions in the small intestine [46].

3.5. Production of Anti-carcinogenic Compounds

In recent years, several processes have been revealed, the most notable of which is the role of certain reactive oxygen species (ROS) and the activation of specific peptide receptors in maintaining intestinal homeostasis. Recent research has suggested that particular gut microorganisms, such as *Lactobacillus* spp., can assist to modulate these processes effectively against colon cancer [8]. Free radicals are highly reactive molecules that damage the tumor-forming cells. Due to its inherent positive capabilities in creating anti-oxidant enzymes, a recent study stressed the relevance of choosing lactic acid bacteria as the progenitor strain. Immune cells *via* G protein-coupled receptors (GPCRs) sense short-chain fatty acids (SCFAs) such as butyrate, which has been reported to influence antigen presentation by DCs and subsequent T cell development. Butyrate has also been shown to limit lymphoma tumour growth by causing cancer cell apoptosis through its histone deacetylase inhibitory action [47, 48]. Butyrate can influence inflammation, epithelial proliferation, and apoptosis when produced by particular members of the *Firmicutes* phylum through the fermentation of dietary fibres and resistant starches [49]. Butyrate was detected by the host colonic receptors GPR109 and GPR43, according to Ganapathy *et al.* [50] and animals lacking GPR109 had enhanced tumour susceptibility and colon carcinogenesis in two separate colon cancer mouse models.

SCFAs metabolites produced by the probiotic *Propionibacterium freudenreichii* also led to apoptosis in CRC cells *in vitro*. Production of SCFAs by *L. fermentum* could inhibit the proliferative activity of CRC [51]. CD8$^+$ T cell activation and tumour regression were improved when non-irradiated antibody-lymph depleted mice were supplemented with ultrapure LPS obtained from irradiated animals. The addition of ultrapure LPS to irradiated animals increased the number and function of the adoptively transplanted cells, resulting in long-term remission of mice with large B16F10 tumours and improved the autoimmune vitiligo. As a result, disrupting the host-microbe homeostatic balance can improve cell-based tumour immunotherapy [52]. *L. acidophilus* DSMZ-EPS-20079 oligosaccharides have anticancer properties against human colon cancer, as evidenced by their regulatory effects on both apoptotic and NF-κB inflammatory pathways [53]. Probiotic yeast *S. cerevisiae* and *S. boulardii* were also reported for their anticancer activity in few studies. The inhibitory role of *K. marxianus* and *P. kudriavzevii* exopolysaccharide (EPSs) on SW-480 (non-metastatic), HT-29 (low-metastatic), and HCT-116 (highly-metastatic) was investigated with human embryonic kidney normal cell line (KDR/293). According to the findings, EPSs significantly enhanced apoptosis by up-regulating pro-apoptotic genes (*BAX*, Caspase-3, and Caspase-8) and down-regulating anti-apoptotic genes (such as *BCL-2*) [54]. Several probiotic bacteria species, including *Lactobacillus acidophilus*, *Lactobacillus casei*, *Lactobacillus delbrueckii*, *Bifidobacterium infantis*, *Bifidobacterium breve*, *Bifidobacterium longum*, and *Streptococcus thermophilus* can create conjugated linoleic acids from linoleic acid. The fatty acids generated by these bacteria exert anti-proliferative and pro-apoptotic effects on colonocytes [55].

3.6. Degradation of Carcinogenic Compounds

Probiotic strain binds to carcinogenic compounds by the cationic exchange between the carcinogenic compounds and the peptidoglycan layer (outer layer) of microbes. Thus, carcinogenic compounds would be eliminated together with the bacteria *via* faeces [56]. Specific chemicals, such as N-nitroso compounds and heterocyclic aromatic amines, can be metabolised and inactivated by some probiotic strains. All of these actions, particularly the degradation of carcinogenetic enzymes, appear to be influenced by the probiotic strain and their viability under intestinal conditions, *viz.* pH, the presence of bile salts, and gastrointestinal enzymes [40]. *In vivo* studies of probiotic *E. faecium* CRL 183 in male Wistar rats reduced the incidence of adenocarcinoma by 40% and decreased the volume of colon tumours generated by 1,2 dimethylhydrazine [57]. *Bifidobacterium longum*, *Lactobacillus acidophilus*, and *Streptococcus salivarius* strains have been shown to bind and release heterocyclic amines and mutagens such as 2-amino-3,4-dimethylimidazo [4,5-f] quinoline (MeIQ), 2-amino-3-methyl-3H-imidazo [4,5-f] quinoline (MHIQ), and 5-phenyl-2-amino- (TrpP2) [58, 59].

3.7. Influence on Harmful Enzymes

β-glucuronidase, a bacterial enzyme with broad substrate specificity, can hydrolyze a variety of glucuronides and leads to the release of carcinogens into the colon, including PAH (*e.g.*, benzo[a]pyrene), a key risk factor for CRC [60]. In the colon, glucosidase breaks down plant glycosides like cycasin, producing aglycones, which are carcinogens. Nitroreductase converts N-nitro compounds (such as nitrobenzenes) to amines, which are usually mutagenic and carcinogenic, while nitrate reductase contributes to the production of highly toxic and carcinogenic nitrite. Colon cancer patients have considerably higher nitroreductase activity than healthy people [61, 62].

4. ANTICANCER ACTIVITY OF PROBIOTICS

Lactic acid bacteria are classified as probiotics, and they play an important role in human health by boosting nutrient absorption, influencing the immune system, and preventing pathogen colonisation. Three *Lactobacillus* strains viz. *Lactobacillus casei* SR1, *Lactobacillus casei* SR2, and *Lactobacillus paracasei* SR4 isolated from human breast milk exhibited higher anticancer activity against the cervix cancer (HeLa cell line) by promoting the upregulation of genes like *BAX, BAD*, caspase3, caspase8, and caspase9 and by downregulating the *BCl2* gene compared to control cells [63]. The anticancer activity of probiotics in colon cancer also includes: (i) negative regulation of inflammatory pathways that promote tumorigenesis, (ii) upregulation of cytokines, which promote tissue repair and anti-tumor responses, (iii) inhibition of biofilm formation and cell proliferation through Toll-like receptors, (iv) binding, degradation and inhibition of mutagens, and (v) host's innate immunity modulation and enhancement *via* secretion of anti-inflammatory molecules [64, 65]. The recent reports on the anticancer activity of probiotic strains are summarized in Table **2**.

Table 2. Recent reports on anticancer activity of probiotic strains.

Probiotic Strains	Anticancer Activity	Reference
Weissella paramesenteroides MN2C2	Exopolysaccharides were effective & highly selective against colon Caco-2, liver HepG-2 and breast MCF-7 malignant cells	[66]
Pediococcus spp.	Induced apoptosis in the cancerous cells by increasing the BAX protein expression and decreasing the Bcl-2 protein expression	[67]
B. adolescentis *B. animalis subsp. lactis* *B. bifidum & B.*	Down-regulated and up-regulated anti-apoptotic & pro-apoptotic genes like BAD, Bcl-2, Caspase-3, Caspase-8, Caspase-9, and Fas-R	[68]
Lactobacillus rhamnosus	Regulated apoptotic mediators (Erb B-2 and Erb B-3)	[69]
Saccharomyces cerevisiae var. *boulardii*	Induced apoptosis in human gastric cancer cells	[70]
Enterococcus faecalis	Exerted anti-proliferative activity on a breast cancer cell line	[71]
Lactobacillus hilgardii	Induced apoptosis in Caco-2 cell line	[72]
Lactobacillus casei	Exerted anti-proliferative activity & extensive apoptosis in prostate cancer cells	[73]
Lactobacillus acidophilus	The mRNA expression levels of apoptosis-related genes were significantly up-regulated and downregulated in the treated cancer cells	[74]
Lactobacillus paracasei	Exerted inhibitory effect of cell wall protein on human cell carcinoma and cell growth	[75]
Kluyveromyces marxianus & *Pichia kudriavzevii*	Inhibited AKT-1, mTOR,& JAK-1 pathways which induce apoptosis in colon cancer	[76]
Lipomyces starkeyi VIT-MN03 & *Saccharomyces fibuligera* VIT-MN04	Exerted anti-proliferative activity on Caco-2 cell line	[77]

Many studies found that the strain *Lactobacillus rhamnosus* GG has a substantial anti-proliferative role and induces apoptosis in *Mus musculus* and human colon cancer as well as lowers the level of IL-8 [78 - 81]. Furthermore, studies showed that probiotic strains such as *L. acidophilus, L. casei, L. fermentum, L. delbrueckii, L. helveticus, L. paracasei, L. pentosus, L. plantarum, L. salivarius, Bifidobacterium lactis, B. adolescentis, Lactococcus lactis, Pediococcus pentosaceus, Streptococcus thermophilus* can reduce the proliferation or induce apoptosis in human colonic cancer cells (Caco-2) [46]. Potential adjuvant effects are also induced by specific cellular components of probiotic lactic acid bacteria, such as modulation of the cell-mediated immune response, activation of reticulo-endothelial system, augmentation of cytokine pathways, and regulation of interleukins and tumour necrosis factors [82]. Fermentation of non-digestible chemicals exerts a positive effect on tumour cells by modulating proliferation and death [47]. Gavresea *et al.* [83] demonstrated that carcinogen 1,2-dimethyly-drazine supplemented rats along with symbiotics (probiotics and prebiotics) had a 100% survival rate, but rats given only carcinogen had a 70% survival rate. In laboratory mice, synbiotics appear to protect against preneoplastic colon lesions. Bacterial carcinogenesis is characterised by the production of numerous toxins that affect the cell cycle, proliferation, differentiation, and death [84].

4.1. Production of Inhibitory Substances By Probiotics

Probiotics have become an essential medicine due to their beneficial effects on the host's health. Several *in vitro* studies and animal models showed that probiotics reduce the risk of gastrointestinal cancer through a variety of mechanisms that includes anti-carcinogenic effects, anti-mutagenic properties, modification of tumour cell differentiation, production of SCFAs, alteration of tumour gene expressions, activation of the host immune system, and inhibition of the bacteria that cause gastrointestinal cancer [20]. Probiotics are used to enhance the levels of cytokines, immunoglobulins, macrophage activation, NK cells' activity, and immunological stimulation against pathogenic bacteria and protozoa [85]. *Lactobacillus* spp. metabolites inactivate cells through altering cell wall components, peptidoglycans, cytoplasmic extracts, and cell-free processes may have anti-proliferative and apoptotic effects on cancer cells. Moreover, it shows an inhibitory effect in HT-29 cancer cell lines, with a rapid apoptotic response and cell cycle suppression in the S phase [86].

SCFAs are the primary metabolites produced by bacterial fermentation of dietary fibre, and they are essential for gut health. SCFAs are also important for regulating different activities, such as anti-inflammatory and immunomodulatory properties. SCFAs have been linked to an antitumor impact because the inflammatory process predisposes the development of cancer and promotes all stages of carcinogenesis. SCFAs promote the proliferation and development of normal intestinal cells in both the large and small intestines. SCFAs may communicate with the gut epithelium and immune cells *via* metabolite-sensing G protein-coupled receptors free fatty acid receptor 3 (FFAR3 or G protein-coupled receptor 41 (GPR41)], FFAR2 (GPR43), and GPR109A or HCAR2 [76]. SCFA molecules can exert various effects, including initiating or inhibiting autophagy, which can decrease cancer cell proliferation or induce apoptosis. SCFAs produced by *Propionibacteria* increase the permeability of the lysosomal membrane in cancer cells that allows CatD to enter the cytosol and protect the cells from apoptosis in the human intestine [86]. In addition, probiotics are known for bacteriocin production, for example, *Bacillus polyfermenticus* bacteriocin inhibits the growth of cancer cells like colon, cervix, breast, and lungs. The down regulation of ErbB2 and ErbB3 expression at the mRNA and protein levels confirmed the anticancer activity of bacteriocin by probiotics. *Bifidobacterium* prevents the growth of colon cancer cells by inhibiting the cell cycle in the G0/G1 phase and raising the activity of the enzyme alkaline phosphatase, a unique marker that is reduced in malignant cells [87].

Exopolysaccharides (EPSs) produced by probiotics have various potential health benefits and functional role in humans and animals. The anticancer activity of polysaccharide is based on the stimulation of immune system cells, primarily T and B lymphocytes, macrophages and the induction of interleukin release by NK cells. The biological activities associated to apoptotic and anti-angiogenic effects of probiotics as anticancer adjuvants have been highlighted by their effects on the expression of c-Myc, c-Fos and vascular endothelial growth factor [88]. Moreover, EPSs are considered to be a safer choice in complex conditions such as cancer and immune-related diseases. Lactic acid bacteria such as *Lactobacillus johnsonii* NCC533, *S. mutans* JC2, *Leuconostoc cittreum* CW28 and *Lactobacillus reuteri* 121 produce inulin (a non-digestible fiber), which enhances the production of butyrate. This could promote enterocytes, inhibition of pathogens, and lower the lumen's pH. Moreover, inulin is used as a vehicle for targeted drug delivery in colon cancer treatment [89, 90]. *Enterococcal* probiotic strains *viz. E. hirae* 20c, *E. faecium* 12a, and L12b produce a proteinaceous substance (anticancer component) that specifically inhibits the human cancer cell lines but not normal cells [91]. In another study, metabiotics produced by the probiotic *Lactobacillus rhamnosus* MD 14 were found to be antigenotoxic and cytotoxic to colon cancer cells [92]. Thus, anticancer compounds from probiotic strains have been considered a promising prospect in recent years.

In addition, some of the bioactive compounds of kefir, such as polysaccharides and peptides, have great potential for inhibition of proliferation and induction of apoptosis in tumor cells. Many studies revealed that kefir acts on different cancers such as CRC, malignant T lymphocytes, breast cancer and lung carcinoma [93]. Gut microbiota products, including toxins, microbial ligands of pattern recognition receptors (PRRs), and metabolites such as butyrate, polyamines, and pyridoxine, are examples of anticancer compounds with potential immunostimulatory characteristics. Probiotics can reduce tumor cell growth by inhibiting bacteria that produce enzymes such as β-glucosidase, β-glucuronidase, and azoreductase that catalyse the conversion of pro-carcinogens to proximal carcinogens. Furthermore, probiotics can eliminate carcinogens such as nitrosamines by inactivating the nitroreductase enzyme, thereby lowering the risk of genotoxic exposure in the colon lumen [94]. The manipulation of cancer-associated gut microbiota was also achieved by faecal microbiota transplantation

(FMT), antibiotic treatment and prebiotics that promote the growth of beneficial bacteria to modify the composition of the gut flora for therapeutic purposes [6]. However, the long-term clinical studies are highly needed to predict the mechanism and safety of probiotics for cancer treatment.

4.2. Efficacy of Probiotics During Cancer Treatment

Gut microbes not only enhance the action of chemotherapy drugs but also reduce the side effects of these medications. In general, individuals with ulcerative colitis (UC) are more likely to develop CRC [95]. Immune checkpoint blockade (ICB) immunotherapy has also been shown to be effective in various malignancies by blocking cytotoxic T-lymphocyte associated protein 4 (CTLA-4) or programmed cell death protein 1 (PD-1)/programmed death ligand 1 (PD-L1) and boosted the antitumor immunity. *Lactobacillus reuteri* administration prevented the onset and progression of colitis by reducing distribution of group 3 innate lymphocytes (ILC3s) caused by ICB-related colitis [96]. The effectiveness and safety of probiotics in preventing radiotherapy-induced diarrhoea (RID) in cervical cancer patients was demonstrated by Qiu *et al.* [95]. The use of probiotics may improve the intestinal tolerance to higher radiation doses and reduce the severity of radiation-induced enteritis. Thus, probiotics may be a promising therapeutic alternative for cervical cancer patients suffering from radiotherapy-induced diarrhoea. In another study, Lin and Shen [96] suggested that probiotics could reduce the incidence of chemo radiotherapy-induced diarrhoea (CRID), especially the CTC grade ≥ 2 or ≥ 3 diarrhoea. Therefore, probiotics have significant efficacy in the prevention of chemo radiotherapy-induced diarrhoea in people with abdominal and pelvic cancer.

Oral mucositis (OM) is a common and annoying side effect of several cancer treatment options, including chemotherapy, radiation, and chemo-radiotherapy. The pain, ulceration, dysphagia and starvation caused by cancer therapy may be prevented and treated using probiotics [97]. The probiotic-derived factors play a significant role in interaction with intestinal epithelial cells. The LGG-derived (*L. rhamnosus* GG) protein can protect intestinal and colonic epithelial cell models from cytokine-induced apoptosis. The P40-induced cytoprotective responses in intestinal epithelial cells, such as reduced cytokine-induced apoptosis, retained barrier function, and increased mucin synthesis, require activation of the epidermal growth factor (EGF) receptor by p40 [98, 99]. Furthermore, p40 enhances IgA class switching in B cells and increases IgA production in the intestine by upregulating EGF-receptor-dependent synthesis of a proliferation-inducing ligand in intestinal epithelial cells [101]. *Bifidobacterium* augments the immunostimulatory effects of CTLA-4 blockade, whereas *B. fragilis* improves the therapeutic benefits of antibodies that target the PD-1/PD-L1 therapeutic axis. Hence, the combination of immunotherapy and probiotics has been considered the best treatment for colon cancer [100, 101].

The gut microbiota is becoming a popular cancer treatment in some of the countries. In Japan, *Clostridium butyricum* MIYARI 588 strain is utilized as a probiotic therapy to treat antibiotic induced dysbiosis [102]. *C. butyricum* therapy (CBT) increases *Bifidobacterium* and reduces intestinal epithelial damage. In a tumor-bearing mouse model, a probiotic strain (*Bifidobacterium*) increased the dendritic cell activity and T-cell–directed antitumor immunity, resulting in improved immune check point blockade (ICB) efficacy. Tomita *et al.* [103] demonstrated that patients with non-small cell lung cancer (NSCLC) treated with probiotic CBT significantly improved the progression-free survival (PFS) and overall survival (OS) when compared to the no-probiotic CBT group. Even in patients who had antibiotic therapy prior to ICB, PFS and OS were significantly improved in the individuals who received the probiotic CBT compared to those who did not receive the CBT. Using a CRC rat model, it was recently demonstrated that *Bifidobacterium infantis* treatment significantly reduced chemotherapy-induced intestinal mucositis. In addition, pro-inflammatory cytokines (IL-6, IL-1, & TNF-α) were found to be lower, whereas the highest regulatory T cell (CD4$^+$CD25$^+$ FOXP3$^+$ cells) response was observed [104].

The healthy intestinal microbiome has a diverse microbial community, which may influence chemotherapeutic response and overall cancer survival. The role of the microbiome in the anticancer activity of chemotherapy drugs has been demonstrated in mouse models [105, 106]. In this aspect, prebiotic and probiotic treatment could be used to maintain variety and improve the chemotherapeutic efficacy before and after chemotherapy. Three meta-analysis studies investigated the relative efficiency of prebiotic, probiotic, and synbiotic therapy, concluding that synbiotics were more beneficial than probiotics or prebiotics alone in preventing post-operative infection problems [107]. Probiotic strains *viz.* *Enterococcus faecalis*, *Saccharomyces boulardii*, *Streptococcus thermopilus*, and *Leuconostoc mesenteroides* have been extensively studied for the efficacy of probiotics during cancer treatment. These strains ensure their efficacy by improving diarrhoea, and intestinal peristalsis, reducing enterocolitis and regulating intestinal immunity [86]. The oral administration of a probiotic mix (*Lactobacilli* and *Bifidobacteria*) showed an effective reduction of diarrhoea and gastrointestinal dysfunctions during irinotecan-based chemotherapy. When CRC patients were co-treated with a symbiotic mix of prebiotics and probiotics, they had a lower risk of developing post-operative irritable bowel syndrome (IBS) [108, 109]. Several clinical trials are on-going to evaluate the safety and efficacy of probiotics administration during anticancer therapy [22].

Radiation-induced enteropathy is a typical consequence of pelvic tumor radiation that has a negative impact on patient quality of life. Probiotics are supposed to help in restoring the healthy bowel microbiota and strengthen the intestinal barrier. Although probiotics are useful in the treatment of radiation-induced enteropathy, Kim *et al.* [110] proved the impact of probiotics on the incidence of chronic radiation-induced enteropathy as well as the safety of probiotics in patients with gynecologic or urologic malignancy. The advantages of probiotics for cancer prevention and treatment are illustrated in Fig. (**4**).

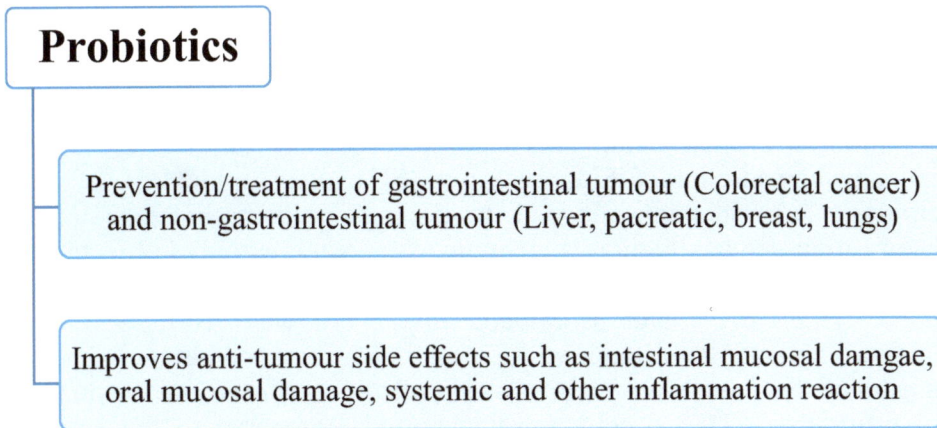

Probiotics

- Prevention/treatment of gastrointestinal tumour (Colorectal cancer) and non-gastrointestinal tumour (Liver, pacreatic, breast, lungs)
- Improves anti-tumour side effects such as intestinal mucosal damgae, oral mucosal damage, systemic and other inflammation reaction

Fig. (4). Beneficial effects of probiotics in cancer treatment.

5. BIOTHERAPEUTIC DRUGS FOR CANCER

Many therapeutic options are available, but the treatment of cancer is still not effective. Chemotherapeutic medicines used to treat cancer pose a significant difficulty because of their non-specificity toward normal cells and the possibility of adverse effects. Also, cancer cells have been found to develop resistance to chemotherapy medicines over time. Therefore, meticulous attempts must be made to make novel and safe anticancer drugs [111]. Thus, future anticancer medicines may incorporate the utilization of commensal-derived microbes or their compounds [6]. Alternative therapeutic techniques have been emphasized by conventional anticancer treatments such as chemotherapy and the developing resistance to anticancer drugs. Engineered probiotics can overcome these restrictions by precisely targeting the tumor cells [112].

The gut microbiota influences drug efficacy through a variety of pathways, including metabolism, immunomodulation, translocation, enzymatic degradation, diversity reduction, and ecological variability. Thus, gut microbiota has emerged as a novel target for improving cancer therapy efficacy while reducing toxicity and side effects [113]. Dietary changes and the use of functional foods (fortified foods with added ingredients to provide specific health-improving benefits, such as antioxidants, omega-3 fatty acids, and glutamine) may help to improve the toxic effects of the treatment, such as nausea, diarrhoea, and constipation, in cancer patients receiving radiotherapy to the abdomino-pelvic region.

A group of experts gathered scientific research with the goal of determining which co-adjuvant foods aid these patients. *Lactobacillus* spp. and *Bifidobacterium* spp. probiotics are considered safe even in neutropenic patients and have been shown to reduce gastrointestinal symptoms [114]. A case study on Japanese women revealed that taking *Lactobacillus casei Shirota* (LcS) in combination with isoflavones from soy was protective against breast cancer risk [115]. Probiotics used with chemotherapy reduced the degree of tumor malignancy compared to 5-Fluorouracil (5-FU) alone, with 40% of animals developing tubular adenoma and 60% developing carcinoma *in situ*, compared to 100% of carcinoma *in situ*, in rats receiving chemotherapy only [116]. In another study, a mixture of *Bifidobacterium bifidum*, *Bifidobacterium longum*, *Bifidobacterium lactis*, and *Bifidobacterium breve* was given to mice after melanoma implantation along with anti-PD-L1 immunotherapy. The study demonstrated that the tumor volume was significantly reduced and the numbers of tumor-infiltrating $CD8^+$ T cells were increased, compared to the anti-PD-L1 therapy alone [104].

In melanoma or sarcoma-bearing mice with decreased gut microbiota, administration of *Akkermansia muciniphila*, alone or in combination with *Enterococcus hirae*, restored the response to anti-PD1 therapy, as seen by reduced tumor size. The increased secretion of IL-12 generally synergizes anti-PD1 therapy, which includes the expansion of $CD4^+$ T cells in mesenteric and tumor-draining lymph nodes [117]. Another study found that patients with head and neck cancer who received cisplatin chemotherapy, radiotherapy and also consumed a probiotic mix containing *B. longum*, *L. lactis*, and *Enterococcus faecium* during the treatment had less severe oral mucositis. Probiotics significantly countered the loss of $CD8^+$, $CD4^+$, and $CD3^+$ T cells caused by anticancer treatments, resulting in an increase in patients' immunity [118]. The administration of probiotics throughout the radiation therapy schedule reduced the enterocolitis occurrence, incidence, and severity of diarrhoea, as well as the frequency of daily bowel movements, and delayed the use of antidiarrheal medicines [119]. In cervical cancer carriers undergoing radiotherapy combined with cisplatin chemotherapy, the severity of diarrhoea and the requirement for anti-diarrheal medicines were considerably reduced in patients who were given *L. acidophilus* with *B. bifidum*-based probiotics before and during radiotherapy [110]. Similarly, in cervical cancer patients who took *L. acidophilus* LA-5 and *B. animalissubsp. lactis* BB-12, throughout the course of their radiotherapy regimen, the incidence and intensity of diarrhoea decreased along with the use of anti-diarrheal medicine and the number of episodes of abdominal pain [120].

The use of probiotics as vectors for medication delivery or gene therapy is another interesting application of probiotics in cancer treatment. As many chemo- and immunotherapeutic medicines have systemic toxicity, the probiotic microorganisms have been designed to deliver the treatment locally at the tumor site [121, 122]. This offers the dual benefit of enhancing pharmacological efficacy while lowering the side effects. Furthermore, probiotic strains have been employed to transfer anticancer proteins to tumor sites, and to inhibit tumor growth [123]. Manipulation of gut microbiota by probiotics may be a viable approach for preventing cancer, improving therapeutic efficacy, and reducing the side effects of current anticancer therapy. The majority of these advantages occurred by modifying the immune and inflammatory responses of the host. The probiotic administration exerts beneficial effects such as enhanced immune system, reduced inflammation, and modulation of apoptosis and proliferation, thereby can prevent cancer and increase the efficacy of therapy as well as decrease the toxicity of therapy in cancer treatment [124]. Cancer immunotherapy combined with effective functionalized nano-systems has also emerged as a promising treatment method. The efficacy of nanomedicine-based cancer immunotherapies and their applications are also being investigated, such as: i) immune checkpoint inhibitors and nanomedicine, ii) CRISPR-Cas nanoparticles (NPs) in cancer immunotherapy, iii) combination cancer immunotherapy with core-shell nanoparticles, iv) biomimetic NPs for cancer immunotherapy, and v) CAR-T cells and cancer nano-immunotherapy [125].

CONCLUSION

The gut microbiota has been linked to cancer and has been found to influence the efficacy of anticancer drugs. Resistance to chemo medicines or immune checkpoint inhibitors (ICIs) is linked to the altered gut microbiota, whereas supplementation with other bacterial species restores the anticancer treatment responses. The importance of probiotics and prebiotics in altering the microbiota, which can influence immune system development and disruption, as well as developing a symbiotic relationship with the host, results in a balanced and effective immune response. Moreover, oral colon-specific delivery methods have emerged as the major therapeutic cargo by creating a substantial influence in the field of modern medicine for local medication delivery in intestinal inflammation. Probiotics have the potential to become a long-term treatment for metabolic problems, such as gastrointestinal malignancies. Especially, oral probiotic therapy is a crucial factor during the management of post-operative problems of GI tract cancers. In the future, we need to define the microbiota's variability *in situ* and in the GI tract. Additional integrative research should also address the interactions among the microbiota, host, and environment to gain a better understanding of how such heterogeneity might result in comparable or distinct functional profiles. Furthermore, the detailed mechanisms of the gut microbiome will provide crucial insights into effective approaches that manipulate the microbiome in the prevention and treatment of various cancers.

CONSENT FOR PUBLICATION

Not applicable.

CONFLICT OF INTEREST

The authors declare no conflict of interest, financial or otherwise.

ACKNOWLEDGEMENT

The authors are thankful to the School of BioSciences and Technology, VIT, Vellore, Tamil Nadu, India, for providing access to get the literatures while writing this book chapter.

REFERENCES

[1] Górska A, Przystupski D, Niemczura MJ, Kulbacka J. Probiotic bacteria: a promising tool in cancer prevention and therapy. Curr Microbiol 2019; 76(8): 939-49.
[http://dx.doi.org/10.1007/s00284-019-01679-8] [PMID: 30949803]

[2] Molska M, Reguła J. Potential mechanisms of probiotics action in the prevention and treatment of colorectal cancer. Nutrients 2019; 11(10): 2453.
[http://dx.doi.org/10.3390/nu11102453] [PMID: 31615096]

[3] Wen H, Yin X, Yuan Z, Wang X, Su S. Comparative analysis of gut microbial communities in children under 5 years old with diarrhea. J Microbiol Biotechnol 2018; 28(4): 652-62.
[http://dx.doi.org/10.4014/jmb.1711.11065] [PMID: 29618180]

[4] Fulbright LE, Ellermann M, Arthur JC. The microbiome and the hallmarks of cancer. PLoS Pathog 2017; 13(9): e1006480.
[http://dx.doi.org/10.1371/journal.ppat.1006480] [PMID: 28934351]

[5] Maldonado Galdeano C, Cazorla SI, Lemme Dumit JM, Vélez E, Perdigón G. Beneficial effects of probiotic consumption on the immune system. Ann Nutr Metab 2019; 74(2): 115-24.
[http://dx.doi.org/10.1159/000496426] [PMID: 30673668]

[6] Zitvogel L, Daillère R, Roberti MP, Routy B, Kroemer G. Anticancer effects of the microbiome and its products. Nat Rev Microbiol 2017; 15(8): 465-78.
[http://dx.doi.org/10.1038/nrmicro.2017.44] [PMID: 28529325]

[7] Li S, Konstantinov SR, Smits R, Peppelenbosch MP. Bacterial biofilms in colorectal cancer initiation and progression. Trends Mol Med 2017; 23(1): 18-30.
[http://dx.doi.org/10.1016/j.molmed.2016.11.004] [PMID: 27986421]

[8]   Chen DS, Mellman I. Elements of cancer immunity and the cancer–immune set point. Nature 2017; 541(7637): 321-30.
[http://dx.doi.org/10.1038/nature21349] [PMID: 28102259]

[9]   Yoshimoto S, Loo TM, Atarashi K, *et al.* Obesity-induced gut microbial metabolite promotes liver cancer through senescence secretome. Nature 2013; 499(7456): 97-101.
[http://dx.doi.org/10.1038/nature12347] [PMID: 23803760]

[10]   Siegel RL, Miller KD, Jemal A. Cancer statistics, 2018. CA Cancer J Clin 2018; 68(1): 7-30.
[http://dx.doi.org/10.3322/caac.21442] [PMID: 29313949]

[11]   Source I. Globocan 2018. International Agency for Research on Cancer. World Health Organization.
https://gco.iarc.fr/today/data/factsheets/populations/356-india-fact-sheets.pdf Accessed on. 2020; 2.

[12]   Ok CY, Young KH. Checkpoint inhibitors in hematological malignancies. J Hematol Oncol 2017; 10(1): 103.
[http://dx.doi.org/10.1186/s13045-017-0474-3] [PMID: 28482851]

[13]   Evrard B, Coudeyras S, Dosgilbert A, *et al.* Dose-dependent immunomodulation of human dendritic cells by the probiotic *Lactobacillus rhamnosus* Lcr35. PLoS One 2011; 6(4): e18735.
[http://dx.doi.org/10.1371/journal.pone.0018735] [PMID: 21533162]

[14]   Dong L, Li J, Liu Y, Yue W, Luo X. Toll-like receptor 2 monoclonal antibody or/and Toll-like receptor 4 monoclonal antibody increase counts of Lactobacilli and *Bifidobacteria* in dextran sulfate sodium-induced colitis in mice. J Gastroenterol Hepatol 2012; 27(1): 110-9.
[http://dx.doi.org/10.1111/j.1440-1746.2011.06839.x] [PMID: 21722182]

[15]   Drago L. Probiotics and colon cancer. Microorganisms 2019; 7(3): 66.
[http://dx.doi.org/10.3390/microorganisms7030066] [PMID: 30823471]

[16]   Chang JH, Shim YY, Cha SK, Reaney MJT, Chee KM. Effect of *Lactobacillus acidophilus* KFRI342 on the development of chemically induced precancerous growths in the rat colon. J Med Microbiol 2012; 61(3): 361-8.
[http://dx.doi.org/10.1099/jmm.0.035154-0] [PMID: 22034161]

[17]   Rook G A W, Brunet LR. Microbes, immunoregulation, and the gut. Gut 2005; 54(3): 317-20.
[http://dx.doi.org/10.1136/gut.2004.053785] [PMID: 15710972]

[18]   Koboziev I, Reinoso Webb C, Furr KL, Grisham MB. Role of the enteric microbiota in intestinal homeostasis and inflammation. Free Radic Biol Med 2014; 68: 122-33.
[http://dx.doi.org/10.1016/j.freeradbiomed.2013.11.008] [PMID: 24275541]

[19]   Dos Reis SA, da Conceição LL, Siqueira NP, Rosa DD, da Silva LL, Peluzio MCG. Review of the mechanisms of probiotic actions in the prevention of colorectal cancer. Nutr Res 2017; 37: 1-19.
[http://dx.doi.org/10.1016/j.nutres.2016.11.009] [PMID: 28215310]

[20]   Javanmard A, Ashtari S, Sabet B, *et al.* Probiotics and their role in gastrointestinal cancers prevention and treatment; an overview. Gastroenterol Hepatol Bed Bench 2018; 11(4): 284-95.
[PMID: 30425806]

[21]   Zhang C, Wang H, Chen T. Interactions between intestinal microflora/probiotics and the immune system. BioMed Res Int 2019; 2019: 1-8.
[http://dx.doi.org/10.1155/2019/6764919] [PMID: 31828119]

[22]   Vivarelli S, Salemi R, Candido S, *et al.* Gut microbiota and cancer: from pathogenesis to therapy. Cancers (Basel) 2019; 11(1): 38.
[http://dx.doi.org/10.3390/cancers11010038] [PMID: 30609850]

[23]   Erdman SE, Poutahidis T. Gut microbiota modulate host immune cells in cancer development and growth. Free Radic Biol Med 2017; 105: 28-34.
[http://dx.doi.org/10.1016/j.freeradbiomed.2016.11.013] [PMID: 27840315]

[24]   Goubet AG, Daillère R, Routy B, Derosa L, M Roberti P, Zitvogel L. The impact of the intestinal

microbiota in therapeutic responses against cancer. C R Biol 2018; 341(5): 284-9.
[http://dx.doi.org/10.1016/j.crvi.2018.03.004] [PMID: 29631891]

[25]   Chen DS, Mellman I. Oncology meets immunology: the cancer-immunity cycle. immunity. 2013; 39(1): 1-0.

[26]   Huynh L, Hipolito C, ten Dijke P. A perspective on the development of TGF-β inhibitors for cancer treatment. Biomolecules 2019; 9(11): 743.
[http://dx.doi.org/10.3390/biom9110743] [PMID: 31744193]

[27]   Nishimura CD, Pulanco MC, Cui W, Lu L, Zang X. PD-L1 and B7-1 cis-interaction: New mechanisms in immune checkpoints and immunotherapies. Trends Mol Med 2021; 27(3): 207-19.
[http://dx.doi.org/10.1016/j.molmed.2020.10.004] [PMID: 33199209]

[28]   Aindelis G, Chlichlia K. Modulation of anti-tumour immune responses by probiotic bacteria. Vaccines (Basel) 2020; 8(2): 329.
[http://dx.doi.org/10.3390/vaccines8020329] [PMID: 32575876]

[29]   Galdeano CM, de Moreno de LeBlanc A, Vinderola G, Bonet MEB, Perdigón G. Proposed model: mechanisms of immunomodulation induced by probiotic bacteria. Clin Vaccine Immunol 2007; 14(5): 485-92.
[http://dx.doi.org/10.1128/CVI.00406-06] [PMID: 17360855]

[30]   Alfaro C, Sanmamed MF, Rodríguez-Ruiz ME, *et al.* Interleukin-8 in cancer pathogenesis, treatment and follow-up. Cancer Treat Rev 2017; 60: 24-31.
[http://dx.doi.org/10.1016/j.ctrv.2017.08.004] [PMID: 28866366]

[31]   Jacouton E, Chain F, Sokol H, Langella P, Bermúdez-Humarán LG. Probiotic strain *Lactobacillus casei* BL23 prevents colitis-associated colorectal cancer. Front Immunol 2017; 8: 1553.
[http://dx.doi.org/10.3389/fimmu.2017.01553] [PMID: 29209314]

[32]   Del Carmen S, de Moreno de LeBlanc A, Levit R, *et al.* Anti-cancer effect of lactic acid bacteria expressing antioxidant enzymes or IL-10 in a colorectal cancer mouse model. Int Immunopharmacol 2017; 42: 122-9.
[http://dx.doi.org/10.1016/j.intimp.2016.11.017] [PMID: 27912148]

[33]   Kuugbee ED, Shang X, Gamallat Y, *et al.* Structural change in microbiota by a probiotic cocktail enhances the gut barrier and reduces cancer *via* TLR2 signaling in a rat model of colon cancer. Dig Dis Sci 2016; 61(10): 2908-20.
[http://dx.doi.org/10.1007/s10620-016-4238-7] [PMID: 27384052]

[34]   Gianotti L, Morelli L, Galbiati F, *et al.* A randomized double-blind trial on perioperative administration of probiotics in colorectal cancer patients. World J Gastroenterol 2010; 16(2): 167-75.
[http://dx.doi.org/10.3748/wjg.v16.i2.167] [PMID: 20066735]

[35]   Iwasaki A, Medzhitov R. Toll-like receptor control of the adaptive immune responses. Nat Immunol 2004; 5(10): 987-95.
[http://dx.doi.org/10.1038/ni1112] [PMID: 15454922]

[36]   Ghoneum M, Felo N, Agrawal S, Agrawal A. A novel kefir product (PFT) activates dendritic cells to induce CD4+T and CD8+T cell responses *in vitro*. Int J Immunopathol Pharmacol 2015; 28(4): 488-96.
[http://dx.doi.org/10.1177/0394632015599447] [PMID: 26384392]

[37]   Mohamadzadeh M, Klaenhammer TR. Specific *Lactobacillus* species differentially activate Toll-like receptors and downstream signals in dendritic cells. Expert Rev Vaccines 2008; 7(8): 1155-64.
[http://dx.doi.org/10.1586/14760584.7.8.1155] [PMID: 18844590]

[38]   Kosaka A, Yan H, Ohashi S, *et al.* *Lactococcus lactis* subsp. *cremoris* FC triggers IFN-γ production from NK and T cells *via* IL-12 and IL-18. Int Immunopharmacol 2012; 14(4): 729-33.
[http://dx.doi.org/10.1016/j.intimp.2012.10.007] [PMID: 23102661]

[39]   Tiptiri-Kourpeti A, Spyridopoulou K, Santarmaki V, *et al.* *Lactobacillus casei* exerts anti-proliferative

effects accompanied by apoptotic cell death and up-regulation of TRAIL in colon carcinoma cells. PLoS One 2016; 11(2): e0147960.
[http://dx.doi.org/10.1371/journal.pone.0147960] [PMID: 26849051]

[40]   Zhu Q, Gao R, Wu W, Qin H. The role of gut microbiota in the pathogenesis of colorectal cancer. Tumour Biol 2013; 34(3): 1285-300.
[http://dx.doi.org/10.1007/s13277-013-0684-4] [PMID: 23397545]

[41]   Goldin BR, Gorbach SL. The effect of milk and *lactobacillus* feeding on human intestinal bacterial enzyme activity. Am J Clin Nutr 1984; 39(5): 756-61.
[http://dx.doi.org/10.1093/ajcn/39.5.756] [PMID: 6424430]

[42]   Verma A, Shukla G. Probiotics *Lactobacillus rhamnosus* GG, *Lactobacillus acidophilus* suppresses DMH-induced procarcinogenic fecal enzymes and preneoplastic aberrant crypt foci in early colon carcinogenesis in Sprague Dawley rats. Nutr Cancer 2013; 65(1): 84-91.
[http://dx.doi.org/10.1080/01635581.2013.741746] [PMID: 23368917]

[43]   Kotzampassi K, Stavrou G, Damoraki G, *et al.* A four-probiotics regimen reduces postoperative complications after colorectal surgery: a randomized, double-blind, placebo-controlled study. World J Surg 2015; 39(11): 2776-83.
[http://dx.doi.org/10.1007/s00268-015-3071-z] [PMID: 25894405]

[44]   Klampfer L. Cytokines, inflammation and colon cancer. Curr Cancer Drug Targets 2011; 11(4): 451-64.
[http://dx.doi.org/10.2174/156800911795538066] [PMID: 21247378]

[45]   Caballero-Franco C, Keller K, De Simone C, Chadee K. The VSL#3 probiotic formula induces mucin gene expression and secretion in colonic epithelial cells. Am J Physiol Gastrointest Liver Physiol 2007; 292(1): G315-22.
[http://dx.doi.org/10.1152/ajpgi.00265.2006] [PMID: 16973917]

[46]   Śliżewska K, Markowiak-Kopeć P, Śliżewska W. The role of probiotics in cancer prevention. Cancers (Basel) 2020; 13(1): 20.
[http://dx.doi.org/10.3390/cancers13010020] [PMID: 33374549]

[47]   Kahouli I, Handiri NR, Malhotra M, Riahi A, Alaoui-Jamali M. Characterization of *L. reuteri* NCIMB 701359 Probiotic Features for Potential Use as a Colorectal Cancer Biotherapeutic by Identifying Fatty Acid Profile and Anti-Proliferative Action against Colorectal Cancer Cells. Drug Des 2016; 5(2): 2169-0138.
[http://dx.doi.org/10.4172/2169-0138.1000131]

[48]   Joglekar P, Segre JA. Building a translational microbiome toolbox. Cell 2017; 169(3): 378-80.
[http://dx.doi.org/10.1016/j.cell.2017.04.009] [PMID: 28431240]

[49]   Ganapathy V, Thangaraju M, Prasad PD, Martin PM, Singh N. Transporters and receptors for short-chain fatty acids as the molecular link between colonic bacteria and the host. Curr Opin Pharmacol 2013; 13(6): 869-74.
[http://dx.doi.org/10.1016/j.coph.2013.08.006] [PMID: 23978504]

[50]   Lan A, Lagadic-Gossmann D, Lemaire C, Brenner C, Jan G. Acidic extracellular pH shifts colorectal cancer cell death from apoptosis to necrosis upon exposure to propionate and acetate, major end-products of the human probiotic *propionibacteria*. Apoptosis 2007; 12(3): 573-91.
[http://dx.doi.org/10.1007/s10495-006-0010-3] [PMID: 17195096]

[51]   Paulos CM, Wrzesinski C, Kaiser A, *et al.* Microbial translocation augments the function of adoptively transferred self/tumor-specific CD8+ T cells *via* TLR4 signaling. J Clin Invest 2007; 117(8): 2197-204.
[http://dx.doi.org/10.1172/JCI32205] [PMID: 17657310]

[52]   El-Deeb NM, Yassin AM, Al-Madboly LA, El-Hawiet A. A novel purified *Lactobacillus acidophilus* 20079 exopolysaccharide, LA-EPS-20079, molecularly regulates both apoptotic and NF-κB inflammatory pathways in human colon cancer. Microb Cell Fact 2018; 17(1): 29.

[http://dx.doi.org/10.1186/s12934-018-0877-z] [PMID: 29306327]

[53] Sambrani R, Abdolalizadeh J, Kohan L, Jafari B. Recent advances in the application of probiotic yeasts, particularly *Saccharomyces*, as an adjuvant therapy in the management of cancer with focus on colorectal cancer. Mol Biol Rep 2021; 48(1): 951-60.
[http://dx.doi.org/10.1007/s11033-020-06110-1] [PMID: 33389533]

[54] Ewaschuk JB, Walker JW, Diaz H, Madsen KL. Bioproduction of conjugated linoleic acid by probiotic bacteria occurs *in vitro* and *in vivo* in mice. J Nutr 2006; 136(6): 1483-7.
[http://dx.doi.org/10.1093/jn/136.6.1483] [PMID: 16702308]

[55] Burns AJ, Rowland IR. Antigenotoxicity of probiotics and prebiotics on faecal water-induced DNA damage in human colon adenocarcinoma cells. Mutat Res 2004; 551(1-2): 233-43.
[http://dx.doi.org/10.1016/j.mrfmmm.2004.03.010] [PMID: 15225596]

[56] Sivieri K, Spinardi-Barbisan ALT, Barbisan LF, *et al.* Probiotic *Enterococcus faecium* CRL 183 inhibit chemically induced colon cancer in male Wistar rats. Eur Food Res Technol 2008; 228(2): 231-7.
[http://dx.doi.org/10.1007/s00217-008-0927-6]

[57] Orrhage K, Sillerström E, Gustafsson JÅ, Nord CE, Rafter J. Binding of mutagenic heterocyclic amines by intestinal and lactic acid bacteria. Mutat Res 1994; 311(2): 239-48.
[http://dx.doi.org/10.1016/0027-5107(94)90182-1] [PMID: 7526189]

[58] Bolognani F, Rumney CJ, Rowland IR. Influence of carcinogen binding by lactic acid-producing bacteria on tissue distribution and *in vivo* mutagenicity of dietary carcinogens. Food Chem Toxicol 1997; 35(6): 535-45.
[http://dx.doi.org/10.1016/S0278-6915(97)00029-X] [PMID: 9225011]

[59] McIntosh FM, Maison N, Holtrop G, *et al.* Phylogenetic distribution of genes encoding β-glucuronidase activity in human colonic bacteria and the impact of diet on faecal glycosidase activities. Environ Microbiol 2012; 14(8): 1876-87.
[http://dx.doi.org/10.1111/j.1462-2920.2012.02711.x] [PMID: 22364273]

[60] Hamer HM, De Preter V, Windey K, Verbeke K. Functional analysis of colonic bacterial metabolism: relevant to health? Am J Physiol Gastrointest Liver Physiol 2012; 302(1): G1-9.
[http://dx.doi.org/10.1152/ajpgi.00048.2011] [PMID: 22016433]

[61] Riaz Rajoka MS, Zhao H, Lu Y, *et al.* Anticancer potential against cervix cancer (HeLa) cell line of probiotic *Lactobacillus casei* and *Lactobacillus paracasei* strains isolated from human breast milk. Food Funct 2018; 9(5): 2705-15.
[http://dx.doi.org/10.1039/C8FO00547H] [PMID: 29762617]

[62] Drago L. Probiotics and colon cancer. Microorganisms 2019; 7(3): 66.
[http://dx.doi.org/10.3390/microorganisms7030066] [PMID: 30823471]

[63] Raman M, Ambalam P, Kondepudi KK, *et al.* Potential of probiotics, prebiotics and synbiotics for management of colorectal cancer. Gut Microbes 2013; 4(3): 181-92.
[http://dx.doi.org/10.4161/gmic.23919] [PMID: 23511582]

[64] Amer MN, Elgammal EW, Atwa NA, Eldiwany AI, Dawoud IE, Rashad FM. Structure elucidation and *in vitro* biological evaluation of sulfated exopolysaccharide from LAB *Weissella paramesenteroides* MN2C2. Journal of Applied Pharmaceutical Science. 2021; 11(5): 022-31.

[65] Jafari-Nasab T, Khaleghi M, Farsinejad A, Khorrami S. Probiotic potential and anticancer properties of *Pediococcus* sp. isolated from traditional dairy products. Biotechnol Rep (Amst) 2021; 29: e00593.
[http://dx.doi.org/10.1016/j.btre.2021.e00593] [PMID: 33598413]

[66] Faghfoori Z, Faghfoori MH, Saber A, Izadi A, Yari Khosroushahi A. Anticancer effects of *bifidobacteria* on colon cancer cell lines. Cancer Cell Int 2021; 21(1): 258.
[http://dx.doi.org/10.1186/s12935-021-01971-3] [PMID: 33980239]

[67] Pakbin B, Pishkhan Dibazar S, Allahyari S, Javadi M, Farasat A, Darzi S. Probiotic *Saccharomyces*

cerevisiae var. *boulardii* supernatant inhibits survivin gene expression and induces apoptosis in human gastric cancer cells. Food Sci Nutr 2021; 9(2): 692-700.
[http://dx.doi.org/10.1002/fsn3.2032] [PMID: 33598154]

[68]   Sharma P, Kaur S, Chadha BS, Kaur R, Kaur M, Kaur S. Anticancer and antimicrobial potential of enterocin 12a from *Enterococcus faecium*. BMC Microbiol 2021; 21(1): 39.
[http://dx.doi.org/10.1186/s12866-021-02086-5] [PMID: 33541292]

[69]   Pourramezan Z, Oloomi M, Kasra-Kermanshahi R. Antioxidant and anticancer activities of *Lactobacillus Hilgardii* strain AG12a. Int J Prev Med 2020; 11(1): 132.
[http://dx.doi.org/10.4103/ijpvm.IJPVM_307_19] [PMID: 33088460]

[70]   Rosa LS, Santos ML, Abreu JP, *et al.* Antiproliferative and apoptotic effects of probiotic whey dairy beverages in human prostate cell lines. Food Res Int 2020; 137: 109450.
[http://dx.doi.org/10.1016/j.foodres.2020.109450] [PMID: 33233128]

[71]   Isazadeh A, Hajazimian S, Shadman B, *et al.* Anti-cancer effects of probiotic *lactobacillus acidophilus* for colorectal cancer cell line caco-2 through apoptosis induction. Ulum-i Daruyi 2020; 27(2): 262-7.
[http://dx.doi.org/10.34172/PS.2020.52]

[72]   Yang LC, Lin SW, Li IC, *et al. Lactobacillus plantarum* GKM3 and *Lactobacillus paracasei* GKS6 supplementation ameliorates bone loss in ovariectomized mice by promoting osteoblast differentiation and inhibiting osteoclast formation. Nutrients 2020; 12(7): 1914.
[http://dx.doi.org/10.3390/nu12071914] [PMID: 32605314]

[73]   Ragavan ML, Das N. *In vitro* studies on therapeutic potential of probiotic yeasts isolated from various sources. Curr Microbiol 2020; 77(10): 2821-30.
[http://dx.doi.org/10.1007/s00284-020-02100-5] [PMID: 32591923]

[74]   Sadeghi-Aliabadi H, Mohammadi F, Fazeli H, Mirlohi M. Effects of *Lactobacillus plantarum* A7 with probiotic potential on colon cancer and normal cells proliferation in comparison with a commercial strain. Iran J Basic Med Sci 2014; 17(10): 815-9.
[PMID: 25729553]

[75]   Orlando A, Refolo MG, Messa C, *et al.* Antiproliferative and proapoptotic effects of viable or heat-killed *Lactobacillus paracasei* IMPC2.1 and *Lactobacillus rhamnosus* GG in HGC-27 gastric and DLD-1 colon cell lines. Nutr Cancer 2012; 64(7): 1103-11.
[http://dx.doi.org/10.1080/01635581.2012.717676] [PMID: 23061912]

[76]   Borowicki A, Michelmann A, Stein K, *et al.* Fermented wheat aleurone enriched with probiotic strains LGG and Bb12 modulates markers of tumor progression in human colon cells. Nutr Cancer 2011; 63(1): 151-60.
[PMID: 21161821]

[77]   Altonsy MO, Andrews SC, Tuohy KM. Differential induction of apoptosis in human colonic carcinoma cells (Caco-2) by *Atopobium*, and commensal, probiotic and enteropathogenic bacteria: Mediation by the mitochondrial pathway. Int J Food Microbiol 2010; 137(2-3): 190-203.
[http://dx.doi.org/10.1016/j.ijfoodmicro.2009.11.015] [PMID: 20036023]

[78]   Lopez M, Li N, Kataria J, Russell M, Neu J. Live and ultraviolet-inactivated *Lactobacillus rhamnosus* GG decrease flagellin-induced interleukin-8 production in Caco-2 cells. J Nutr 2008; 138(11): 2264-8.
[http://dx.doi.org/10.3945/jn.108.093658] [PMID: 18936229]

[79]   Kumar M, Kumar A, Nagpal R, *et al.* Cancer-preventing attributes of probiotics: an update. Int J Food Sci Nutr 2010; 61(5): 473-96.
[http://dx.doi.org/10.3109/09637480903455971] [PMID: 20187714]

[80]   Gavresea F, Vagianos C, Korontzi M, *et al.* Beneficial effect of synbiotics on experimental colon cancer in rats. Turk J Gastroenterol 2018; 29(4): 494-501.
[http://dx.doi.org/10.5152/tjg.2018.17469] [PMID: 30249566]

[81]   Bonnet M, Buc E, Sauvanet P, *et al.* Colonization of the human gut by E. coli and colorectal cancer

risk. Clin Cancer Res 2014; 20(4): 859-67.
[http://dx.doi.org/10.1158/1078-0432.CCR-13-1343] [PMID: 24334760]

[82]   Ghasemian A, Eslami M, Shafiei M, Najafipour S, Rajabi A. Probiotics and their increasing importance in human health and infection control. Rev Med Microbiol 2018; 29(4): 153-8.
[http://dx.doi.org/10.1097/MRM.0000000000000147]

[83]   Eslami M, Yousefi B, Kokhaei P, *et al.* Importance of probiotics in the prevention and treatment of colorectal cancer. J Cell Physiol 2019; 234(10): 17127-43.
[http://dx.doi.org/10.1002/jcp.28473] [PMID: 30912128]

[84]   Carretta MD, Quiroga J, López R, Hidalgo MA, Burgos RA. Participation of short chain fatty acids and their receptors in gut inflammation and colon cancer. Front Physiol 2021; 12: 662739.
[http://dx.doi.org/10.3389/fphys.2021.662739] [PMID: 33897470]

[85]   Louis P, Hold GL, Flint HJ. The gut microbiota, bacterial metabolites and colorectal cancer. Nat Rev Microbiol 2014; 12(10): 661-72.
[http://dx.doi.org/10.1038/nrmicro3344] [PMID: 25198138]

[86]   Ismail B, Nampoothiri KM. Exposition of antitumour activity of a chemically characterized exopolysaccharide from a probiotic *Lactobacillus plantarum* MTCC 9510. Biologia (Bratisl) 2013; 68(6): 1041-7.
[http://dx.doi.org/10.2478/s11756-013-0275-2]

[87]   Patel S, Majumder A, Goyal A. Potentials of exopolysaccharides from lactic Acid bacteria. Indian J Microbiol 2012; 52(1): 3-12.
[http://dx.doi.org/10.1007/s12088-011-0148-8] [PMID: 23449986]

[88]   Zannini E, Waters DM, Coffey A, Arendt EK. Production, properties, and industrial food application of lactic acid bacteria-derived exopolysaccharides. Appl Microbiol Biotechnol 2016; 100(3): 1121-35.
[http://dx.doi.org/10.1007/s00253-015-7172-2] [PMID: 26621802]

[89]   Sharma M, Chandel D, Shukla G. Antigenotoxicity and cytotoxic potentials of metabiotics extracted from isolated probiotic, *Lactobacillus rhamnosus* MD 14 on Caco-2 and HT-29 human colon cancer cells. Nutr Cancer 2020; 72(1): 110-9.
[http://dx.doi.org/10.1080/01635581.2019.1615514] [PMID: 31266374]

[90]   Sharma P, Kaur S, Kaur R, Kaur M, Kaur S. Proteinaceous secretory metabolites of probiotic human commensal *Enterococcus hirae* 20c, *E. faecium* 12a and L12b as antiproliferative agents against cancer cell lines. Front Microbiol 2018; 9: 948.
[http://dx.doi.org/10.3389/fmicb.2018.00948] [PMID: 29867856]

[91]   Sharifi M, Moridnia A, Mortazavi D, Salehi M, Bagheri M, Sheikhi A. Kefir: a powerful probiotics with anticancer properties. Med Oncol 2017; 34(11): 183.
[http://dx.doi.org/10.1007/s12032-017-1044-9] [PMID: 28956261]

[92]   Prasanna PHP, Grandison AS, Charalampopoulos D. *Bifidobacteria* in milk products: An overview of physiological and biochemical properties, exopolysaccharide production, selection criteria of milk products and health benefits. Food Res Int 2014; 55: 247-62.
[http://dx.doi.org/10.1016/j.foodres.2013.11.013]

[93]   Rabbenou W, Ullman TA. Risk of colon cancer and recommended surveillance strategies in patients with ulcerative colitis. Gastroenterol Clin North Am 2020; 49(4): 791-807.
[http://dx.doi.org/10.1016/j.gtc.2020.08.005] [PMID: 33121696]

[94]   Wang T, Zheng N, Luo Q, *et al.* Probiotics *Lactobacillus reuteri* abrogates immune checkpoint blockade-associated colitis by inhibiting group 3 innate lymphoid cells. Front Immunol 2019; 10: 1235.
[http://dx.doi.org/10.3389/fimmu.2019.01235] [PMID: 31214189]

[95]   Qiu G, Yu Y, Wang Y, Wang X. The significance of probiotics in preventing radiotherapy-induced diarrhea in patients with cervical cancer: A systematic review and meta-analysis. Int J Surg 2019; 65:

61-9.
[http://dx.doi.org/10.1016/j.ijsu.2019.03.015] [PMID: 30928672]

[96] Lin S, Shen Y. The efficacy and safety of probiotics for prevention of chemoradiotherapy-induced diarrhea in people with abdominal and pelvic cancer: A systematic review and meta-analysis based on 23 randomized studies. Int J Surg 2020; 84: 69-77.
[http://dx.doi.org/10.1016/j.ijsu.2020.10.012] [PMID: 33080416]

[97] Shu Z, Li P, Yu B, Huang S, Chen Y. The effectiveness of probiotics in prevention and treatment of cancer therapy-induced oral mucositis: A systematic review and meta-analysis. Oral Oncol 2020; 102: 104559.
[http://dx.doi.org/10.1016/j.oraloncology.2019.104559] [PMID: 31923856]

[98] Yan F, Cao H, Cover TL, *et al.* Colon-specific delivery of a probiotic-derived soluble protein ameliorates intestinal inflammation in mice through an EGFR-dependent mechanism. J Clin Invest 2011; 121(6): 2242-53.
[http://dx.doi.org/10.1172/JCI44031] [PMID: 21606592]

[99] Yang LC, Lin SW, Li IC, *et al. Lactobacillus plantarum* GKM3 and *Lactobacillus paracasei* GKS6 supplementation ameliorates bone loss in ovariectomized mice by promoting osteoblast differentiation and inhibiting osteoclast formation. Nutrients 2020; 12(7): 1914.
[http://dx.doi.org/10.3390/nu12071914] [PMID: 32605314]

[100] Wang Y, Liu L, Moore DJ, *et al.* An LGG-derived protein promotes IgA production through upregulation of APRIL expression in intestinal epithelial cells. Mucosal Immunol 2017; 10(2): 373-84.
[http://dx.doi.org/10.1038/mi.2016.57] [PMID: 27353252]

[101] Sivan A, Corrales L, Hubert N, *et al.* Commensal *Bifidobacterium* promotes antitumor immunity and facilitates anti–PD-L1 efficacy. Science 2015; 350(6264): 1084-9.
[http://dx.doi.org/10.1126/science.aac4255] [PMID: 26541606]

[102] Vétizou M, Pitt JM, Daillère R, *et al.* Anticancer immunotherapy by CTLA-4 blockade relies on the gut microbiota. Science 2015; 350(6264): 1079-84.
[http://dx.doi.org/10.1126/science.aad1329] [PMID: 26541610]

[103] Tomita Y, Ikeda T, Sakata S, *et al.* Association of probiotic *clostridium butyricum* therapy with survival and response to immune checkpoint blockade in patients with lung cancer. Cancer Immunol Res 2020; 8(10): 1236-42.
[http://dx.doi.org/10.1158/2326-6066.CIR-20-0051] [PMID: 32665261]

[104] Mi H, Dong Y, Zhang B, *et al. Bifidobacterium infantis* ameliorates chemotherapy-induced intestinal mucositis *via* regulating T cell immunity in colorectal cancer rats. Cell Physiol Biochem 2017; 42(6): 2330-41.
[http://dx.doi.org/10.1159/000480005] [PMID: 28848081]

[105] Viaud S, Saccheri F, Mignot G, *et al.* The intestinal microbiota modulates the anticancer immune effects of cyclophosphamide. science. 2013; 342(6161): 971-6.

[106] Iida N, Dzutsev A, Stewart CA, *et al.* Commensal bacteria control cancer response to therapy by modulating the tumor microenvironment. science 2013; 342(6161): 967-70.

[107] Scott AJ, Merrifield CA, Younes JA, Pekelharing EP. Pre-, pro- and synbiotics in cancer prevention and treatment—a review of basic and clinical research. Ecancermedicalscience 2018; 12: 869.
[http://dx.doi.org/10.3332/ecancer.2018.869] [PMID: 30263060]

[108] Mego M, Chovanec J, Vochyanova-Andrezalova I, *et al.* Prevention of irinotecan induced diarrhea by probiotics: A randomized double blind, placebo controlled pilot study. Complement Ther Med 2015; 23(3): 356-62.
[http://dx.doi.org/10.1016/j.ctim.2015.03.008] [PMID: 26051570]

[109] Flesch AT, Tonial ST, Contu PDC, Damin DC. Perioperative synbiotics administration decreases postoperative infections in patients with colorectal cancer: a randomized, double-blind clinical trial.

Rev Col Bras Cir 2017; 44(6): 567-73.
[http://dx.doi.org/10.1590/0100-69912017006004] [PMID: 29267553]

[110] Kim YJ, Yu J, Park SP, Lee SH, Kim YS. Prevention of radiotherapy induced enteropathy by probiotics (PREP): protocol for a double-blind randomized placebo-controlled trial. BMC Cancer 2021; 21(1): 1032.
[http://dx.doi.org/10.1186/s12885-021-08757-w] [PMID: 34530750]

[111] Roy S, Trinchieri G. Microbiota: a key orchestrator of cancer therapy. Nat Rev Cancer 2017; 17(5): 271-85.
[http://dx.doi.org/10.1038/nrc.2017.13] [PMID: 28303904]

[112] Heap JT, Theys J, Ehsaan M, *et al.* Spores of *Clostridium* engineered for clinical efficacy and safety cause regression and cure of tumors *in vivo.* Oncotarget 2014; 5(7): 1761-9.
[http://dx.doi.org/10.18632/oncotarget.1761] [PMID: 24732092]

[113] Ma W, Mao Q, Xia W, Dong G, Yu C, Jiang F. Gut microbiota shapes the efficiency of cancer therapy. Front Microbiol 2019; 10: 1050.
[http://dx.doi.org/10.3389/fmicb.2019.01050] [PMID: 31293523]

[114] Serna-Thomé G, Castro-Eguiluz D, Fuchs-Tarlovsky V, *et al.* Use of functional foods and oral supplements as adjuvants in cancer treatment. Rev Invest Clin 2018; 70(3): 136-46.
[http://dx.doi.org/10.24875/RIC.18002527] [PMID: 29943769]

[115] Toi M, Hirota S, Tomotaki A, *et al.* Probiotic beverage with soy isoflavone consumption for breast cancer prevention: a case-control study. Curr Nutr Food Sci 2013; 9(3): 194-200.
[http://dx.doi.org/10.2174/15734013113099990001] [PMID: 23966890]

[116] Genaro SC, Lima de Souza Reis LS, Reis SK, Rabelo Socca EA, Fávaro WJ. Probiotic supplementation attenuates the aggressiveness of chemically induced colorectal tumor in rats. Life Sci 2019; 237: 116895.
[http://dx.doi.org/10.1016/j.lfs.2019.116895] [PMID: 31610204]

[117] Routy B, Le Chatelier E, Derosa L, *et al.* Gut microbiome influences efficacy of PD-1–based immunotherapy against epithelial tumors. Science 2018; 359(6371): 91-7.
[http://dx.doi.org/10.1126/science.aan3706] [PMID: 29097494]

[118] Jiang C, Wang H, Xia C, *et al.* A randomized, double-blind, placebo-controlled trial of probiotics to reduce the severity of oral mucositis induced by chemoradiotherapy for patients with nasopharyngeal carcinoma. Cancer 2019; 125(7): 1081-90.
[http://dx.doi.org/10.1002/cncr.31907] [PMID: 30521105]

[119] Delia P, Sansotta G, Donato V, *et al.* Use of probiotics for prevention of radiation-induced diarrhea. World J Gastroenterol 2007; 13(6): 912-5.
[http://dx.doi.org/10.3748/wjg.v13.i6.912] [PMID: 17352022]

[120] Chitapanarux I, Chitapanarux T, Traisathit P, Kudumpee S, Tharavichitkul E, Lorvidhaya V. Randomized controlled trial of live *lactobacillus acidophilus* plus *bifidobacterium bifidum* in prophylaxis of diarrhea during radiotherapy in cervical cancer patients. Radiat Oncol 2010; 5(1): 31.
[http://dx.doi.org/10.1186/1748-717X-5-31] [PMID: 20444243]

[121] Gurbatri CR, Lia I, Vincent R, *et al.* Engineered probiotics for local tumor delivery of checkpoint blockade nanobodies. Sci Transl Med 2020; 12(530): eaax0876.
[http://dx.doi.org/10.1126/scitranslmed.aax0876] [PMID: 32051224]

[122] Song Q, Zheng C, Jia J, *et al.* A probiotic spore-based oral autonomous nanoparticles generator for cancer therapy. Adv Mater 2019; 31(43): 1903793.
[http://dx.doi.org/10.1002/adma.201903793] [PMID: 31490587]

[123] He L, Yang H, Tang J, *et al.* Intestinal probiotics *E. coli* Nissle 1917 as a targeted vehicle for delivery of p53 and Tum-5 to solid tumors for cancer therapy. J Biol Eng 2019; 13(1): 58.
[http://dx.doi.org/10.1186/s13036-019-0189-9] [PMID: 31297149]

[124] Panebianco C, Latiano T, Pazienza V. Microbiota manipulation by probiotics administration as emerging tool in cancer prevention and therapy. Front Oncol 2020; 10: 679.
[http://dx.doi.org/10.3389/fonc.2020.00679] [PMID: 32523887]

[125] Lakshmanan VK, Jindal S, Packirisamy G, *et al.* Nanomedicine-based cancer immunotherapy: recent trends and future perspectives. Cancer Gene Ther 2021; 28(9): 911-23.
[http://dx.doi.org/10.1038/s41417-021-00299-4] [PMID: 33558704]

CHAPTER 3

Probiotics Based Anticancer Immunity in Skin Cancer

Engkarat Kingkaew[1] and **Somboon Tanasupawat**[1,*]

[1] *Department of Biochemistry and Microbiology, Faculty of Pharmaceutical Sciences, Chulalongkorn University, Bangkok, Thailand*

Abstract: Cancer, a condition caused by unregulated cell proliferation, has elevated the global mortality rate that was rising on a daily basis. The treatments for cancer have numerous adverse effects on patients' lives. To enhance this treatment, probiotics and their metabolites (postbiotics) play an important role in the prevention and treatment of cancer. The mechanisms behind probiotic anti-tumor and/or anti-cancer actions are not yet comprehended. Numerous studies demonstrate that probiotics are useful in cancer prevention and treatment. The majority of which are involved in balancing microbiota, producing essential compounds containing beneficial effects and anti-tumor and cancer activity, preventing pathogen infection, modulating the host immunity, reducing inflammation, and in alleviating the severity of some risk factors. Few studies advise that they should not be used, emphasizing the risk of infection to patients. This chapter provides an overview of skin cancer, skin microbiome, gut microbiome, and its implications in skin cancer, as well as probiotic and postbiotic therapeutic approaches.

Keywords: Lactic acid bacteria, Microbiome, Probiotics, Postbiotics, Skin cancer.

1. INTRODUCTION

Cancer, a condition caused by unregulated cell proliferation, affects millions of people each year and is recognized as one of humanity's worst major health problems [1]. As a result, scientific researchers are aiming to develop a wide range of cancer therapies nowadays. In recent years, there has been a major surge in the investigation of the use of probiotics as an adjuvant to conventional cancer therapies [2]. FAO/WHO defines probiotics as "living microorganisms that provide health advantages on the host when administered in suitable doses." [3, 4]. Probiotics confer benefits in numerous ways, including dropping gut pH,

---

* **Corresponding author Somboon Tanasupawat:** Department of Biochemistry and Microbiology, Faculty of Pharmaceutical Sciences, Chulalongkorn University, Bangkok, Thailand; E-mail: somboon.t@chula.ac.th

Mitesh Kumar Dwivedi, Alwarappan Sankaranarayanan & Sanjay Tiwari (Eds.)

preventing pathogen colonization, and modulating the host immune response [5]. Probiotics also prevent and treat cancer by controlling the intestinal microbiota, strengthening the colon, boosting the function of the intestinal barrier, regulating enzymes and metabolisms of gut bacteria, and blocking carcinogenic compounds, producing essential compounds containing anti-proliferative activity, and reducing inflammation [6, 7]. Therefore, probiotics could be a promising tool for skin cancer therapy. However, further study about how to supplement these probiotics and their appropriate dosage is required [8].

2. SKIN CANCERS

Based on the world's earliest records, cancer has been a serious health concern since 3,000 B.C., and its incidence continues to climb to this day [9]. Due to the multiple physiological, social, material, and spiritual threats it poses, cancer is difficult to treat. Globally, around one million new cases of cancer are diagnosed each year [10]. It arises as a consequence of the uncontrolled growth of abnormal cells (neoplasia) in any region of the body. As these cells proliferate, they produce a tumor-like mass [1]. In fact, invasion, metastasis, and uncontrolled growth must be present in the cell in order to speak of cancer [10]. If a normal cell acquires these malign features, it appears to reach the subsequent stage of carcinogenesis. These four phases are as follows: Phase 1 (initiation, progressing extremely gradually, also recognized as the latent stage), Phase 2 (promotion, rapidly growing cell groups, promoters are impactful), Phase 3 (progression, operating independently of the surrounding tissue, genetic mutations are irreversible), and Stage 4 (invasion and metastasis, complicated to treat) [1]. Interfering with cells in the beginning stages of mutation may prevent the development of cancer. Therefore, a clinical diagnosis devoid of risk factors is necessary for each patient. Individuals having a family history of cancer are regarded to be more susceptible [9]. There are currently efforts to create treatment options for some types of cancer. It is well acknowledged that cancer is a disease that varies from person to person. Chemotherapy, radiation therapy, and medical techniques are frequently employed in cancer treatment and are the key factors. Nevertheless, the previously described therapies might have a negative impact on one's quality of life [1]. Cancer, a condition defined by uncontrolled cell proliferation, kills millions of people each year and is one of humanity's most serious health issues [10]. As a result, various researchers are continually working to develop multiple cancer therapy options.

Cancer of the skin is the most prevalent type of human skin. More than 4 million cases of non-melanoma (*i.e.*, Basal Cell Carcinoma (BCC) and Squamous Cell Carcinoma (SCC)) are diagnosed annually in the United States [11, 12]. In the

United States, these cancers affect more people than all other forms of cancer combined, posing a significant threat to public health [13]. Therefore, a full knowledge of the processes behind skin cancer is necessary for the development of adequate preventative and treatment methods and the optimal allocation of medical resources. Currently, there is a major emphasis on a study on the involvement of the immune system in the pathogenesis and development of skin cancer in order to develop innovative therapeutic strategies [12].

2.1. Classification of Skin Cancer

The most common cancer is skin cancer, which encompasses both non-melanoma and melanoma [14]. Non-melanoma skin cancer accounts for roughly 30% of all malignancies, and its prevalence is rising significantly [15]. BCC is the most widespread kind of skin cancer (75-80% of cases) and also the most common type of cancer in people [16]. SCC is the second most common form of skin cancer in the United States, behind BCC, with around one million cases each year. This kind of cancer might grow on healthy tissue or preexisting problems like actinic keratosis or an old burn scar. SCC risk factors include exposure to ultraviolet (UV) radiation, light skin, age, male gender, persistent lesions, radiation treatment, the presence of oncogenic viruses (*i.e.*, human papillomavirus (HPV)), environmental exposures, and immunosuppression [15, 17, 18]. Immunosuppressive therapy, whether physiological or pharmacological, is related to a higher cancer risk relative to the general population, suggesting the importance of immune system disorders in the genesis and development of skin cancer [19].

Melanoma represents the most lethal form of skin cancer and places a substantial load on the healthcare system. Melanoma, unlike other malignancies, affects youthful, more socially active individuals with a median age of 57 at diagnosis. Hereditary and environmental factors contribute to the development of skin cancers. Despite ongoing research to create innovative therapeutic modalities, the prospects for those with severe illnesses remain dismal [20]. In the general population, cutaneous lymphoma, Kaposi sarcoma, Merkel cell carcinoma (MCC), skin adnexal tumors, and skin sarcoma are the most prevalent forms of skin cancer [21]. MCC, a neuroendocrine epidermal tumor, is a unique and aggressive form of skin cancer. Merkel cell polyomavirus (MCPyV) is responsible for the majority of cases, however other risk factors including advanced age, UV exposure, and immunosuppressive therapy have also been documented [22].

2.2. Pathophysiology of Skin Cancer

Frequent skin cancer is subdivided into invasive melanoma and non-melanoma skin cancers (NMSCs). This category consists of keratinocyte cancers such as basal cell carcinoma (BCC) and squamous cell carcinoma (SCC) [23]. Melanoma and NMSCs may be caused by various risk factors, including genetic mutation, immunosuppression, and exposure to environmental risk factors, such as ultraviolet (UV) radiation [24]. UV exposure is classified as a "carcinogenic factor" and is the most important factor for skin carcinogenesis. Because it is both a mutagen and a non-specific mutagenic agent, it has both the characteristics of a tumor activator and a tumor promoter [25]. Exposed skin to UV light may experience oxidative damage. UVB and UVA radiation may stimulate the production of reactive oxygen or nitrogen species (ROS/RNS) in the skin [26]. UV-induced ROS/RNS production increases and alters the structure and function of genes and proteins, leading to skin damage [27]. Furthermore, immunosurveillance mechanisms and the immunoediting framework provided a greater understanding of cutaneous immunology. The altered expression of (tumor-associated) antigens, such as reduced or limited MHC-1 expression, alters the tumor cells' immunogenicity, resulting in cancer development [12].

Furthermore, the role of skin pathogens in skin carcinogenesis is interesting and has yet to be established. Thus, the next possible explanation is described. After birth, the skin begins to colonize with a diversity of resident commensal bacteria and temporary pathogens [28]. Significantly, various variables impact the kind and amount of bacteria, involving host characteristics such as age (infancy, adolescent), sex (pregnant), culture, hygiene practice, behavioral exposures, use of skin medications and/or products, and systemic diseases [28 - 30]; Hereditary factors, like primary immunodeficiency disorders, may lead to immunodeficiency disorders [31]; specific cutaneous characteristics such as anatomic area, moisture content, pH, and skin diseases include ulcers, abscesses, and chronic dermatitis [30 - 33]; and environmental factors [34, 35]. Thus, if these factors are changed into inappropriate conditions, tt will play a crucial role in activating inflammation, leading to the development of tumors and cancer. Interestingly, probiotics have also been shown to reduce human low-density lipoprotein oxidation and to confer systemic antioxidant protection [36, 37]. It has been found that probiotics and their metabolites are a promising therapeutic approach for epidermal oxidative stress and the cancer prevention, as described in the next topic [38].

3. SKIN MICROBIOME AND SKIN CANCER

As people get older, malignancies become more common. Viruses and ultraviolet have been extensively studied in relation to skin cancer. Skin cancer incidence was recently revealed to be reduced in germ-free rats. Consequently, it is believed that dysbiosis skin microbiome may have a role in the formation of a range of skin cancers. Nevertheless, it is ambiguous whether progression is caused by tumor cells or microbial dysbiosis [39]. The correlation between the microbiome and cancer is a relatively recent and understudied theory, especially regarding skin cancer. Several studies have shown that the gut microbiota is involved in tumor genesis and/or progression. In addition, the gut microbiota seems vital in immunotherapy responses, which may be extended to the skin microbiome [40, 41].

Some of this research implies that dysbiosis may be a cancer promoter. Several studies have investigated the correlation between a variety of skin cancers and bacterial skin microbiome dysbiosis in inflammatory diseases involving interleukin-17 (IL-17) secretion (signature pro-inflammatory cytokines of the CD4$^+$ T helper 17 (Th17) cells) [42], such as psoriasis, acne and skin cancer [42 - 45]. In addition, SCC and actinic keratosis have recently been linked to a rise in some *Staphylococcus aureus* isolates and a reduction in skin commensals [46]. Due to the immune system's tolerance for commensal bacteria, the microbiome does not provoke a pro-inflammatory response under ordinary situations, hence sustaining homeostasis [41]. For instance, when these functions are interrupted or pathogens penetrate this well-balanced system, dysregulation develops and the immune system is triggered against the microbiota, resulting in inflammatory responses [47, 48] or adapting the localized immune reaction, which may stimulate tumor development in the gut [40, 41]. Intestinal inflammation has also been shown to raise the probability of microbiota generating mutagens that cause DNA damage, hence driving tumor and cancer growth [49].

For skin cancer studies, many bacteria live on the skin. The most prevalent skin commensal bacterial genera in healthy and normal skin are *Corynebacterium, Micrococcus, Propionibacterium,* and *Staphylococcus* [50, 51]. Notably, *Staphylococcus epidermidis* is more prevalent in the interfollicular epidermis, whilst *Cutibacterium acnes* (formerly *Propionibacterium acnes*) is observed predominantly in the pilosebaceous units [52, 53]. Several *S. epidermidis* strains synthesize antimicrobial peptides [54], while *Cb. acnes* produces lipases [55], which limit the pathogenic growth such as Group A *Streptococcus* (GAS) and *S. aureus* [52]. Additionally, Mrázek, Mekadim [56] investigated pigs and discovered that the biodiversity differed dramatically between normal skin and cancerous skin. Researchers found *Fusobacterium* and *Trueperella* species with in microbiomes of melanoma specimens, as well as a greater number of *Staphylococcus* and *Streptococcus* rather than in the microbiome of normal skin. Based on this study, it is feasible to conclude that *Fusobacteria* may be linked to the formation of tumors. As a potential mechanism, the researchers postulated a tumor-based immune evasion. Due to *F. nucleatum* could bind to different tumor types, the association of the Fap2 (fusobacterial protein) with the inhibiting receptor TIGIT of immunity cells (also named T cell immunoreceptor with Ig and ITIM domains) protects malignancies from the immune system, limiting natural killer (NK) cell cytotoxicity [56, 57]. In addition, Merkel cell polyomavirus (MCPyV), a virus presumed to be a permanent resident of the skin, has been linked to an increased risk of developing Merkel cell cancer (MCC) [43]. According to recent research, the skin microbiota could inhibit tumor development [58]. The investigation identifies a isolate of *S. epidermidis* that was found in the skin microbiota and it could synthesize 6-N-hydroxyaminopurine (6-HAP), a chemical that inhibits the activity of DNA polymerase [58]. The growth of tumor cell lines was limited by 6-HAP, but it had no effect on normal keratinocytes. A 6-HAP intravenous infusion inhibited the growth of melanoma in mice without producing systemic harm. Colonization of mice with S. epidermidis isolates releasing 6-HAP lowered chronically UV exposure skin damage as well as tumor formation compared to the colonization of mice with a control strain that did not synthesize 6-HAP [58]. *S. epidermidis* isolates synthesizing 6-HAP were discovered in the skin metagenome of several healthy human volunteers, indicating that certain people's microbiomes may protect them from skin cancer [58]. These results suggest a unique role for commensal skin bacteria in the host's defense against UV-induced cancerous skin. Wang and Choi proposed an *in vitro* study in which human melanocytes are co-cultured with commensal skin bacteria (*i.e.*, *Cb. acnes* and *S. epidermidis*). After UVB irradiation, commensal *S. epidermidis* and their lipoic acid (LPA or TLR2 ligand, which has special anti-inflammatory effect on keratinocyte cells, strengthening UVB tolerance) enhance melanocyte survival. This action is caused by an increase in TRAF1, CASP5, CASP14, and TP73 expression; *Cb. acnes*, on the other hand, stimulates apoptosis in UVB-irradiated melanocytes *via* TNF-α production. It is possible that the seemingly contradictory effects may be explained by variations in the location and concentration of *Cb. acnes* in normal skin. *Cb. acnes* is commonly found in hair follicles, where the environment is essential for stem cell maintenance. Since DNA damage in these cells may cause serious mutations, *Cb. acnes* may have evolved in the follicular environment to protect stem cell health. *In contrast, S. epidermidis* seems to be more abundant in dry regions of the body, particularly the interfollicular epidermis. As mentioned earlier, lipoteichoic acid (LTA) aids melanocytes in avoiding UVB-induced apoptosis, that is essential for preserving normal inter-follicular melanocytes under sunlight exposure and limiting their conversion into tumor cells [59]. Further investigations which corroborate this concept include findings from the intestinal microbiome suggesting bacteria could inhibit the growth of tumor *via* synthesizing short-chain fatty acids (SCFAs) [60,

61]. Besides that, skin microbiota may synthesize *cis*-urocanic acid *via* decomposing L-histidine that helps in the suppression of immunity caused through UV radiation as well as limits melanoma formation [58].

There have only been a few of human inquiries to our knowledge. One research looked at the link between the microbiota on the skin and the risk of developing skin cancer. Despite the fact that the sample was limited, they showed no significant variations in the variety or quantity of genera between the microbiomes of skin melanomas and melanocytic nevi (15 melanoma17 nevi and) [62].

In terms of non-melanoma skin cancer, a present investigation looked at the microbial community of actinic keratosis (AK) and SCC in immunocompetent males, either longitudinally or cross-sectionally [46]. *Malassezia* and *Cutibacterium* were more generally reported in healthy perilesional regions, while *Staphylococcus* was frequent in SCC and AK, with the *S. aureus* isolates predominating. In particular, 11 of *S. aureus* Operational Taxonomic Units (OTUs) were found in participants; 6 of them were substantially related to SCCs, with OTUs 50 and 216 present in every patients, indicating their unique participation in the development from AK to SCC [46]. The mentioned observations have recently been proven, with an excess of *S. aureus* seen in SCC and AK samples compared to basal cell carcinoma specimens. As a result of the reduction in *Malassezia* in SCCs, it was hypothesized that yeast may act as a defense against over-colonization of *S. aureus* [63]. In actinic keratosis and BCCs, protective reactive oxygen species (ROS) are also lowered [64, 65]. This suggests that skin commensals such as *S. epidermidis* and *Cb. acnes* may also protect the host from the DNA damage caused by UV radiation.

Recent research highlighted the role of the intestinal microbiota in the response to anti-PD-1 immunotherapy in patients with metastatic melanoma, based on the local possible pathogen influence of the skin microbiota on the promotion and/or growth of skin cancer. There was remarkable correlation between the occurrence of certain bacteria, including *Enterococcus faecium*, *Collinsella aerofaciens* as well as *Bifidobacterium longum*, and a positive clinical response to treatment [66]. The transplantation of feces from responders into germ-free (GF) mice improved tumor regulation, elevated T cell responses, and increased the efficacy of anti-P--L1 therapy, as shown by this study. According to these results, the beneficial commensal microbiota could be responsible for regulating anti-tumor immunity in people with cancer [66]. Moreover, dermal probiotic therapies are recommended to lower the incidence of skin cancer due to enhanced immunosurveillance and alleviate inflammation. In fact, probiotics have capacity to alter tumor *via* modulating immunity responses, potentially contributing to medicinal benefits

[43]. Notwithstanding, further study is required to completely comprehend the skin microbiota feature in skin cancer.

4. GUT MICROBIOME AND ITS IMPLICATIONS IN SKIN CANER

Patients with cancer are commonly exposed to dysbiosis of the intestinal microbiota as a consequence of treatments that affect the diversity and immunity of these bacteria [67]. Consequently, the gut microbiota and immunomodulation are altered and the inflammation occurs as described in above section. Though the association between skin cancer and this dysbiosis is ambiguous, the association with cancer in principle has been studied to a restricted scope. In murine models, for example, colorectal cancer (CRC) is related to a rise of *Bacteroides fragilis*. Furthermore, a changing gut microbiota increases the chance of developing CRC [68]. Moreover, the study of Guo, Liu [69] suggested that *Helicobacter pylori* is related to an elevated risk of pancreatic cancer. This could be due to a disrupted gut microbiota, that has been correlated with *Helicobacter*-associated disorders [70]. Further investigation is necessary, nevertheless, to examine the association between skin cancer and gut dysbiosis. Lastly, it is unclear if the formation of tumor is a result of microbial dysbiosis.

5. PROBIOTIC BASED THERAPEUTIC APPROACHES

5.1. Probiotics and their Beneficial Roles

According to the report of Salminen, Collado [71], probiotics are "live microorganisms that, when administered in adequate amounts, confer a health benefit on the host". Probiotics can be derived from a variety of genera and species [72]. Lactic acid bacteria (LAB; *Bifidobacterium*, *Lactobacillus*, *Enterococcus*, and *Streptococcus* species), *Escherichia coli*, *Bacillus* and *Propionibacterium* species are used as probiotics [3]. The probiotics in the human gastrointestinal environment interact strongly with nutrition and host cells. This is a quite sophisticated biological system, yet it is absolutely necessary for maintaining the homeostasis of the intestines and for human growth. The probiotic, as a result of the metabolic processes it engages in, has a crucial role in the body's nutrition and metabolism [4]. In addition to this, it has a considerable influence on the maturation and operation of several systems, including the immune system. Probiotics and the host cells that they associate with have a number of mutual benefits as a result of their connection. The primary roles of probiotics in the host are as follows:

1. Involvement in the construction of the gastrointestinal wall.
2. Enhancing colonization resistance.
3. Synthesis of short chain fatty acid.
4. Synthesis vitamins (*i.e.*, K and B group).
5. Interaction with the immune system of the mucous membranes.
6. Xenobiotics destruction.

Therefore, the most important functions of probiotics are to protect against gastrointestinal infections, to modulate the immune system, to lower serum cholesterol and blood pressure, to inhibit the development of cancer, to improve nutritional utilization and bioavailability metabolism, and to promote overall metabolic health [73, 74]. Notably, dysbiosis refers to the microbial imbalance that can cause the several diseases. It could be alleviated by the ingestion of pro- and pre-biotics (indigestible substrates) that affect the microbiota in a positive way for the prophylaxis and even medication of some diseases. It is well acknowledged that the intestinal microbiota impacts human health and that probiotics have an effect on it.

5.2. Probiotics and Microorganisms of The Skin

The microflora of the skin is crucial for the metabolism of skin proteins, free fatty acids, and sebum, as well as the competitive exclusion of pathogens that are invasive and cause disease in the skin [38]. The scientific investigation into the make-up and operation of the skin's microflora has recently been given new life. It has emerged as one of the most fascinating and rapidly expanding subfields in human cutaneous physiology [75]. This normal skin microbiota is considered to be related to pathogen competitive exclusion, a function that probiotics could be able to improve [76]. It has been shown that some probiotics may assist to modify the cutaneous microbiota, as well as the lipid barrier and the skin immune system, which ultimately leads to the maintenance of normal skin homeostasis [38]. Cutaneous immunosurveillance is necessary not only to defend the body from infective pathogens, but also to recognize and eradicate mutated cells, that can lead to skin carcinomas [77, 78]. Because of the harsh circumstances that exist on the skin, a few number of gram-positive bacteria have managed to thrive there [79]. On the skin, resident bacterial species such as *Propionibacteria* (*Cb. acnes, P. avidum*, and *P. granulosum*), coagulase-negative *Staphylococci* (*S. epidermidis*), *Micrococci*, *Corynebacteria*, and *Acinetobacter*, as well as transient species such as *S. aureus, Escherichia coli, Pseudomonas aeroguinosa*, and *Bacillus* spp. are present [80]. A recent study that used 16S rRNA gene survey methodologies indicated that the human skin microbiota is far more sophisticated than what was observed in prior studies [81]. It has been discovered that *S.*

epidermidis is the most frequently found flora on the skin [81]. In addition, the occurrence of this species might influence the function of the skin barrier and/or the maturation of innate immune responses in human skin. To a host that is "normal and healthy," the native microflora may be "useful," but to a host that has compromised skin integrity, the natural microflora may be toxic [80]. There is certain evidence to suggest that the adaptive immune system is the one that is stimulated by the skin microbiota, as opposed to the non-adaptive immune system. In this respect, it has been shown that bacteria on the skin are bound with immunoglobulins, which are most likely generated by the secretions of the eccrine sweat glands [82]. Several physical factors affect the quantity of bacteria species found on human skin (*i.e.*, the quantity and size of follicles and glands, function, the flow of secretions, the integrity of barrier function, skin pH, and osmotic) and biochemical factors (*i.e.*, soluble micronutrients obtained from sebum—such as amino acids and lipids; sweat—such as vitamins and lactate, and amino acids—as well as those synthesized as a consequence of the microbiologically metabolic activity on the skin; *e.g.*, lantibiotics produced by *Staphylococcus* spp., bacteriocins, Methanethiol, acids and enzymes) [80]. The cutaneous pH has the potential to have an effect on the bacterial populations that are found on the surface of the skin, which in turn has an effect on the local microflora and helps to regulate epidermal permeability, barrier equilibrium, and stratum corneum integrity [83]. High stratum corneum pH has been linked to various cutaneous conditions, including acute eczema, atopic dermatitis, and seborrheic dermatitis. In these conditions, an increase in pH may have a detrimental impact on cutaneous functioning, which may cause the illnesses to become more severe and result in more severe clinical symptoms [38]. Therefore, the integration of probiotics into metabolic processes that include fermentation in order to generate lactic acid and acquire energy [84, 85] could be an attractive strategy.

5.3. Role of Probiotics' Metabolites (Postbiotics) in Cancer Prevention

Probiotics produce several metabolites, which are called postbiotics such as exopolysaccharides (EPSs), short-chain fatty acids (SCFAs), bacteriocins, and cell wall components. These contain cytotoxic activity and can be applied for cancer treatment [86, 87]. The roles of postbiotics in skin cancer prevention and skin beneficial effects are shown in Table **1**.

5.3.1. Exopolysaccharides (EPSs)

Exopolysaccharides are biopolymers and characterized as homopolysaccharides (*i.e.* identical monosaccharide units) or heteropolysaccharides (*i.e.* different monosaccharide units) based on their composition (*i.e.* different monosaccharides). Their production is extremely isolate specific, and the amount that they produce may vary based on variables like as the composition of the medium and the incubation conditions [88, 89]. These attributes have a direct bearing on the different sugar compositions that are accountable for anti-proliferative effects; on the other hand, monosaccharide composition, protein content, molecular mass, the location of glycosidic linkages, and substituent groups all have an effect on anticancer activity [90]. Their particular anticancer mechanisms are unclear, although some have been reported, including tumorigenesis prevention, activation of cancer cell death, indirect stimulation of macrophages to enhance phagocytosis, and acceleration of pro-inflammatory factor and interferon-gamma (IFN-γ) production. Nevertheless, due to their massive quantity, EPSs are unable to penetrate cells, hence their function must be performed through recognition by cell surface receptors [88, 90, 91].

5.3.2. Short-chain Fatty Acids (SCFAs) and Lipids

SCFAs are synthesized from LAB and non-LAB. These SCFAs activate the secretion of anti-inflammatory cytokines, inhibit inflammatory pathways, improve the antioxidant system, activate cellular apoptosis, and suppress proliferation [87, 92, 93]. The anticancer activity of conjugated linoleic acid (CLA) is based on structural differences between isomers, such as the location and cis-trans configuration of the conjugated double bonds. Conjugated fatty acids may have stronger tumor-suppressing effects, with the mechanism focusing on lipid peroxidation, apoptosis activation, and modified cellular phospholipid composition, according to the findings of several research investigations [94].

5.3.3. Bacteriocins

Bacteriocins are ribosomal peptides. They are typically cationic peptides that have the ability to generate holes on cytoplasmic membranes, which leads to important components from the inside of the cell leaking out [95]. Even though the mechanism against cancer cells has not been completely understood, cell surface characteristics between cancer cells and normal cells could be used to describe it. Negative charges are predominant on cancerous cells owing to larger quantities of anionic phosphatidylserine, O-glycosylated mucins, sialylated gangliosides, and heparin sulfates than normal cell membranes, which are neutral in charge [89, 96]. Therefore, bacteriocins can attach to negatively charged cancer cells and show an anti-proliferative effect [97].

5.3.4. Cell-wall Compounds

The D-configuration of amino acids in peptidoglycan, such as alanine (Ala), glutamine (Gln), and asparagine (Asn), has been demonstrated to have remarkable cytotoxicity and to boost the host innate immunity [89, 98, 99]. The S-layer protein (SlpA) is an additional component of the cell wall. These proteins are organized into arrays of single polypeptides that are non-covalently bound to the bacterial cell's outer layer. They have a wide range of biological activities, including the activation of immune responses, the modulation of dendritic cells (DCs) and T-cell functions, and the induction of pro- and anti-inflammatory cytokines [99, 100].

Table. (1). The beneficial roles of postbiotics and bacteriocins in skin cancer prevention and/or skin beneficial effects.

Postbiotics	Beneficial Features	References
Lipoteichoic acids of *Lb. rhamonosus* GG	1)Stimulating interferon-gamma (IFN-γ) and enhancing T-helper cell (Th) and cytotoxic T cell (CTL) activity. 2) Delaying in the tumor development. 3) Rising IgA⁺ and activating dendritic cells.	[101], [102]
*Bifidobacterium animalis*01 protein and selenium (Se) (Pro-Se)	Acting as an antioxidant agent.	[103]
Extracellular polysaccharide (EPS) of *Bacillus coagulans* RK-02	Showing antioxidant and free radical scavenging activities.	[104]
Crude extracts of *Lb. brevis*	Suppressing the expression of NOS activity and IFN-g/PGE2 generation, matrix metalloproteinase(MMP)activity in lipopolysaccharide (LPS)-activated macrophages in cell culture.	[105]
Bf. longum lysates	Preventing the secretion of neuromediators involved in sensitivity phenomena, reducing neurogenic inflammation frequently associated with sensitive skin symptoms, enhancing skin barrier function, and defending neurons from external stimuli.	[106]
Short chain fatty acids (SCFAs) derived from LAB (*i.e.*, *Lactobacillus* spp.) and non-LAB (*i.e.*, *Clostridium butyricum*)	1) Stimulating the release of anti-inflammatory cytokines, 2) Inhibiting inflammatory pathways, improving the antioxidant system, 3) Inducing cellular apoptosis 4) Suppressing proliferative activity 5) Relieving chemotherapy-induced diarrhoea	[87], [92], [93], [107]
Bacteriocins		

(Table 1) cont.....

Postbiotics	Beneficial Features	References
Nisin	1) Inducing cell death and cell-cycle arrest 2) Suppressing cell proliferation 3) Synergizing with chemotherapeutic drugs, such as doxorubicin against skin cancers 4) Stimulating the interleukin-12 (IL-12; an interleukin that have an vital role in Th1-type immune response against cancer) 5) Regulating the pro-inflammatory cytokine	[108 - 113]
Nisin A	Activating human keratinocyte HaCaT activity, decreasing LPS-induced pro-inflammatory cytokine levels (*i.e.*, TNF-α), and accelerating wound repairing	[114]
Plantaricin EF	Reducing the inflammation	[115], [116]
Salivaricin LHM	Alleviating the inflammation	[115], [116]

Table. (2). The beneficial roles of probiotics in cancer prevention and/or skin beneficial effects.

Probiotics	Features	References
Genetically engineered *Bf. bifidum* BGN4	Strong stimulating interleukin-10 (IL-10; a potent anti-inflammatory factor and has a key function in the inhibition of tumorigenesis) production to confer anti-inflammatory effects and cancer immunotherapy	[117], [118]
Bf. infantis CCRC 14633 and *Bf. longum* B6	1) Synthesizing and elevating riboflavin (vitamin B2) levels in 48-h soy milk fermentation	[119]
Bf. longum ATCC 15708 and *Lb. acidophilus* ATCC 4356	1) Lessening, preventing, and allviating skin irritation and irritative skin diseases. 2) Acting as antioxidant compounds in *in vitro* and *in vivo* studies	[120], [121]
Bf. Lactis CNCM I-3446 and *Lb. paracasei* CNCM I-2116	Reducing neurosensitivity in female patients with reactive skin	[122]
Lb. fermentum	1) Involving in generating antioxidant compounds (*i.e.*, glutathione), which can reduce the inflammation 2) Alleviating inflammation in mice model	[123]
Arginine deiminase activity positive strains of *Lb. brevis*	1) Inducing apoptosis 2) Reducing nitric oxide production, leading to alleviating inflammatory condition	[124]
Fermented dairy product containing *Lb. casei, Lb. bulgaricus*, and *Streptococcus thermophilus*	1) Reducing transepidermal dehydration 2) Enhancing stratum corneum barrier	[125]
Lb. helveticus	Enhancing synthesis of the differentiation-related factor profilaggrin (a building block of a moisturizing component that regulates normal epidermal moisture and resilience)	[126]

(Table 2) cont.....

Probiotics	Features	References
Lb. johnsonii	1) Enhancing the rehabilitation of the skin immunity 2) Defending the cutaneous immune system against UVB exposure-associated immunosuppressive effects (in hairless mice model)	[127], [128]

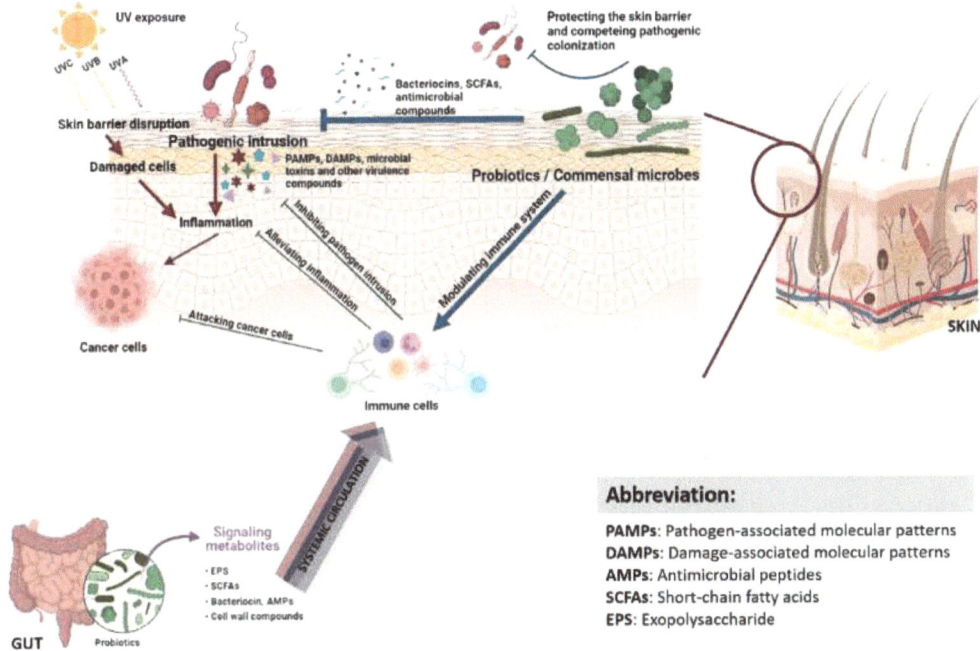

Fig. (1). Proposed anti/preventative-skin cancer mechanisms of probiotics and skin commensal microbes. The composition of skin microbes can be influenced by a crosstalk between the disturbed skin barrier, UV exposure, and skin commensal. The changes in skin microbiota, along with damage-associated molecular patterns (DAMPs), pathogen-associated molecular patterns (PAMPs), microbial toxins and other virulence factors, can cause chronic skin inflammation and cellular damage, which can contribute to the beginning and development of skin cancer. The probiotics and skin commensal microbes can prevent or treat disease. They can manage this by passively inhabiting an environment identical to that of pathogens, preventing them from invading the skin. They can also compete against pathogens by producing antimicrobial compounds. Besides, they may modulate the immune system, directing it to treat disease-causing organisms or enhancing immune tolerance, which can alleviate the severity of inflammatory diseases. Furthermore, probiotics (in gut) are primarily responsible for their cancer prevention and treatment. By improving the physicochemical situation of the colon, elevating the feature of the intestinal barrier, controlling the gut microbiota, and altering the intestinal bacterial enzymes and metabolism, carcinogens are degraded and inflammation is reduced [6, 7]. In addition, probiotic byproducts and immune mediators from the gut may enter the systemic circulation and suppress skin cancer growth indirectly.

5.4. Role of Probiotics in the Prevention of Skin Cancer

Probiotics are recently applied and supplemented in cancer treatment as previously described by Górska, Przystupski [2]. Nevertheless, the mechanisms underlying the antitumor properties and advanced knowledge of probiotics are currently being studied and are incompletely understood. The probiotics are related to a variety of pathways that are considered to be important in this process. Some of these pathways are involved in [10]: (1) Modulating the microbiota by preventing undesirable microorganisms that produce cancer-associated compounds, (2) Stimulation of immunomodulatory cells and inhibition of pathogens by the synthesis of antimicrobial compounds, (3) Decrease of genotoxicity and DNA damage, and (4) Synthesis of essential metabolites. The proposed mechanism of anti/prevention-skin cancer by probiotics and skin commensal microbes is shown in Fig. (**1**). Moreover, the roles of probiotics in skin cancer prevention and skin beneficial effects are shown in Table **2**.

CONCLUSION

In conclusion, microbiota has a vital role in dermatology and can be used as a therapeutic target. Recent investigations on the therapeutic effects of probiotics are promising. They might have possible roles in the prevention and treatment of skin cancer, such as limiting pathogens, regulating immunity, lowering inflammation, and producing vital compounds containing skin beneficial effects and anti-proliferative activity for tumors and/or cancer of the skin. Nevertheless, the studies on the issue acknowledge that more evidence is required to verify the effectiveness of probiotics in the prevention and treatment of skin cancer. While clinical usage of probiotics has already established a safety profile, long-term safety evidence is inadequate. Concerningly, few reports associate probiotics with infections and other serious adverse effects in immunocompromised patients. As a consequence of this, more significant sample numbers and higher power clinical studies are necessary in order to evaluate the safety of such use of probiotics.

CONSENT FOR PUBLICATION

Not applicable.

CONFLICT OF INTEREST

The authors declare no conflict of interest, financial or otherwise.

ACKNOWLEDGEMENT

Declared none.

REFERENCES

[1]   Şener D, Bulut HN, Güneş Bayir A. Probiotics and Relationship Between Probiotics and Cancer Types. Bezmialem Sci 2021; 9(4): 490-7.

[http://dx.doi.org/10.14235/bas.galenos.2021.5375]

[2]   Górska A, Przystupski D, Niemczura MJ, Kulbacka J. Probiotic Bacteria: A Promising Tool in Cancer Prevention and Therapy. Curr Microbiol 2019; 76(8): 939-49.
        [http://dx.doi.org/10.1007/s00284-019-01679-8] [PMID: 30949803]

[3]   Pandey KR, Naik SR, Vakil BV. Probiotics, prebiotics and synbiotics- a review. J Food Sci Technol 2015; 52(12): 7577-87.
        [http://dx.doi.org/10.1007/s13197-015-1921-1] [PMID: 26604335]

[4]   Aureli P, Capurso L, Castellazzi AM, *et al.* Probiotics and health: An evidence-based review. Pharmacol Res 2011; 63(5): 366-76.
        [http://dx.doi.org/10.1016/j.phrs.2011.02.006] [PMID: 21349334]

[5]   Williams NT. Probiotics. Am J Health Syst Pharm 2010; 67(6): 449-58.
        [http://dx.doi.org/10.2146/ajhp090168] [PMID: 20208051]

[6]   Chandel D, Sharma M, Chawla V, Sachdeva N, Shukla G. Isolation, characterization and identification of antigenotoxic and anticancerous indigenous probiotics and their prophylactic potential in experimental colon carcinogenesis. Sci Rep 2019; 9(1): 14769.
        [http://dx.doi.org/10.1038/s41598-019-51361-z] [PMID: 31611620]

[7]   Liong MT. Probiotics: a critical review of their potential role as antihypertensives, immune modulators, hypocholesterolemics, and perimenopausal treatments. Nutr Rev 2007; 65(7): 316-28.
        [http://dx.doi.org/10.1111/j.1753-4887.2007.tb00309.x] [PMID: 17695372]

[8]   Valeriano VD, Parungao-Balolong MM, Kang DK. *In vitro* evaluation of the mucin-adhesion ability and probiotic potential of *Lactobacillus mucosae* LM1. J Appl Microbiol 2014; 117(2): 485-97.
        [http://dx.doi.org/10.1111/jam.12539] [PMID: 24807045]

[9]   Baykara O. Current Modalities in Treatment of Cancer. Balıkesır Health Sci J 2016; 5: 154-65.

[10]   Kahraman M, Karahan AG. Tumor Suppressor Effects of Probiotics Turk bull hyg exp biol 2018; 75(4): 421-.

[11]   Rogers HW, Weinstock MA, Feldman SR, Coldiron BM. Incidence estimate of nonmelanoma skin cancer (keratinocyte carcinomas) in the US population, 2012. JAMA Dermatol 2015; 151(10): 1081-6.
        [http://dx.doi.org/10.1001/jamadermatol.2015.1187] [PMID: 25928283]

[12]   Rangwala S, Tsai KY. Roles of the immune system in skin cancer. Br J Dermatol 2011; 165(5): 953-65.
        [http://dx.doi.org/10.1111/j.1365-2133.2011.10507.x] [PMID: 21729024]

[13]   Karimkhani C, Boyers LN, Dellavalle RP, Weinstock MA. It's time for "keratinocyte carcinoma" to replace the term "nonmelanoma skin cancer". J Am Acad Dermatol 2015; 72(1): 186-7.
        [http://dx.doi.org/10.1016/j.jaad.2014.09.036] [PMID: 25497921]

[14]   Apalla Z, Nashan D, Weller RB, Castellsagué X. Skin cancer: epidemiology, disease burden, pathophysiology, diagnosis, and therapeutic approaches. Dermatol Ther (Heidelb) 2017; 7(S1) (Suppl. 1): 5-19.
        [http://dx.doi.org/10.1007/s13555-016-0165-y] [PMID: 28150105]

[15]   Burton KA, Ashack KA, Khachemoune A. Cutaneous squamous cell carcinoma: a review of high-risk and metastatic disease. Am J Clin Dermatol 2016; 17(5): 491-508.
        [http://dx.doi.org/10.1007/s40257-016-0207-3] [PMID: 27358187]

[16]   Chung S. Basal cell carcinoma. Arch Plast Surg 2012; 39(2): 166-70.
        [http://dx.doi.org/10.5999/aps.2012.39.2.166] [PMID: 22783519]

[17]   Gurudutt VV, Genden EM. Cutaneous squamous cell carcinoma of the head and neck. J Skin Cancer 2011; 2011: 1-10.
        [http://dx.doi.org/10.1155/2011/502723] [PMID: 21461387]

[18]   Que SKT, Zwald FO, Schmults CD. Cutaneous squamous cell carcinoma. J Am Acad Dermatol 2018;

78(2): 237-47.
[http://dx.doi.org/10.1016/j.jaad.2017.08.059] [PMID: 29332704]

[19] Gerlini G, Romagnoli P, Pimpinelli N. Skin cancer and immunosuppression. Crit Rev Oncol Hematol 2005; 56(1): 127-36.
[http://dx.doi.org/10.1016/j.critrevonc.2004.11.011] [PMID: 15978830]

[20] Ali Z, Yousaf N, Larkin J. Melanoma epidemiology, biology and prognosis. Eur J Cancer, Suppl 2013; 11(2): 81-91.
[http://dx.doi.org/10.1016/j.ejcsup.2013.07.012] [PMID: 26217116]

[21] Ridky TW. Nonmelanoma skin cancer. J Am Acad Dermatol 2007; 57(3): 484-501.
[http://dx.doi.org/10.1016/j.jaad.2007.01.033] [PMID: 17512631]

[22] Schadendorf D, Lebbé C, zur Hausen A, *et al.* Merkel cell carcinoma: Epidemiology, prognosis, therapy and unmet medical needs. Eur J Cancer 2017; 71: 53-69.
[http://dx.doi.org/10.1016/j.ejca.2016.10.022] [PMID: 27984768]

[23] Grosu-Bularda A, Lăzărescu L, Stoian A, Lascăr I. Immunology and skin cancer Arch Clin Cases 2018; 5(3).

[24] Carr S, Smith C, Wernberg J. Epidemiology and risk factors of melanoma. Surg Clin North Am 2020; 100(1): 1-12.
[http://dx.doi.org/10.1016/j.suc.2019.09.005] [PMID: 31753105]

[25] D'Orazio J, Jarrett S, Amaro-Ortiz A, Scott T. UV radiation and the skin. Int J Mol Sci 2013; 14(6): 12222-48.
[http://dx.doi.org/10.3390/ijms140612222] [PMID: 23749111]

[26] Xu Y, Fisher GJ. Ultraviolet (UV) light irradiation induced signal transduction in skin photoaging. J Dermatol Science Suppl 2005; 1(2): S1-8.
[http://dx.doi.org/10.1016/j.descs.2005.06.002]

[27] Rittié L, Fisher GJ. UV-light-induced signal cascades and skin aging. Ageing Res Rev 2002; 1(4): 705-20.
[http://dx.doi.org/10.1016/S1568-1637(02)00024-7] [PMID: 12208239]

[28] Rosenthal M, Goldberg D, Aiello A, Larson E, Foxman B. Skin microbiota: Microbial community structure and its potential association with health and disease. Infect Genet Evol 2011; 11(5): 839-48.
[http://dx.doi.org/10.1016/j.meegid.2011.03.022] [PMID: 21463709]

[29] Bouslimani A, Porto C, Rath CM, *et al.* Molecular cartography of the human skin surface in 3D. Proc Natl Acad Sci USA 2015; 112(17): E2120-9.
[http://dx.doi.org/10.1073/pnas.1424409112] [PMID: 25825778]

[30] Pereira SG, Moura J, Carvalho E, Empadinhas N. Microbiota of chronic diabetic wounds: ecology, impact, and potential for innovative treatment strategies. Front Microbiol 2017; 8: 1791.
[http://dx.doi.org/10.3389/fmicb.2017.01791] [PMID: 28983285]

[31] Oh J, Freeman AF, Park M, *et al.* The altered landscape of the human skin microbiome in patients with primary immunodeficiencies. Genome Res 2013; 23(12): 2103-14.
[http://dx.doi.org/10.1101/gr.159467.113] [PMID: 24170601]

[32] Oh J, Byrd AL, Park M, Kong HH, Segre JA, Program NCS. Temporal stability of the human skin microbiome. Cell 2016; 165(4): 854-66.
[http://dx.doi.org/10.1016/j.cell.2016.04.008] [PMID: 27153496]

[33] Schommer NN, Gallo RL. Structure and function of the human skin microbiome. Trends Microbiol 2013; 21(12): 660-8.
[http://dx.doi.org/10.1016/j.tim.2013.10.001] [PMID: 24238601]

[34] Clemente JC, Pehrsson EC, Blaser MJ, *et al.* The microbiome of uncontacted Amerindians. Sci Adv 2015; 1(3): e1500183.

[http://dx.doi.org/10.1126/sciadv.1500183] [PMID: 26229982]

[35]   Leung MHY, Tong X, Wilkins D, Cheung HHL, Lee PKH. Individual and household attributes influence the dynamics of the personal skin microbiota and its association network. Microbiome 2018; 6(1): 26.
[http://dx.doi.org/10.1186/s40168-018-0412-9] [PMID: 29394957]

[36]   Peguet-Navarro J, Dezutter-Dambuyant C, Buetler T, *et al.* Supplementation with oral probiotic bacteria protects human cutaneous immune homeostasis after UV exposure-double blind, randomized, placebo controlled clinical trial. Eur J Dermatol 2008; 18(5): 504-11.
[PMID: 18693151]

[37]   Bouilly-Gauthier D, Jeannes C, Maubert Y, *et al.* Clinical evidence of benefits of a dietary supplement containing probiotic and carotenoids on ultraviolet-induced skin damage. Br J Dermatol 2010; 163(3): 536-43.
[http://dx.doi.org/10.1111/j.1365-2133.2010.09888.x] [PMID: 20545689]

[38]   Cinque B, La Torre C, Melchiorre E, Marchesani G, Zoccali G, Palumbo P, *et al.* Use of probiotics for dermal applications. Probiotics 2011; pp. 221-41.

[39]   Vergara D, Simeone P, Damato M, Maffia M, Lanuti P, Trerotola M. The cancer microbiota: EMT and inflammation as shared molecular mechanisms associated with plasticity and progression. JOncol 2019 2019.

[40]   Yu Y, Champer J, Beynet D, Kim J, Friedman AJ. The role of the cutaneous microbiome in skin cancer: lessons learned from the gut. J Drugs Dermatol 2015; 14(5): 461-5.
[PMID: 25942663]

[41]   Russo E, Taddei A, Ringressi MN, Ricci F, Amedei A. The interplay between the microbiome and the adaptive immune response in cancer development. Therap Adv Gastroenterol 2016; 9(4): 594-605.
[http://dx.doi.org/10.1177/1756283X16635082] [PMID: 27366226]

[42]   Zhao J, Chen X, Herjan T, Li X. The role of interleukin-17 in tumor development and progression. J Exp Med 2020; 217(1): e20190297.
[http://dx.doi.org/10.1084/jem.20190297] [PMID: 31727782]

[43]   Sherwani MA, Tufail S, Muzaffar AF, Yusuf N. The skin microbiome and immune system: Potential target for chemoprevention? Photodermatol Photoimmunol Photomed 2018; 34(1): 25-34.
[http://dx.doi.org/10.1111/phpp.12334] [PMID: 28766918]

[44]   Chen X, Cai G, Liu C, *et al.* IL-17R–EGFR axis links wound healing to tumorigenesis in Lrig1[+] stem cells. J Exp Med 2019; 216(1): 195-214.
[http://dx.doi.org/10.1084/jem.20171849] [PMID: 30578323]

[45]   Wu L, Chen X, Zhao J, *et al.* A novel IL-17 signaling pathway controlling keratinocyte proliferation and tumorigenesis *via* the TRAF4–ERK5 axis. J Exp Med 2015; 212(10): 1571-87.
[http://dx.doi.org/10.1084/jem.20150204] [PMID: 26347473]

[46]   Wood DLA, Lachner N, Tan JM, *et al.* A natural history of actinic keratosis and cutaneous squamous cell carcinoma microbiomes. MBio 2018; 9(5): e01432-18.
[http://dx.doi.org/10.1128/mBio.01432-18] [PMID: 30301852]

[47]   Wu S, Rhee KJ, Albesiano E, *et al.* A human colonic commensal promotes colon tumorigenesis *via* activation of T helper type 17 T cell responses. Nat Med 2009; 15(9): 1016-22.
[http://dx.doi.org/10.1038/nm.2015] [PMID: 19701202]

[48]   Yoshimoto S, Loo TM, Atarashi K, *et al.* Obesity-induced gut microbial metabolite promotes liver cancer through senescence secretome. Nature 2013; 499(7456): 97-101.
[http://dx.doi.org/10.1038/nature12347] [PMID: 23803760]

[49]   Arthur JC, Perez-Chanona E, Mühlbauer M, *et al.* Intestinal inflammation targets cancer-inducing activity of the microbiota. Science 2012; 338(6103): 120-3.
[http://dx.doi.org/10.1126/science.1224820] [PMID: 22903521]

[50]   Human Microbiome Project C. Structure, function and diversity of the healthy human microbiome. Nature 2012; 486(7402): 207-14.
[http://dx.doi.org/10.1038/nature11234] [PMID: 22699609]

[51]   Grice EA, Kong HH, Conlan S, *et al.* Topographical and temporal diversity of the human skin microbiome. Science 2009; 324(5931): 1190-2.
[http://dx.doi.org/10.1126/science.1171700] [PMID: 19478181]

[52]   Christensen GJM, Brüggemann H. Bacterial skin commensals and their role as host guardians. Benef Microbes 2014; 5(2): 201-15.
[http://dx.doi.org/10.3920/BM2012.0062] [PMID: 24322878]

[53]   Costello EK, Lauber CL, Hamady M, Fierer N, Gordon JI, Knight R. Bacterial community variation in human body habitats across space and time. Science 2009; 326(5960): 1694-7.
[http://dx.doi.org/10.1126/science.1177486] [PMID: 19892944]

[54]   Bastos M, Ceotto H, Coelho M, Nascimento J. *Staphylococcal* antimicrobial peptides: relevant properties and potential biotechnological applications. Curr Pharm Biotechnol 2009; 10(1): 38-61.
[http://dx.doi.org/10.2174/138920109787048580] [PMID: 19149589]

[55]   Gribbon EM, Cunliffe WJ, Holland KT. Interaction of *Propionibacterium acnes* with skin lipids *in vitro*. J Gen Microbiol 1993; 139(8): 1745-51.
[http://dx.doi.org/10.1099/00221287-139-8-1745] [PMID: 8409917]

[56]   Mrázek J, Mekadim C, Kučerová P, *et al.* Melanoma-related changes in skin microbiome. Folia Microbiol (Praha) 2019; 64(3): 435-42.
[http://dx.doi.org/10.1007/s12223-018-00670-3] [PMID: 30554379]

[57]   Wen J, Mao X, Cheng Q, Liu Z, Liu F. A pan-cancer analysis revealing the role of TIGIT in tumor microenvironment. Sci Rep 2021; 11(1): 22502.
[http://dx.doi.org/10.1038/s41598-021-01933-9] [PMID: 34795387]

[58]   Nakatsuji T, Chen TH, Butcher AM, *et al.* A commensal strain of *Staphylococcus epidermidis* protects against skin neoplasia. Sci Adv 2018; 4(2): eaao4502.
[http://dx.doi.org/10.1126/sciadv.aao4502] [PMID: 29507878]

[59]   Wang Z, Choi JE, Wu CC, Di Nardo A. Skin commensal bacteria *Staphylococcus epidermidis* promote survival of melanocytes bearing UVB-induced DNA damage, while bacteria *Propionibacterium acnes* inhibit survival of melanocytes by increasing apoptosis. Photodermatol Photoimmunol Photomed 2018; 34(6): 405-14.
[http://dx.doi.org/10.1111/phpp.12411] [PMID: 29974533]

[60]   Tang Y, Chen Y, Jiang H, Robbins GT, Nie D. G-protein-coupled receptor for short-chain fatty acids suppresses colon cancer. Int J Cancer 2011; 128(4): 847-56.
[http://dx.doi.org/10.1002/ijc.25638] [PMID: 20979106]

[61]   Archer SY, Meng S, Shei A, Hodin RA. p21WAF1 is required for butyrate-mediated growth inhibition of human colon cancer cells. Proc Natl Acad Sci USA 1998; 95(12): 6791-6.
[http://dx.doi.org/10.1073/pnas.95.12.6791] [PMID: 9618491]

[62]   Salava A, Aho V, Pereira P, *et al.* Skin microbiome in melanomas and melanocytic nevi. Eur J Dermatol 2016; 26(1): 49-55.
[http://dx.doi.org/10.1684/ejd.2015.2696] [PMID: 26680010]

[63]   Madhusudhan N, Pausan MR, Halwachs B, *et al.* Molecular profiling of keratinocyte skin tumors links *Staphylococcus aureus* overabundance and increased human β-defensin-2 expression to growth promotion of squamous cell carcinoma. Cancers (Basel) 2020; 12(3): 541.
[http://dx.doi.org/10.3390/cancers12030541] [PMID: 32111012]

[64]   Andersson T, Ertürk Bergdahl G, Saleh K, *et al.* Common skin bacteria protect their host from oxidative stress through secreted antioxidant RoxP. Sci Rep 2019; 9(1): 3596.
[http://dx.doi.org/10.1038/s41598-019-40471-3] [PMID: 30837648]

[65]   Allhorn M, Arve S, Brüggemann H, Lood R. A novel enzyme with antioxidant capacity produced by the ubiquitous skin colonizer *Propionibacterium acnes*. Sci Rep 2016; 6(1): 36412.
[http://dx.doi.org/10.1038/srep36412] [PMID: 27805044]

[66]   Matson V, Fessler J, Bao R, *et al.* The commensal microbiome is associated with anti–PD-1 efficacy in metastatic melanoma patients. Science 2018; 359(6371): 104-8.
[http://dx.doi.org/10.1126/science.aao3290] [PMID: 29302014]

[67]   Frosali S, Pagliari D, Gambassi G, Landolfi R, Pandolfi F, Cianci R. How the Intricate Interaction among Toll-Like Receptors, Microbiota, and Intestinal Immunity Can Influence Gastrointestinal Pathology. J Immunol Res 2015; 2015: 1-12.
[http://dx.doi.org/10.1155/2015/489821] [PMID: 26090491]

[68]   Chen J, Domingue JC, Sears CL. Microbiota dysbiosis in select human cancers: Evidence of association and causality. Semin Immunol 2017; 32: 25-34.
[http://dx.doi.org/10.1016/j.smim.2017.08.001] [PMID: 28822617]

[69]   Wu J, Guo Y, Liu W. *Helicobacter pylori* infection and pancreatic cancer risk: A meta-analysis. J Cancer Res Ther 2016; 12(8) (Suppl.): 229.
[http://dx.doi.org/10.4103/0973-1482.200744] [PMID: 28230023]

[70]   Pichon M, Burucoa C. Impact of the Gastro-Intestinal Bacterial Microbiome on *Helicobacter*-Associated Diseases. Healthcare (Basel) 2019; 7(1): 34.
[http://dx.doi.org/10.3390/healthcare7010034] [PMID: 30813360]

[71]   Salminen S, Collado MC, Endo A, Hill C, Lebeer S, Quigley EMM, *et al.* The International Scientific Association of Probiotics and Prebiotics (ISAPP) consensus statement on the definition and scope of postbiotics. Nat Rev Gastroenterol Hepatol 2021; 1-19.

[72]   Sanders ME, Akkermans LMA, Haller D, *et al.* Safety assessment of probiotics for human use. Gut Microbes 2010; 1(3): 164-85.
[http://dx.doi.org/10.4161/gmic.1.3.12127] [PMID: 21327023]

[73]   Butel MJ. Probiotics, gut microbiota and health. Med Mal Infect 2014; 44(1): 1-8.
[http://dx.doi.org/10.1016/j.medmal.2013.10.002] [PMID: 24290962]

[74]   Tripathi MK, Giri SK. Probiotic functional foods: Survival of probiotics during processing and storage. J Funct Foods 2014; 9: 225-41.
[http://dx.doi.org/10.1016/j.jff.2014.04.030]

[75]   Cogen AL, Nizet V, Gallo RL. Skin microbiota: a source of disease or defence? Br J Dermatol 2008; 158(3): 442-55.
[http://dx.doi.org/10.1111/j.1365-2133.2008.08437.x] [PMID: 18275522]

[76]   Ouwehand AC, Båtsman A, Salminen S. Probiotics for the skin: a new area of potential application? Lett Appl Microbiol 2003; 36(5): 327-31.
[http://dx.doi.org/10.1046/j.1472-765X.2003.01319.x] [PMID: 12680947]

[77]   Euvrard S, Kanitakis J, Claudy A. Skin cancers after organ transplantation. N Engl J Med 2003; 348(17): 1681-91.
[http://dx.doi.org/10.1056/NEJMra022137] [PMID: 12711744]

[78]   Woods GM, Malley RC, Muller HK. The skin immune system and the challenge of tumour immunosurveillance. Eur J Dermatol 2005; 15(2): 63-9.
[PMID: 15757812]

[79]   Leyden JJ, McGinley KJ, Nordstrom KM, Webster GF. Skin Microflora. J Invest Dermatol 1987; 88(s3) (Suppl.): 65s-72s.
[http://dx.doi.org/10.1111/1523-1747.ep12468965] [PMID: 3102625]

[80]   Krutmann J. Pre- and probiotics for human skin. J Dermatol Sci 2009; 54(1): 1-5.
[http://dx.doi.org/10.1016/j.jdermsci.2009.01.002] [PMID: 19203862]

[81]   Grice EA, Kong HH, Renaud G, *et al*. A diversity profile of the human skin microbiota. Genome Res 2008; 18(7): 1043-50.
[http://dx.doi.org/10.1101/gr.075549.107] [PMID: 18502944]

[82]   Metze D, Kersten A, Jurecka W, Gebhart W. Immunoglobulins coat microorganisms of skin surface: a comparative immunohistochemical and ultrastructural study of cutaneous and oral microbial symbionts. J Invest Dermatol 1991; 96(4): 439-45.
[http://dx.doi.org/10.1111/1523-1747.ep12469908] [PMID: 2007782]

[83]   Feingold KR. Thematic review series: Skin Lipids. The role of epidermal lipids in cutaneous permeability barrier homeostasis. J Lipid Res 2007; 48(12): 2531-46.
[http://dx.doi.org/10.1194/jlr.R700013-JLR200] [PMID: 17872588]

[84]   Farmer S. Topical compositions containing probiotic *bacillus* bacteria, spores, and extracellular products and uses thereof. Google Patents 2005.

[85]   Chiba K. Development of cosmetic ingredients using lactic acid bacteria Cosmet stage 2007; 1: 35-42.

[86]   Chuah LO, Foo HL, Loh TC, *et al*. Postbiotic metabolites produced by *Lactobacillus plantarum* strains exert selective cytotoxicity effects on cancer cells. BMC Complement Altern Med 2019; 19(1): 114.
[http://dx.doi.org/10.1186/s12906-019-2528-2] [PMID: 31159791]

[87]   Lamichhane P, Maiolini M, Alnafoosi O, *et al*. Colorectal Cancer and Probiotics: Are Bugs Really Drugs? Cancers (Basel) 2020; 12(5): 1162.
[http://dx.doi.org/10.3390/cancers12051162] [PMID: 32380712]

[88]   Angelin J, Kavitha M. Exopolysaccharides from probiotic bacteria and their health potential. Int J Biol Macromol 2020; 162: 853-65.
[http://dx.doi.org/10.1016/j.ijbiomac.2020.06.190] [PMID: 32585269]

[89]   Nataraj BH, Ali SA, Behare PV, Yadav H. Postbiotics-parabiotics: the new horizons in microbial biotherapy and functional foods. Microb Cell Fact 2020; 19(1): 168.
[http://dx.doi.org/10.1186/s12934-020-01426-w] [PMID: 32819443]

[90]   Jiang B, Tian L, Huang X, *et al*. Characterization and antitumor activity of novel exopolysaccharide APS of *Lactobacillus plantarum* WLPL09 from human breast milk. Int J Biol Macromol 2020; 163: 985-95.
[http://dx.doi.org/10.1016/j.ijbiomac.2020.06.277] [PMID: 32629060]

[91]   Zhou Y, Cui Y, Qu X. Exopolysaccharides of lactic acid bacteria: Structure, bioactivity and associations: A review. Carbohydr Polym 2019; 207: 317-32.
[http://dx.doi.org/10.1016/j.carbpol.2018.11.093] [PMID: 30600013]

[92]   Legesse Bedada T, Feto TK, Awoke KS, Garedew AD, Yifat FT, Birri DJ. Probiotics for cancer alternative prevention and treatment. Biomed Pharmacother 2020; 129: 110409.
[http://dx.doi.org/10.1016/j.biopha.2020.110409] [PMID: 32563987]

[93]   Sivamaruthi BS, Kesika P, Chaiyasut C. The role of probiotics in colorectal cancer management. Evid Based Complementary Altern Med 2020.
[http://dx.doi.org/10.1155/2020/3535982]

[94]   Ren Q, Yang B, Zhu G, *et al*. Antiproliferation Activity and Mechanism of c9, t11, c15-CLNA and t9, t11, c15-CLNA from *Lactobacillus plantarum* ZS2058 on Colon Cancer Cells. Molecules 2020; 25(5): 1225.
[http://dx.doi.org/10.3390/molecules25051225] [PMID: 32182796]

[95]   Mokoena MP. Lactic acid bacteria and their bacteriocins: classification, biosynthesis and applications against uropathogens: a mini-review. Molecules 2017; 22(8): 1255.
[http://dx.doi.org/10.3390/molecules22081255] [PMID: 28933759]

[96]   Kaur S, Kaur S. Bacteriocins as potential anticancer agents. Front Pharmacol 2015; 6: 272.
[http://dx.doi.org/10.3389/fphar.2015.00272] [PMID: 26617524]

[97]   Juretić D, Golemac A, Strand DE, *et al.* The Spectrum of Design Solutions for Improving the Activity-Selectivity Product of Peptide Antibiotics against Multidrug-Resistant Bacteria and Prostate Cancer PC-3 Cells. Molecules 2020; 25(15): 3526.
[http://dx.doi.org/10.3390/molecules25153526] [PMID: 32752241]

[98]   Fichera GA, Fichera M, Milone G. Antitumoural activity of a cytotoxic peptide of *Lactobacillus casei* peptidoglycan and its interaction with mitochondrial-bound hexokinase. Anticancer Drugs 2016; 27(7): 609-19.
[http://dx.doi.org/10.1097/CAD.0000000000000367] [PMID: 27101258]

[99]   Minj J, Chandra P, Paul C, Sharma RK. Bio-functional properties of probiotic *Lactobacillus*: current applications and research perspectives. Crit Rev Food Sci Nutr 2020; 1-18.
[PMID: 32519883]

[100]   Prado Acosta M, Goyette-Desjardins G, Scheffel J, Dudeck A, Ruland J, Lepenies B. S-Layer From *Lactobacillus brevis* Modulates Antigen-Presenting Cell Functions *via* the Mincle-Syk-Card9 Axis. Front Immunol 2021; 12: 602067.
[http://dx.doi.org/10.3389/fimmu.2021.602067] [PMID: 33732234]

[101]   Weill FS, Cela EM, Paz ML, Ferrari A, Leoni J, Maglio DHG. Lipoteichoic acid from *Lactobacillus rhamnosus GG* as an oral photoprotective agent against UV-induced carcinogenesis. Br J Nutr 2013; 109(3): 457-66.
[http://dx.doi.org/10.1017/S0007114512001225] [PMID: 22874095]

[102]   Yazdi MH, Soltan Dallal MM, Hassan ZM, *et al.* Oral administration of *Lactobacillus acidophilus* induces IL-12 production in spleen cell culture of BALB/c mice bearing transplanted breast tumour. Br J Nutr 2010; 104(2): 227-32.
[http://dx.doi.org/10.1017/S0007114510000516] [PMID: 20193099]

[103]   Shen Q, Zhang B, Xu R, Wang Y, Ding X, Li P. Antioxidant activity *in vitro* of the selenium-contained protein from the Se-enriched *Bifidobacterium* animalis 01. Anaerobe 2010; 16(4): 380-6.
[http://dx.doi.org/10.1016/j.anaerobe.2010.06.006] [PMID: 20601030]

[104]   Kodali VP, Sen R. Antioxidant and free radical scavenging activities of an exopolysaccharide from a probiotic bacterium. Biotechnol J 2008; 3(2): 245-51.
[http://dx.doi.org/10.1002/biot.200700208] [PMID: 18246578]

[105]   Riccia DND, Bizzini F, Perilli MG, *et al.* Anti-inflammatory effects of *Lactobacillus brevis* (CD2) on periodontal disease. Oral Dis 2007; 13(4): 376-85.
[http://dx.doi.org/10.1111/j.1601-0825.2006.01291.x] [PMID: 17577323]

[106]   Guéniche A, Bastien P, Ovigne JM, *et al. Bifidobacterium* longum lysate, a new ingredient for reactive skin. Exp Dermatol 2010; 19(8): e1-8.
[http://dx.doi.org/10.1111/j.1600-0625.2009.00932.x] [PMID: 19624730]

[107]   Tian Y, Li M, Song W, Jiang R, Li Y. Effects of probiotics on chemotherapy in patients with lung cancer. Oncol Lett 2019; 17(3): 2836-48.
[http://dx.doi.org/10.3892/ol.2019.9906] [PMID: 30854059]

[108]   Preet S, Bharati S, Panjeta A, Tewari R, Rishi P. Effect of nisin and doxorubicin on DMBA-induced skin carcinogenesis—a possible adjunct therapy. Tumour Biol 2015; 36(11): 8301-8.
[http://dx.doi.org/10.1007/s13277-015-3571-3] [PMID: 26002579]

[109]   Norouzi Z, Salimi A, Halabian R, Fahimi H. Nisin, a potent bacteriocin and anti-bacterial peptide, attenuates expression of metastatic genes in colorectal cancer cell lines. Microb Pathog 2018; 123: 183-9.
[http://dx.doi.org/10.1016/j.micpath.2018.07.006] [PMID: 30017942]

[110]   Lu X. Impact of IL-12 in Cancer. Curr Cancer Drug Targets 2017; 17(8): 682-97.
[PMID: 28460617]

[111]   Moein M, Imani Fooladi AA, Mahmoodzadeh Hosseini H. Determining the effects of green chemistry

synthesized Ag-nisin nanoparticle on macrophage cells. Microb Pathog 2018; 114: 414-9.
[http://dx.doi.org/10.1016/j.micpath.2017.12.034] [PMID: 29241764]

[112]   Małaczewska J, Kaczorek-Łukowska E, Wójcik R, Rękawek W, Siwicki AK. *In vitro* immunomodulatory effect of nisin on porcine leucocytes. J Anim Physiol Anim Nutr (Berl) 2019; 103(3): 882-93.
[http://dx.doi.org/10.1111/jpn.13085] [PMID: 30916834]

[113]   Preet S, Pandey SK, Kaur K, Chauhan S, Saini A. Gold nanoparticles assisted co-delivery of nisin and doxorubicin against murine skin cancer. J Drug Deliv Sci Technol 2019; 53: 101147.
[http://dx.doi.org/10.1016/j.jddst.2019.101147]

[114]   Mouritzen MV, Andrea A, Qvist K, Poulsen SS, Jenssen H. Immunomodulatory potential of Nisin A with application in wound healing. Wound Repair Regen 2019; 27(6): 650-60.
[http://dx.doi.org/10.1111/wrr.12743] [PMID: 31287619]

[115]   Heeney DD, Zhai Z, Bendiks Z, *et al. Lactobacillus plantarum* bacteriocin is associated with intestinal and systemic improvements in diet-induced obese mice and maintains epithelial barrier integrity *in vitro*. Gut Microbes 2019; 10(3): 382-97.
[http://dx.doi.org/10.1080/19490976.2018.1534513] [PMID: 30409105]

[116]   Mahdi LH, Jabbar HS, Auda IG. Antibacterial immunomodulatory and antibiofilm triple effect of Salivaricin LHM against *Pseudomonas aeruginosa* urinary tract infection model. Int J Biol Macromol 2019; 134: 1132-44.
[http://dx.doi.org/10.1016/j.ijbiomac.2019.05.181] [PMID: 31136751]

[117]   Hong N, Ku S, Yuk K, Johnston TV, Ji GE, Park MS. Production of biologically active human interleukin-10 by *Bifidobacterium bifidum* BGN4. Microb Cell Fact 2021; 20(1): 16.
[http://dx.doi.org/10.1186/s12934-020-01505-y] [PMID: 33468130]

[118]   Oft M. IL-10: master switch from tumor-promoting inflammation to antitumor immunity. Cancer Immunol Res 2014; 2(3): 194-9.
[http://dx.doi.org/10.1158/2326-6066.CIR-13-0214] [PMID: 24778315]

[119]   Hou JW, Yu RC, Chou CC. Changes in some components of soymilk during fermentation with *bifidobacteria*. Food Res Int 2000; 33(5): 393-7.
[http://dx.doi.org/10.1016/S0963-9969(00)00061-2]

[120]   Gueniche A. Use of probiotic microorganisms to limit skin irritation. Google Patents 2013.

[121]   Lin MY, Chang FJ. Antioxidative effect of intestinal bacteria *Bifidobacterium longum* ATCC 15708 and *Lactobacillus acidophilus* ATCC 4356. Dig Dis Sci 2000; 45(8): 1617-22.
[http://dx.doi.org/10.1023/A:1005577330695] [PMID: 11007114]

[122]   Gueniche A, Benyacoub J, Breton L, Bureau-Franz I, Blum S, Leclaire J, Eds. 2007.

[123]   Peran L, Camuesco D, Comalada M, *et al. Lactobacillus fermentum*, a probiotic capable to release glutathione, prevents colonic inflammation in the TNBS model of rat colitis. Int J Colorectal Dis 2006; 21(8): 737-46.
[http://dx.doi.org/10.1007/s00384-005-0773-y] [PMID: 16052308]

[124]   De Simone C. Use of bacteria endowed with arginine deiminase to induce apoptosis and/or reduce an inflammatory reaction and pharmaceutical or dietetic compositions containing such bacteria. Google Patents 2003.

[125]   Puch F, Samson-Villeger S, Guyonnet D, Blachon JL, Rawlings AV, Lassel T. Consumption of functional fermented milk containing borage oil, green tea and vitamin E enhances skin barrier function. Exp Dermatol 2008; 17(8): 668-74.
[http://dx.doi.org/10.1111/j.1600-0625.2007.00688.x] [PMID: 18318715]

[126]   Baba H, Masuyama A, Takano T. Short communication: Effects of *Lactobacillus helveticus*-fermented milk on the differentiation of cultured normal human epidermal keratinocytes. J Dairy Sci 2006; 89(6): 2072-5.

[http://dx.doi.org/10.3168/jds.S0022-0302(06)72275-5] [PMID: 16702271]

[127] Gueniche A, Benyacoub J, Blum S, Breton L, Castiel I. Probiotics for skin benefits Nutritional Cosmetics. Elsevier 2009; pp. 421-39.
[http://dx.doi.org/10.1016/B978-0-8155-2029-0.50029-6]

[128] Guéniche A, Benyacoub J, Buetler TM, Smola H, Blum S. Supplementation with oral probiotic bacteria maintains cutaneous immune homeostasis after UV exposure. Eur J Dermatol 2006; 16(5): 511-7.
[PMID: 17101471]

CHAPTER 4

Probiotics-based Anticancer Immunity In Colon Cancer

Sujitra Techo¹, Engkarat Kingkaew² and Somboon Tanasupawat²,*

¹ *Mahidol University, Nakhonsawan Campus, Nakhonsawan, Thailand*

² *Department of Biochemistry and Microbiology, Faculty of Pharmaceutical Sciences, Chulalongkorn University, Bangkok, Thailand*

Abstract: Probiotics are live microorganisms, which confer a health benefit to the host after administering them in adequate amounts. Health benefits of probiotics include antimicrobial activity and gastrointestinal infections, effectiveness against diarrhoea and *Helicobacter pylori* infection, improvement in lactose metabolism, reduction in serum cholesterol, inflammatory bowel disease, immune system stimulation, anti-mutagenic properties, and anti-carcinogenic properties. Since probiotics exhibit a positive health impact, many researchers pay attention to the role of probiotics in the enhancement of the immunological response of the host and also in colon cancer prevention and treatment. Probiotic strains, either live or dead cells, belong to the genera *Lactobacillus* and *Bifidobacterium,* which are typically evaluated for their immunomodulatory effect on the immune system. These strains can improve the immunological response both *in vitro* and *in vivo*. Many mechanisms of probiotics in the prevention and treatment of colon cancer have been proposed. Several studies demonstrate that probiotics and synbiotics exert an anti-carcinogenic effect on colon cancer cells *(in vitro)* as well as in clinical trials *(in vivo)*. These studies illustrate that probiotics and synbiotics are applied as adjunctive or alternative therapeutic agents for colon cancer management.

Keywords: Colon cancer, Immunomodulatory effect, Lactic acid bacteria, *Lactobacillus*, *Bifidobacterium*, Probiotics, Preventive effect.

1. INTRODUCTION

One hundred trillion microorganisms residing in the gastrointestinal tract (GIT), which are known as gut microbiota, provide essential health benefits to their host, especially by regulating immune homeostasis [1]. Non-specific and specific immune system components' development is stimulated by the GIT microbiota

---
* **Corresponding author Somboon Tanasupawat:** Department of Biochemistry and Microbiology, Faculty of Pharmaceutical Sciences, Chulalongkorn University, Bangkok, Thailand; E-mail: somboon.T@chula.ac.th

Mitesh Kumar Dwivedi, Alwarappan Sankaranarayanan & Sanjay Tiwari (Eds.)

just after birth and during the entire life and it functions as an anti-infectious barrier by suppressing the adherence of pathogenic microorganisms and subsequent cellular substratum colonization and by the production of bacteriocins and other toxic metabolites [2]. Gut microbiota dysbiosis has been associated with many disorders, including inflammatory bowel disease (IBD), obesity, asthma, psychiatric illnesses, and cancers [3]. Probiotics are defined as live microorganisms, which, when administered in adequate amounts, confer a health benefit to the host [4]. Health benefits of probiotics include antimicrobial activity and gastrointestinal infections, effectiveness against diarrhoea, improvement in lactose metabolism, reduction in serum cholesterol, immune system stimulation, anti-mutagenic properties and anti-carcinogenic properties. *Helicobacter pylori* bacterium has been recognized as an important cause of chronic gastritis and peptic ulcer and is a risk factor for gastric carcinoma [5]. Therefore, many investigations have focused on probiotics that exert the anti-*H. pylori* activity. *Lb. fermentum* P43-01 produced bacteriocin-like compounds which showed a broad spectrum of antimicrobial activities against *H. pylori* strains isolated from patients [6]. Due to the several advantages of probiotics to host's health, researchers have paid attention to them. Many researchers report about the immunomodulatory activity of probiotics on the immune system. These useful microorganisms in both live and inactivated forms can enhance the immune responses in colon cancer cells [16 - 22]. In addition, the application of probiotics or synbiotics in mice models resulted in the improvement of anti-inflammatory activity and reduction of proinflammatory cytokines levels [20, 23 - 28]. Numerous research works showed that probiotics and synbiotics exert preventive effects against cancer carcinogenesis in *in vitro* and *in vivo* models [17, 28, 30 - 41]. Moreover, several clinical studies have illustrated that probiotics or synbiotics can be used as alternative or adjunctive therapeutic substances in patients with colon cancer [42 - 49]. This chapter summarizes the updated knowledge of the effect of probiotics on the modulation of immune responses in both *in vitro* and *in vivo* models. The mechanisms of probiotics related to the prevention and treatment of colon cancer are also described. Furthermore, the scientific evidences associated with the preventive and treatment effects of probiotics/synbiotics in cell lines, animal models and clinical trials are also reviewed.

2. PROBIOTICS AND THEIR SELECTION

A United Nations and World Health Organization Expert Panel defines the term "probiotics" as *live microorganisms, which, when administered in adequate amounts, confer a health benefit to the host* [4]. Microorganisms typically used as probiotics belong to the heterogeneous genera of lactic acid bacteria (LAB) [*Lactobacillus (Lb.)*, *Enterococcus (E.)*, *Streptococcus (S.)*, *Lactococcus (Lc.)*,

Pediococcus (*P.*), and *Leuconostoc* (*Ln.*), and *Bifidobacterium* (*B.*)]. Moreover, some strains of *Bacillus, Escherichia* and yeast are also included as probiotic microorganisms (Table **1**) [7 - 9].

Table. (1). List of microorganisms used as probiotics [8, 9].

Lactobacillus (Lb.)	Bifidobacterium (B.)	Other LAB	Other microorganisms
Lb. fermentum	*B. longum*	*S. thermophilus*	*Bacillus subtilis*
Lb. reuteri	*B. bifidum*	*S. diacetylactis*	*Bacillus clausii*
Lb. mesenteroides	*B. animali*	*S. intermedius*	*Escherichia coli* strain Nissle
Lb. plantarum	*B. adolescentis*	*P. acidilactici*	*Saccharomyces cerevisiae*
Lb. rhamnosus	*B. breve*	*E. faecium*	*Saccharomyces bourlardii*
Lb. casei	*B. infantis*	*Lc. lactis*	-
Lb. paracasei	*B. lactis*	*Ln. mesenteroides*	-
Lb. johnsonii	*B. thermophilum*	-	-
Lb. acidophilus	-	-	-
Lb. lactis	-	-	-
Lb. crispatus	-	-	-
Lb. delbrueckii	-	-	-
Lb. farciminis	-	-	-
Lb. gasseri	-	-	-

The selection of probiotic strains is based on safety, functional properties and technological compatibility. Microorganisms that are used as probiotics should meet the terms of GRAS (Generally Recognized as Safe) in the United States and QPS (Qualified Presumption of Safety) status, considering the European Food Safety Authority (EFSA). The safety aspect of probiotic cultures includes the absence of pathogenicity and antibiotic resistance [10]. Probiotic strains must be identified to the strain level by phenotypic and genotypic characterization and then their safety assessment from historical evidence or experimental trial is carried out. LAB are known as GRAS and many *Lactobacillus* and *Bifidobacterium* species are intestinal gut microbiota. However, the safety assessment is still required because some LAB strains are associated with opportunistic infections [11]. Functional or probiotic properties are crucial criteria for which the probiotic strains must be evaluated. Microorganisms which are classified as probiotics must have basic properties such as resistance to gastric juices, exposure to bile, proliferation and colonization at the digestive tract.

Moreover, modulation of the immune response of the host, production of antimicrobial substances, antagonistic activity against pathogenic bacteria, anti-mutagenic, anti-carcinogenic, anti-cholesterol, anti-depressant, anti-anxiety, anti-obesity, anti-diabetic properties and secretion of functional molecules, are the desirable features that have a positive effect on human health. For technological aspect, probiotic cultures are developed as medical or pharmaceutical products for human use; therefore, the cultures must survive and maintain their properties during processing, storage and also throughout the distribution of the products [9]. Selection of probiotic microorganisms require *in vitro* tests followed by studies in the animal models. After desirable results are obtained, the human studies by clinical studies (phase 1), individual patient studies (phase 2) and finally large-scale human studies (phase 3) are carried out [12].

3. COLON CANCER

Colon cancer is the second leading cause of cancer-associated fatality around the world [13]. More than 1 million people annually are diagnosed with colon cancer, and it is responsible for the death of more than 500,000 persons. World Health Organization (WHO) reported that there will be 17 million people deaths, 27 million new cases of cancer, and 75 million people living with the disease by the year 2030 [14]. According to molecular genetics, colon cancer is the most understood complex cancer. Colon carcinogenesis starts from the occurrence of specific types of neoplastic polyps in colonic mucosa and then develops into carcinomas, as illustrated by epidemiologic, clinical, pathologic, and molecular genetic findings [15]. The dietary pattern of people has been changed and includes high-fat and low-fiber diets. Factors such as aging, genomic instability, obesity, diabetes, atherosclerosis and gut microbiota are linked with an increased risk of colon cancer [14].

4. IMMUNOMODULATORY EFFECT OF PROBIOTICS

Many strains of probiotics have shown their immunomodulatory effect on the immune system. The action of probiotics on the intestinal mucosal immune response is well established in either *in vitro* and *in vivo* models, as shown in Tables **2** and **3**. Most strains used in the experiment are the members of *Lactobacillus* and *Bifidobacterium* in both live and dead cells. Furthermore, synbiotics (probiotics mixed with prebiotics) are also used to evaluate their immunomodulatory effects, especially in *in vivo* studies.

Probiotic microorganisms can modulate an intestinal mucosal immune response. The level of interleukin-8 (IL-8, a pro-inflammatory cytokine) in the HT-29 model was reduced when pre-incubated with *B. longum* and *Lb. bulgaricus* LB10. Nuclear factor-κB (NF-κB, p65) in the epithelia was secreted by Tumor necrosis factor-α (TNF-α) stimulation. Decreased expression of NF-κB p65 occurred in cells treated with *B. longum* and *Lb. bulgaricus* LB10 [16]. *B. adolescentis* SPM0212, in a dose-dependent manner, inhibited TNF-α production, which may be beneficial in human intestinal tracts for immune reinforcement [17]. Pathogenic ligands and flagellin could stimulate IL-8 production in intestinal epithelial cells. Pretreatment of Caco-2 cell line with either live *Lb. rhamnosus* GG (LGG) or UV-inactivated LGG resulted in 66 and 59% reduction of IL-8 level, compared with the flagellin group. Moreover, both live and UV-inactivated LGG could prevent flagellin-induced NF-κB nuclear translocation. Inhibitor of κB (IκB) was also increased by both live and UV-inactivated LGG. Moreover, ubiquitinated-IκB (Ub-IκB) expression was reduced by only UV-inactivated LGG. The study concluded that UV-inactivated and live (LGG) were efficient to decrease the IL-8 production in the intestinal epithelium and other mechanisms in different pathways, such as changes in cytoplasmic IκB, by which it inhibits the NF-κB nuclear translocation [18]. Human β-defensins (HBD), including HBD-1, HBD-2 and HBD-3 play a role in the defense of epithelial sites. These defensins are expressed either constitutively or upregulated in response to microbial or pro-inflammatory stimuli. HBD-2 mRNA expression and HBD-2 secretion were significantly induced in a dose- [16±1.4 pg/ml and 31.5±2.3 pg/ml at Multiplicity of Infection (MOI) 10 and 50, respectively] and time-dependent manner, when Caco-2 cells were pre-incubated with *Lb. plantarum*. The interleukin-23 (IL-23) secretion (850±5.4 pg/ml) and IL-23 mRNA expression were increased when LPS was added to the cells for 48 h and decreased when LPS was co-cultured with *Lb. plantarum* (330±4.2 pg/ml) [19]. The probiotic formulation VSL#3 (*B. infantis*, *Lb. acidophilus*, *S. thermophilus* and *Lb. rhamnosus* GG CGMCC 1.2134) stimulated the epithelial production of TNF-α and activated NF-κB *in vitro* [20]. *Lb. plantarum* Lp62 isolated from cocoa fermentation inhibited IL-8 production by *Salmonella typhi*-stimulated HT-29 cells and prevented the adhesion of pathogens to these epithelial cells. In addition, a strain could modulate TNF-α, IL1-β, and IL-17 secretion by J774 macrophages and also induce increased IL-10 secretion by mononuclear cells [21]. The multi-species probiotics (MSP; *Lb. rhamnosus* RO-11, *Lb. casei* RO-215, *Lb. plantarum* RO-1012, *Lb. helveticus* RO-52, *B. longum* BB536, *B.breve* RO-70, *P. acidilactici* RO-1001 and *Lc. lactis* RO-1058) modulated the cytokine production by human peripheral blood mononuclear cells (PBMC) and affected the cross-talk between PBMCs and HT-29 cancer cells. The production of TNF-α, IL-1β, IL-6, and IL-10 was increased in not-stimulated PBMCs incubated with MSP. No alteration of IL-6, interferon-γ (IFN-γ), and IL-1Ra levels were observed. The stimulatory effect of MSP on lipopolysaccharide (LPS)-promoted PBMCs was less pronounced for TNF-α, IL-

1β, and IFN-γ, and the IL-6 production was decreased; phorbol 12-myristate 13-acetate (PMA)-induced IL-2 and IFN-γ secretion was also inhibited. The addition of MSP to co-cultures of PBMCs and HT-29 cancer cells led to a remarkable increase in TNF-α and IL-1β secretion, with no change in remaining cytokines [22].

Furthermore, yoghurt consumption had a positive effect on health and on the improvement of the mucosal immune system. BALB/c mice were used to investigate the effect of yoghurt consumption on the immunoregulatory mechanisms involved in the inhibition of tumor growth. Yoghurt containing *Lb. delbrueckii* subsp. *bulgaricus* and *S. thermophilus* increased the number of apoptotic cells and induced the IFN-γ and TNF-α cytokine release, along with their production being regulated by an increase in IL-10. Yoghurt may exert anti-tumor activity by a decrease in the inflammatory immune response mediated by IgA^+ increase, apoptosis induction and IL-10 release [23]. Further, the effect of probiotics (*Lb. rhamnosus* GG & *B. lactis* Bb12; PRO), prebiotics (inulin-based enriched with oligofructose; PRE) and synbiotics (combination of probiotics and prebiotics; SYN) on the immune system of azoxymethane (AOM)-induced rats were investigated. Natural killer (NK) cell-like cytotoxicity was significantly reduced in the AOM treatment of control, PRO and PRE groups. The AOM-induced suppression of NK cell-like cytotoxicity was prevented by SYN supplementation in Peyer's patches (PP) as compared with control rats. SYN and PRE supplementations stimulated the IL-10 production in PP in these rats and in mesenteric lymph nodes (MLNs) of rats not treated with AOM. IFN-γ production in PP was also decreased by PRO supplementation [24].

Furthermore, daily intake of *Lb. casei* strain *Shirota* exerted a positive effect on NK-cells' activity. In the middle-aged volunteers, the consumption of yoghurt containing *Lb. casei* strain *Shirota* resulted in a significantly increased NK cells' activity in 3 weeks after the start of intake, and then the elevated NK cells' activity remained for the next 3 weeks. In the elderly volunteer group, NK cells' activity significantly decreased in the control group, 3 weeks after the start of intake; however, the intake of *Lb. casei* strain *Shirota* maintained the NK cells' activity [25].

Probiotic microorganisms generally display anti-inflammatory effects. The multiple probiotic formulations VSL#3 containing *B. infantis, Lb. acidophilus, S. thermophilus* and *Lb. rhamnosus* GG CGMCC 1.2134 prevented the beginning of intestinal inflammation by local stimulation of epithelial innate immune responses (*i.e.*, increased production of epithelial-derived TNF-α and restoration of epithelial barrier function in SAMP mice) [20]. Rats orally received *Lb. rhamnosus* GG CGMCC 1.2134 (LGG) showed significantly reduced tumor incidence, multiplicity and volume in the group treated by 1,2-dimethylhydrazine (DMH) compared to the DMH cancer control group. Moreover, the LGG-treated group exhibited a reduction in the expression of β-catenin and the inflammatory proteins NFκB-p65, cyclooxygenase-2 (COX-2) and TNF-α, the anti-apoptotic protein Bcl-2, whereas the expression of the pro-apoptotic proteins Bax, casp3 and p53 were increased as compared to the DMH group [26]. *Lb. casei* 393 could promote optimal control of the immune response. Administration of *Lb. casei* 393 two weeks before the DMH treatment diminished the pro-inflammatory effect of DMH, and maintained the levels of the three cytokines (IFN-γ, TNF-α & IL-10) as well as colon histology. Moreover, a probiotic strain showed the preventive effect in DMH-treated mice, which increased IL-17A synthesis and regulatory T cells (Tregs) percentages, further indicating a tumor-protecting role [27]. A probiotic mixture could also inhibit the growth of CT26 tumors and induced an immune response in BALB/c mice model. The research study reported that *B. longum*, *B. bifidum*, *Lb. acidophilus*, *Lb. plantarum*, together with resistant dextrin, isomaltooligosaccharides, fructose oligosaccharides and stachyose, reduced the tumor volume of mice that received the probiotic mixture as compared to the control group. Mice treated with the probiotic mixture displayed more apoptotic cells and infiltration of immune cells compared to the control mice. An increased number of CD8+ T cells in the tumor and spleen tissues were also found in mice treated with the probiotic mixture [28].

Table. (2). Immunomodulatory effects of probiotics explored through *in vitro* studies.

Probiotics	Colony forming unit (CFU)	Cell lines	Results	References
B. longum *Lb. bulgaricus* LB10	1×10^8 CFU/ml 1×10^8 CFU/ml	HT29	IL-8 secretion ↓ NF-κB p65 ↓	[16]
B. adolescentis SPM0212	No data	HT-29SW 480Caco-2	Inhibited TNF-α production	[17]
Live or UV-inactivated *Lb. rhamnosus* GG	10^{11} CFU/L	Caco-2	IL-8, NF-κB, Ub-IκB↓ IκB ↑	[18]
Lb. plantarum	No data	Caco-2	HBD-2 mRNA expression and HBD-2 secretion ↑ IL-23 secretion and IL-23 mRNA expression ↑	[19]
B. infantis *Lb. acidophilus* *S. thermophilus* *Lb. rhamnosus* GG CGMCC 1.2134	50×10^9 CFU/day	Epithelial cells	Stimulated epithelial production of TNF-α and activated NF-κB	[20]

(Table 2) cont.....

Probiotics	Colony forming unit (CFU)	Cell lines	Results	References
Lb. plantarum Lp62	10^9 CFU/ml	HT-29	Inhibited IL-8 production Modulated TNF-α, IL1-β, and IL-17 secretion IL-10 secretion ↑	[21]
Lb. rhamnosus RO-11 *Lb. casei* RO-215 *Lb. plantarum* RO-1012 *Lb. helveticus (acidophilus)* RO-52 *B. longum* BB536 *B. breve* RO-70 *P. acidilactici* RO-1001 *Lc. lactis* RO-1058	No data	HT-29	TNF-α and IL-1β secretion ↑	[22]

Table. (3). Immunomodulatory effects of probiotics explored through *in vivo* studies.

Probiotics/synbiotics	Dose/Colony forming unit (CFU)	Results	References
Lb. delbrueckii subsp. *bulgaricus* *S. thermophilus*	10^8 CFU/ml	Apoptosis, IgA$^+$ and IL-10↑	[23]
Lb. rhamnosus GG *B. lactis* Bb12 PRE (inulin-based enriched with oligofructose)	No data	Suppressed NK cell-like cytotoxicity IFN-γ production ↓	[24]
Lb. casei strain *Shirota*	4×10^{10} live cells/bottle	NK-cell activity in middle-aged volunteers ↑ NK-cell activity in elderly volunteers ↓	[25]
B. infantis *Lb. acidophilus* *S. thermophilus*	50×10^9 CFU/day	Stimulated epithelial production of TNF-α and activated NF-κB	[20]
Lb. rhamnosus GG CGMCC 1.2134	1×10^9 CFU/ml	Tumor incidence, multiplicity and volume ↓ β-catenin, NF-κB p65, COX-2 and TNFα and Bcl-2 ↓ Bax, casp3 and p53 ↑	[26]
Lb. casei 393	1×10^6 CFU/100 μl	IL-17A↑ Treg percentages ↑	[27]

(Table 3) cont.....

Probiotics/synbiotics	Dose/Colony forming unit (CFU)	Results	References
B. longum, B. bifidum, Lb. acidophilus, Lb. plantarum, resistant dextrin, isomaltooligosaccharides, fructose oligosaccharides and stachyose	30×10^9 CFU/g	Tumor volume ↓ Apoptotic cells and infiltration of immune cells ↑ Number of CD8$^+$ T cells ↑	[28]

5. MECHANISMS OF PROBIOTICS IN THE PREVENTION AND/OR TREATMENT OF COLON CANCER

The exact mechanisms by which LAB acts upon colon cancer cells are unknown, but several mechanisms have been proposed including (A) enhancement of the host's responses, (B) suppression of the enzymatic activity of pathogenic bacteria, (C) regulation of proliferation and apoptotic response of colon cancer cells, (D) protecting the intestinal mucosal barrier of host, and (E) inhibition of carcinogenic agents [29]. The putative mechanism of prevention and treatment of colorectal cancer (CRC) by probiotics is shown in Fig. (1).

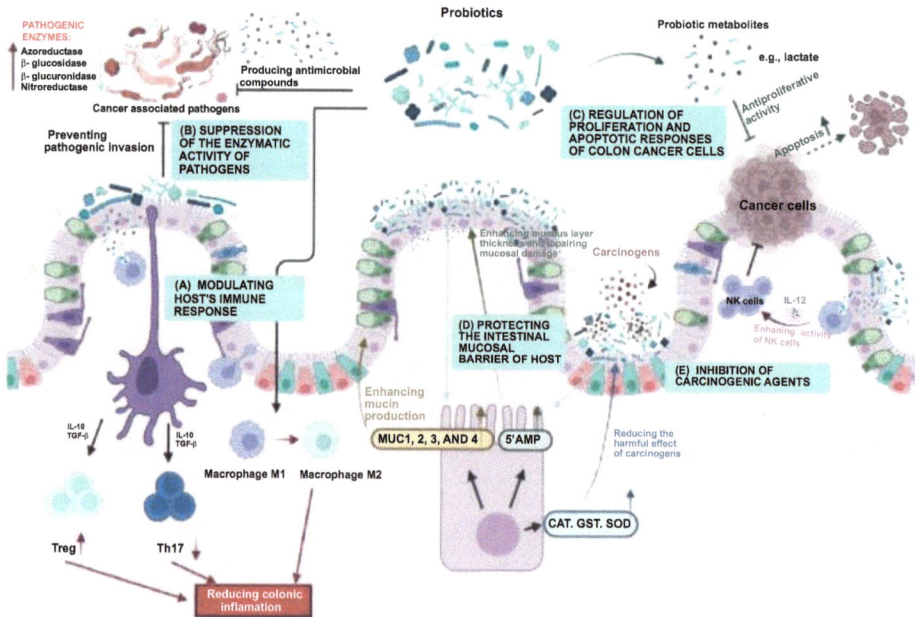

Fig. (1). Putative mechanisms of probiotics in the prevention and treatment of colorectal cancer (CRC). (A) Modulating host's immune response; (B) Suppression of the enzymatic activity of pathogens; (C) Regulation of proliferation and apoptotic responses of colon cancer cells; (D) Protecting the intestinal mucosal barrier of host, and (E) Inhibition of carcinogenic agents.

5.1. Enhancement of The Host's Immune Response

Probiotic modulation affects the host immunity. Chronic and uncontrolled inflammation is key in the pathogenesis and progression of cancer. Probiotics show beneficial immunomodulatory effects to alleviate colonic inflammation [*e.g.*, activating DCs to secrete primary anti-inflammatory cytokines (*e.g.*, IL-10 & TGF-β), reducing Th17 cells, increasing Treg expression and shifting macrophage to M2 subtype] or enhance anti-tumor immunity (*e.g.*, by inducing IL-12 production that enhances the activity of NK cells) [30]. In addition, their metabolites, such as short-chain fatty acids (SCFAs), lead to Treg cells' differentiation (an important role in limiting the inflammatory response of the intestine through the production of IL-10) by inhibition of histone deacetylase (HDAC) resulting in inhibition and reduction of the number of inflammatory cytokines [29]. Besides, butyrate could suppress the COX-2 expression in cancer tissues; consequently, it could prevent the adverse effects of prostaglandins on the mucosal layer [31]. Moreover, the study of Wu H.-J. & Wu E [1]. found that some *Lactobacillus* species can also boost Treg cells' activity, NK cells' activity as well as the antibacterial phagocytic activity of neutrophils in the peripheral blood.

5.2. Suppression of the Enzymatic Activity of Pathogenic Bacteria

An imbalance in the intestinal microbiota causes the release of large numbers of β-glucuronidase, β-glucosidase, azoreductase, and nitroreductase enzymes, as well as the formation of carcinogenic compounds. Toxic metabolites produced by these enzymes include aromatic amines, altered secondary bile salts, hydrogen sulfide, carcinogenic aglycone, acetaldehyde, and free oxygen radicals [29]. Probiotics can suppress these cancer-associated enzymes. Firstly, probiotics inhibit pathogenic bacteria colonization *via* synthesizing antimicrobial compounds, reducing luminal pH, and/or directly interacting with pathogens (*e.g.*, competing for nutrients and location, forming co-aggregates). Secondly, probiotics can enhance the synthesis of antimicrobial peptides such as (LL37) cathelicidin and defensin and promote mucin secretion to prevent pathogenic invasion [30]. Due to this, the pathogens are lowered and pathogenic bacteria's enzymatic activities, including β-glucuronidase, β-glucosidase, azoreductase, and nitroreductase, are also suppressed. *Lb. rhamnosus* GG suppressed the activity of β-glucuronidase. In addition, oral administration of *B. bifidum* and *Lb. acidophilus* for 3 weeks was able to lower the nitroreductase activity [29].

5.3. Regulation of Proliferation and Apoptotic Responses of Colon Cancer Cells

One of the major strategies of tumor cell death in CRC is apoptosis [29]. Probiotic metabolites such as SCFAs (*e.g.*, acetate, lactate, & butyrate) exhibit anti-proliferative activity, which leads to apoptosis in CRC cells [29]. The mechanism of *Lb. rhamnosus* GG in inhibiting the proliferation of HT-29 cell lines, Caco-2 (colorectal cancer cell line), and SW480 (CRC cell line) was also affected by induction of apoptosis and cell cycle arresting [32]. *Lb. fermentum* NCIMB 5221 produced more butyric and acetic acid and revealed the potentially anti-proliferative activity against CRC [33]. Besides, *Lc. lactis* NK34 (10^6 CFU/well) inhibited the proliferation of several CRC cells, including DLD-1, HT-29, and LoVo cell lines [34]. Furthermore, *P. pentosaceus* GS4 synthesized conjugated linoleic acid (CLA), which limited the proliferation of HCT-116 (colon cancer cell line) and induced apoptosis [35]. The cytoplasmic lysate and *Lactobacillus* cell wall increased apoptosis and impeded cell cycle progression in the S phase of HT-29 and LT-97 cell lines [29].

5.4. Protection of Intestinal Mucosal Barrier of Host

When the intestinal mucosa's integrity and barrier function are impaired, allergens become more permeable, and trigger an immunological stress response and inflammation. The inflammatory response begins at a specific location and the mucosa around it. When pathogenic bacteria reach the intestinal epithelium, it damages the epithelial barrier, leading to an increased risk of CRC [36]. Probiotics and their metabolites protect the intestinal tract by blocking HDACs and raising the expression and synthesis of mucins such as MUC1, MUC3, and MUC4. SCFAs help to improve the function and survival of epithelial ducts by activating 5′adenosine monophosphate-activated protein kinase, another vital element in maintaining hypoxia-inducible factor (HIF) through the SCFAs [29]. Some species of *Bifidobacterium* exhibited the ability to enhance epithelial integrity and prevent disruption of the epithelial barrier induced by TNF-α [37]. *Lactobacillus* strains improved the integrity of tight junctions and the intestinal barrier [38]. In a mice inflammatory model, *Lb. rhamnosus* CNCM I-3690 maintained the intestinal barrier functions by inducing the expression of genes associated with healthy gut permeability, regulating goblet cells and the mucus layer, and counteracting changes in the local and systemic lymphocytes [39].

5.5. Inhibition of Carcinogenic Agents

The β-glucuronidase, β-glucosidase, azoreductase, and nitroreductase of pathogens play roles in CRC development and carcinogen production. Probiotics can inhibit carcinogenic agents (heterocyclic aromatic amines [HCA]-and N-nitroses), which are major mutagens that cause carcinogenic mutations in these intestinal cells, through two mechanisms: binding and deactivation. Probiotics also prevent the adverse effect of carcinogens by enhancing the expression of antioxidant enzymes and inactivating carcinogen-deactivating agents such as glutathione-S-transferase (GST), glutathione reductase (GR), glutathione peroxidase (GPx), superoxide dismutase (SOD), and catalase (CAT) [29]. Antioxidants comparable to 100 mg of vitamin C were produced by *P. pentosaceus* 16:1, *Lb. plantarum* 2592, and *Lb. paracasei* F19. Further, to inhibit tumor formation, the antioxidant capability may limit peroxidation and free radicals [40]. Besides, LAB inhibited the activity of carcinogenic compounds such as DMH, N–methyl–N'–nitro-N–nitrosoguanidyne (MNNG), by up taking reactive intermediates, synthesizing compounds that deactivate carcinogens and antioxidant enzymes, for example, SOD, GST, GR, GPx, and CAT [36]. Furthermore, the "drive-passenger" theory, in which DNA damage to epithelial cells and tumor induction, as well as the encouragement of pathogenic bacteria proliferation, offers a suitable environment for tumor growth. *Helicobacter pylori* is one such example of a pathogen and is defined as a cancer-causing agent [29, 41]. The study of Techo *et al.* [6] found that candidate probiotic *Lb. fermentum* P43-01 showed an inhibitory effect on *H. pylori* MS83 and BK364.

6. PROBIOTICS USED FOR COLON CANCER PREVENTION AND/OR TREATMENT

Probiotics and synbiotics express beneficial effects on host's health *via* many mechanisms, as mentioned above. They are employed for colon cancer prevention and treatment. Numerous *in vitro* and *in vivo* researches and clinical trials suggest that probiotics and synbiotics exert an anti-carcinogenic effect on colon cancer cells, as presented in Tables **4**, **5** and **6**.

Table. (4). The use of probiotics/ synbiotics for colon cancer prevention (cell line models).

Probiotics / Synbiotics	Colony forming unit (CFU)	Cell lines	Result	References
B. adolescentis SPM0212	No data	HT-29, SW 480, Caco-2	Inhibited the proliferation of three human colon cancer cell lines	[17]
Lb. acidophilus CL1285 *Lb. casei* LBC80R	10^6 to 10^9 CFU/ml	CRL-2134	Increased apoptosis-induction capacity of 5-FU	[42]
Lb. rhamnosus GG *B. lactis* Bb12 Wheat aleurone	Each 3×10^8 CFU/ml	HT-29, LT-97	Increased apoptosis and up-regulated the genes involved in cell growth and apoptosis (p21 & WNT2B)	[43]

(Table 4) cont.....

Probiotics / Synbiotics	Colony forming unit (CFU)	Cell lines	Result	References
Lb. paracasei IMPC2.1 *Lb. rhamnosus* GG	10^8 CFU/ml	DLD-1	Both viable or heat-killed cells inhibited growth and increased apoptosis of cell lines	[44]
Lc. lactis NK34	10^6 CFU/well	DLD-1, HT-29, LoVo	Strong inhibition of cell proliferation (>77% cytotoxicity)	[34]
Live *Lb. casei* ATCC 393 and its extract	10^9 CFU/ml	CT26, HT-29	Increased significant concentration- and time-dependent anti-proliferative effect	[45]
B. longum, B. bifidum, Lb. acidophilus, Lb. plantarum, resistant dextrin, isomaltooligosaccharides, fructose oligosaccharides and stachyose	30×10^9 CFU/g	CT26	Inhibited the invasion, migration, and proliferation ability	[28]

Table. (5). The use of probiotics /synbiotics for colon cancer prevention (animal models' studies).

Probiotics /Synbiotics	Dose/Colony forming unit	Inductive substance	Result	References
Lb. plantarum, Lc. lactis, Lc. Lactis SOD⁺ and *Lb. plantarum* SOD⁺	10^9 CFU/day	TNBS	Reduced macroscopic, microscopic damage and MPO activity	[46]
Lc. lactis NZ and *Lc. lactis* KAT	No data	DMH	Increased catalase activities and reduced H_2O_2 levels Less extent of colonic damage and inflammation	[47]
Lb. acidophilus KFRI342	2×10^9 CFU/ml, 3 times/week	DMH	Inhibited DMH-induced symptoms in live rats	[48]
Lb. salivarius Ren	Two doses of 5×10^8 and 1×10^{10} CFU/kg body weight for 15 weeks	DMH	Increased SCFAs levels, decreased azoreductase activity, reduced the number of aberrant crypt foci by 40% and suppressed epithelial proliferation.	[49]

(Table 5) cont.....

Probiotics /Synbiotics	Dose/Colony forming unit	Inductive substance	Result	References
Live and dead nano-sized *Lb. plantarum*	Low dose 4×10^9 CFU/kg/day High dose 4×10^{11} CFU/kg/day	DSS and azoxymethane	Reduced inflammatory markers, mediated the expression of cell cycle and apoptotic markers and elevated fecal IgA levels	[50]
Lb.salivarius Ren	5×10^{10} CFU/kg body weight per day	DMH	Decreased cancer incidence (87.5% to 25%) Promoted reversion of the gut microbiota close to the healthy state	[51]
Lb. casei ATCC 393	10^6 CFU, twice a week for 2 weeks	DMH	Reduced the number of DMH-induced aberrant crypt foci, the levels of putrescine, and the expression of ornithine decarboxylase	[52]
B. longum, B. bifidum, Lb. acidophilus, Lb. plantarum, resistant dextrin, isomaltooligosaccharides, fructose oligosaccharides and stachyose	30×10^9 CFU/g	No data	Inhibited the growth of CT26 tumors	[28]

Table. (6). The use of probiotics/synbiotics for preoperative and postoperative surgery in patients (clinical trials).

Probiotics /Synbiotics, Dose	No. of patients (intervention group/control group)	Treatment duration	Result	References
One sachet containing *P. pentosaceus* 5-33:3, *Leu. Mesenteroides* 32-77:1, *Lb. paracasei* subsp. *paracasei*19, *Lb. plantarum* 2362 (each bacterium10^{10} CFU) + 2.5 g beta-glucan, 2.5 g inulin, 2.5 g pectin, 2.5 g resistant starch One sachet, twice daily	28/20	Three days before the scheduled operation date	Increased IL-6 cytokine Increased fibrinogen at 24 h postoperatively	[53]

(Table 6) cont.....

Probiotics /Synbiotics, Dose	No. of patients (intervention group/control group)	Treatment duration	Result	References
One tablet containing *Lb. rhamnosus* R0011, *Lb. acidophilus* R0052 (2×10^9 CFU) One tablet, twice a day	28/32	Twelve weeks	Significantly decreased proportion of patients suffering from irritable bowel symptoms (0 week vs. 12 weeks; 67.9% vs. 45.7%, $p = 0.03$) Improved CRC-related FACT (baseline vs.12 weeks: 19.79±4.66 vs. 21.18±3.67, $p = 0.04$) Fatigue-related FACT (baseline vs. 12 weeks: 43.00 (36.50–45.50) vs. 44.50 (38.50–49.00), $p = 0.02$) PHQ-9 scores (0 weeks vs. 12 weeks; 3.00 (0–8.00) vs. 1.00 (0-3.00), $p = 0.01$)	[54]
Lb. acidophilus LA-5 1.75×10^9CFU, *Lb. plantarum* 0.5×10^9CFU, *B. lactis* BB-12 1.75×10^9CFU and *S. boulardii* 1.5×10^9 CFU per capsule One capsule, twice a day	84/80	One day before operation and continuing for another 15 days postoperatively	Significantly decreased the rate of all postoperative major complications (28.6 vs. 48.8% of the placebo arm, p 0.010, odds ratio 0.42) Gene expression of SOCS3 was positively related to TNF gene expression and of circulating IL-6	[55]
A capsule consists of *Lb. plantarum* CGMCC no.1258$\geq10^{11}$CFU/g, *Lb. acidophilus*-117.0$\times10^{10}$CFU/g and *B. longum*-88$\geq5.0\times10^{10}$ CFU/g 2 g/day, at a total daily dose of 2.6×10^{14} CFU	66/68	Six days preoperatively and 10 days postoperatively	Decreased incidence of infectious complications Reduced concentration of serum zonulin and plasma endotoxin	[56]

(Table 6) cont.....

Probiotics /Synbiotics, Dose	No. of patients (intervention group/control group)	Treatment duration	Result	References
One sachet containing *Lb. acidophilus* (BCMC™12130), *Lb. casei* (BCMC™12313), *Lb. lactis* (BCMC™12451), *B. bifidum* (BCMC™02290), *B. longum* (BCMC™02120), and *B. infantis* (BCMC™02129) One sachet, twice daily	20/20	One sachet in the morning and one sachet in the evening for a consecutive 7 days prior to surgery	Faster return of normal gut function with a median of108.5 h (80-250 h) Shorten the duration of hospital stay at a median of 6.5 days (4-30 days)	[57]
One sachet containing *Lb. acidophilus* NCFM, *Lb. rhamnosus* HN001, *Lb. paracasei* LPC-37, *B. lactis* HN019 (each bacterium 10^9 CFU) + 6 g fructo-oligosaccharide (FOS), Two sachets, twice a day	49/42	Five days before the surgical procedure and for 14 days after the surgery	Reduced postoperative infection rates in patients	[58]
Two daily tablets totaling 1.4×10^{10} CFU *B. lactis* Bl-04 + 7×10^9 CFU *Lb. acidophilus* NCFM + 0.63 g inulin	8/7	Started at the second revisit to the clinic and continued until the day of surgery (average length of the intervention was 31 ± 28 days; range 8-78 days)	Significantly increased butyrate-producing bacteria in the tumor, non-tumor mucosa and faecal microbiota Reduced CRC-associated genera in the faecal microbiota of patients	[59]
One dose comprising of *Lb. acidophilus* NCFM, *Lb. rhamnosus* HN001, *Lb.casei* LPC-37, and *B. lactis* HN019 at 10^9 CFU + 6 g of fructooligosaccharide Twice a day	36/37	Seven days before the date of the surgical procedure	Significantly reduced IL-6 levels (163.2 ± 19.5 vs. 138.8 ± 12.5, $p < 0.001$) and CRP levels (10 ± 5.2 vs. 7.17 ± 3.2, $p < 0.001$)	[60]

B. adolescentis SPM0212 had the efficacy to inhibit harmful faecal enzymes and showed an anticancer effect. The proliferation of three human colon cancer cell lines, including HT-29, SW 480, and Caco-2, was inhibited by this strain. It inhibited the TNF-α production and changed the cellular morphology. Harmful faecal enzyme activities, including β-glucuronidase, β-glucosidase, tryptophanase, and urease in the faeces of rat fed with *B. adolescentis* SPM0212, were reduced [17]. Further, to increase apoptosis, a CRC cell line in the presence of 5-fluorouracil (5-FU;a chemotherapeutic drug used for the treatment of metastatic CRC), the potential of *Lb. acidophilus* CL1285 and *Lb. casei* LBC80R were investigated. Live and irradiation-inactivated LAB increased the apoptotic efficacy of the 5-FU by 40%. Some LAB could enhance the apoptosis-induction capacity of the 5-FU. The study demonstrated that LAB could be used as an adjuvant treatment during anticancer chemotherapy [42]. Prebiotics help to increase the population of *Bifidobacteria* and *Lactobacilli* in the gut by modulating microflora's metabolism. The wheat aleurone fermented with faecal slurries with the addition of *Lb. rhamnosus* GG and *B. lactis* Bb12 increased apoptosis and upregulated the genes involved in cell growth and apoptosis (*p21* and *WNT2B*) in HT-29 and LT-97 human colon cells [43]. Both viable and heat-killed cells of two probiotic strains *Lb. paracasei* IMPC2.1 and *Lb. rhamnosus* GG inhibited the growth and induced apoptosis of CRC cell line (DLD-1). The dead cells of probiotics can be used as an effective component of functional food [44]. Probiotic *Lc. lactis* NK34, which is generally used as a fermentation starter in dairy products, was assessed for its anti-anticancer and anti-inflammatory activities. A probiotic strain showed the strong inhibition of proliferation against DLD-1, HT-29 and LoVo cell lines at 77.23%, 97.05%, and 97.64%, respectively when cancer cells were treated with 10^6 CFU/well of bacteria. Moreover, a probiotic also displayed anti-inflammatory activity in lipopolysaccharide-induced RAW 264.7 cells. The production of nitric oxide (NO) and pro-inflammatory cytokines (TNF-α, IL-18, & COX-2) were reduced [34]. Live *Lb.casei* ATCC 393 and its extract raised a significant concentration- and time-dependent anti-proliferative effect on murine (CT26) and human (HT29) colon carcinoma cell lines. Moreover, decreased viability of colon cancer cells treated with 10^9 CFU/mL *Lb. casei* for 24 hours was found by 78% for HT29 and 52% for CT26 cells. In addition, live *Lb. casei* induced apoptotic cell death in both cell lines as revealed by annexin V and propidium iodide staining [45]. Synbiotics, a combination between probiotics and prebiotics, exhibited anti-proliferative activity against mouse colon cancer CT26 cells. Moreover, the probiotic mixture containing *B. longum*, *B. bifidum*, *Lb. acidophilus*, *Lb. plantarum*, resistant dextrin, isomaltooligosaccharides, fructose oligosaccharides and stachyose, significantly inhibited the proliferation, invasion, and migration ability of CT26 cells as compared to the control cells [28].

Decreasing the level of reactive oxygen species (ROS) such as superoxide radical, hydrogen peroxide (H_2O_2) is also an approach for colon cancer prevention. The effect of intra-colonic infusion of bovine superoxide dismutase (SOD) and the administration of live recombinant *Lc. lactis* or *Lb. plantarum* (10^9 CFU/d, producing or not producing SOD) for 4 days in rats before and after 2,4,6-trinitrobenzenesulphonicacid (TNBS) treatment was investigated. The study showed that macroscopic and microscopic damages were induced, and myeloperoxidase (MPO) activity and intense immunostaining for nitrotyrosine were increased in TNBS-treated rats. These parameters and microscopic damages were also reduced by *Lc. lactis*, *Lc. lactis* SOD$^+$, and *Lb. plantarum* SOD$^+$, but not by *Lb. plantarum* [46]. Catalase activity in intestinal fluids and blood samples from mice was slightly increased, whereas H_2O_2 was decreased, when DMH-treated mice received the catalase-producing *Lc. lactis* strain. Furthermore, DMH-treated mice received the catalase-producing *Lc. lactis* had a significantly lesser extent of colonic damage and inflammation compared to the group that administrated the non-catalase-producing *Lc. lactis* or the group that did not receive bacterial supplementation [47].

Furthermore, the effect of *Lb. acidophilus* KFRI342 isolated from Kimchi on the early development of cancer in animal models was examined. All rats used in the study were allocated into three groups, including the control group that received a high-fat diet (HF), a second group that received a high-fat diet containing the carcinogen (HFC), and a final group that received a high-fat diet containing the carcinogen and *Lb. acidophilus* KFRI342 (HFCL). The number of *Escherichia coli* in faecal samples, the enzyme activities of β-glucuronidase and β-glucosidase, and plasma triglyceride concentration in HFCL group were decreased as compared to the HF and HFC groups. The ratio of aberrant crypts to aberrant crypt foci incidence and the number of aberrant crypts of the rat that consumed *Lb. acidophilus* were reduced [48]. Male F344 rats were induced by DMH and administered two doses of *Lb. salivarius* Ren (LS) at 5×10^8 and 1×10^{10} CFU/kg body weight for 15 weeks. LS-treated group had discrimination of colonic microflora structures. The number of *Prevotella*-related strain was increased, and the level of *Bacillus* related strain was decreased in LS-treated rats. These alterations were accompanied by increasing in SCFAs levels and decreasing in azoreductase activity. LS treatment also reduced the number of precancerous lesions (aberrant crypt foci; ACF) by 40% and suppressed epithelial proliferation [49]. The chemopreventive effect of dead nano-sized *Lb. plantarum* (nLp) and live *Lb. plantarum* (pLp) on colon carcinogenesis was studied using Balb/c mice induced by dextran sulfate sodium (DSS) and azoxymethane. The study showed that in comparison to mice-treated with pLp, less weight-loss, longer colons, lower colon weight/length ratios, and fewer colonic tumors were observed in mice-treated with nLp. In addition, the administration of nLp significantly reduced the expression of inflammatory markers, mediated the expression of cell cycle and apoptotic markers in colon tissues, and elevated the fecal IgA levels more than that of the pLp [50]. Oral administration of *Lb. salivarius* Ren effectively suppressed DMH-induced colonic carcinogenesis in rats. Rats fed with a dose of 5×10^{10} CFU/kg body weight per day had a significant reduction in cancer incidence (87.5% to 25%). Gut microbiota in DMH-induced rats was significantly changed close to the healthy state and the adverse effects were also reduced [51]. The protective role of *Lactobacillus casei* ATCC 393 in DMH-induced mouse model of colon carcinogenesis has also been reported. *Lb.*

casei ATCC 393 at 10^6 CFU was fed orally twice a week for 2 weeks before DMH administration. The administration of a probiotic strain significantly reduced the number of DMH-induced aberrant crypt foci, the levels of putrescine, and the expression of ornithine decarboxylase [52]. The administration of probiotic mixture consisted of *B. longum, B. bifidum, Lb. acidophilus, Lb. plantarum*, resistant dextrin, isomaltooligosaccharides, fructose oligosaccharides and stachyose resulted in significantly smaller tumor volume of mice than that of the control group. In the tumor tissues, mice fed with probiotic mixture showed more apoptotic cells and infiltration of immune cells. Moreover, mice fed with probiotic mixture had increased number of $CD8^+$ T cells in the tumor and spleen tissues [28].

The use of prebiotics and probiotics in patients, instead of mechanical bowel cleaning (a routine procedure for elective colorectal surgery), was carried out by a double-blind randomized placebo-controlled trial. The investigation demonstrated that patients who received synbiotics had significantly higher levels of IL-6 at 72 h after administration and had an increase of fibrinogen at 24 h postoperatively [53]. Probiotics can improve bowel symptoms and quality of life [assessed by using the Functional Assessment of Cancer Therapy (FACT) Measurement System (version 4)] in CRC survivors. A significant decrease in the ratio of patients suffering from irritable bowel symptoms was detected (0 week vs. 12 weeks; 67.9% vs. 45.7%, $p = 0.03$). The study suggested that CRC-related FACT (baseline vs.12 weeks: 19.79±4.66 vs. 21.18±3.67, $p = 0.04$) and fatigue-related FACT (baseline vs. 12 weeks: 43.00(36.50–45.50) vs. 44.50 (38.50–49.00), $p = 0.02$) and PHQ-9 scores (0 weeks vs. 12 weeks; 3.00 (0–8.00) vs. 1.00 (0–3.00), $p = 0.01$) were improved [54]. Patients who received probiotics had a significantly decreased rate of all postoperative major complications (28.6 vs. 48.8% of the placebo arm, $p= 0.010$). The study found a reduced rate of postoperative pneumonia (2.4 *vs.* 11.3%, $p= 0.029$) of surgical site infections (7.1 *vs.* 20.0%, $p=0.020$) and of anastomotic leakage (1.2 *vs.* 8.8%, $p=0.031$). Gene expression of *SOCS3* was positively associated with the *TNF* gene expression and circulating IL-6 levels in the probiotic group [55]. Colorectal liver metastases (CLM) occur frequently, and postoperative intestinal infection is a common complication. Patients with CLM, and control groups were given probiotics orally for 6 days preoperatively and 10 days postoperatively, respectively. The incidence of infectious complications in the probiotics group was lower than in the control group. Probiotics could also reduce the concentration of serum zonulin ($P = 0.004$) and plasma endotoxin ($P< 0.001$) [56]. Probiotic administration is advantageous as a pre-surgical nutritional supplement to assist in bowel recovery and promote the return of normal gut function following abdominal surgery. Patients diagnosed with CRC and intended to undergo surgery were randomized to receive either probiotics (n = 20) or placebo (n = 20) for 7 days prior to the elective surgery. The probiotic-received group had a significantly faster return of normal gut function with a median of 108.5 h (80–250 h) which was 48 h earlier than the placebo group at a median of 156.5 h (94–220 h; $p = 0.022$). The duration of hospital stay in the probiotic-treated group was also shorter at a median of 6.5 days (4-30 days), as compared to the placebo group at 13 days (5-25 days; $p = 0.012$) [57].

The preoperative administration of synbiotics reduced the postoperative infection rates in patients with CRC. Only one patient (2%) in the synbiotic group showed surgical site infection, whereas nine patients (21.4%) in the control group had the same symptom ($p=0.002$). Three cases of intra-abdominal abscess and four cases of pneumonia in the control group were observed, whereas no infections were observed in patients receiving the synbiotics ($p=0.001$) [58]. Probiotics can modify the colonic microbiota in patients with colon cancer. An increased abundance of butyrate-producing bacteria, especially *Faecalibacterium* and *Clostridiales* spp. was found in the tumor, non-tumor mucosa and faecal microbiota of probiotic-treated patients. CRC-associated genera such as *Fusobacterium* and *Peptostreptococcus* were found to be reduced in the faecal microbiota of patients that received probiotics [59]. Significant decrease in the IL-6 levels (163.2±19.5 *vs.* 138.8±12.5, $P<0.001$) and C-reactive protein (CRP) (10±5.2 *vs.* 7.17±3.2, $P<0.001$) were observed after 7 days of synbiotic administration. Patients receiving synbiotics (2.8%) had lower postoperative infectious complications than that of the control group (18.9%) ($P=0.02$). Patients administered with synbiotics (1.42±0.5d) had an antibiotic usage period shorter than that of the control group (3.74±4.3d) ($P<0.001$). The mean hospital length of stay in the symbiotic group (3±1d) was shorter than that of the control group (4±18 d) ($P<0.001$). Three deaths were reported in the control group and none in the synbiotic group ($P=0.115$) [60].

CONCLUSION

Probiotics have received increased medical significance since the functional attributes of probiotics exert positive effects on human health. Most probiotic strains are members of *Lactobacillus* and *Bifidobacterium* species. Several *in vitro* and animal model studies have shown improvement of host immune response. Moreover, several mechanisms involved in colon cancer prevention, and *in vitro* and *in vivo* treatment and clinical practices have been demonstrated. These increasing evidences suggest that probiotics and/or synbiotics can be applied as adjunctive therapeutic agents to patients obtaining chemotherapy, due to their enhanced therapeutic effect of the drug used for treating cancer. Probiotics and/or synbiotics at the appropriate dosages are also used as an alternative therapy for patients diagnosed with colon cancer and those who plan for surgery. Although probiotics exhibit a beneficial effect on the host, the large-scale evaluation, safety assessment, and their side effects should also be evaluated.

CONSENT FOR PUBLICATION

Not applicable.

CONFLICT OF INTEREST

The authors declare no conflict of interest, financial or otherwise.

ACKNOWLEDGEMENTS

Declared none.

REFERENCES

[1]   Wu HJ, Wu E. The role of gut microbiota in immune homeostasis and autoimmunity. Gut Microbes 2012; 3(1): 4-14.
        [http://dx.doi.org/10.4161/gmic.19320] [PMID: 22356853]

[2]   Lazar V, Ditu LM, Pircalabioru GG, *et al.* Aspects of gut microbiota and immune system interactions in infectious diseases, immunopathology and cancer. Front Immunol 2018; 9: 1830.
        [http://dx.doi.org/10.3389/fimmu.2018.01830] [PMID: 30158926]

[3]   Yu AQ, Li L. The potential role of probiotics in cancer prevention and treatment. Nutr Cancer 2016; 68(4): 535-44.
        [http://dx.doi.org/10.1080/01635581.2016.1158300] [PMID: 27144297]

[4]   FAO/WHO. (2002). Guidelines for the evaluation of probiotics in food, Food and Agriculture Organization of the United Nations and World Health Organization Working Group Report, London, Ontario: 1-11.

[5]   Hamilton-Miller JMT. The role of probiotics in the treatment and prevention of *Helicobacter pylori* infection. Int J Antimicrob Agents 2003; 22(4): 360-6.
        [http://dx.doi.org/10.1016/S0924-8579(03)00153-5] [PMID: 14522098]

[6]   Techo S, Visessanguan W, Vilaichone R, Tanasupawat S. Characterization and antibacterial activity against *Helicobacter pylori* of lactic acid bacteria isolated from Thai fermented rice noodle. Probiotics Antimicrob Proteins 2019; 11(1): 92-102.
        [http://dx.doi.org/10.1007/s12602-018-9385-z] [PMID: 29362990]

[7]   Saarela M, Mogensen G, Fondén R, Mättö J, Mattila-Sandholm T. Probiotic bacteria: safety, functional and technological properties. J Biotechnol 2000; 84(3): 197-215.
        [http://dx.doi.org/10.1016/S0168-1656(00)00375-8] [PMID: 11164262]

[8]   Saad N, Delattre C, Urdaci M, Schmitter JM, Bressollier P. An overview of the last advances in probiotic and prebiotic field. Lebensm Wiss Technol 2013; 50(1): 1-16.
        [http://dx.doi.org/10.1016/j.lwt.2012.05.014]

[9]   De Melo Pereira GV, de Oliveira Coelho B, Magalhães Júnior AI, Thomaz-Soccol V, Soccol CR. How to select a probiotic? A review and update of methods and criteria. Biotechnol Adv 2018; 36(8): 2060-76.
        [http://dx.doi.org/10.1016/j.biotechadv.2018.09.003] [PMID: 30266342]

[10]   Javanmard A, Ashtari S, Sabet B, *et al.* Probiotics and their role in gastrointestinal cancers prevention

and treatment; an overview. Gastroenterol Hepatol Bed Bench 2018; 11(4): 284-95.
[PMID: 30425806]

[11]   Binda S, Hill C, Johansen E, *et al.* Criteria to qualify microorganisms as "probiotic" in foods and dietary supplements. Front Microbiol 2020; 11: 1662.
[http://dx.doi.org/10.3389/fmicb.2020.01662] [PMID: 32793153]

[12]   Shewale RN, Sawale PD, Khedkar CD, Singh A. Selection criteria for probiotics: a review. Int J Probiotics Prebiotics 2014; 9(1): 17-22.

[13]   Yaghoubi A, Khazaei M, Avan A, Hasanian SM, Soleimanpour S. The bacterial instrument as a promising therapy for colon cancer. Int J Colorectal Dis 2020; 35(4): 595-606.
[http://dx.doi.org/10.1007/s00384-020-03535-9] [PMID: 32130489]

[14]   Kumar KS, Sastry N, Polaki H, Mishra V. Colon cancer prevention through probiotics: an overview. J Cancer SciTher 2015; 7: 081-92.

[15]   Cappell MS. Pathophysiology, clinical presentation, and management of colon cancer GastroenterolClin N Am 2008; 37: 1-24.

[16]   Bai AP, Ouyang Q, Zhang W, Wang CH, Li SF. Probiotics inhibit TNF-α-induced interleukin-8 secretion of HT29 cells. World J Gastroenterol 2004; 10(3): 455-7.
[http://dx.doi.org/10.3748/wjg.v10.i3.455] [PMID: 14760780]

[17]   Kim Y, Lee D, Kim D, *et al.* Inhibition of proliferation in colon cancer cell lines and harmful enzyme activity of colon bacteria by *Bifidobacterium adolescentis* SPM0212. Arch Pharm Res 2008; 31(4): 468-73.
[http://dx.doi.org/10.1007/s12272-001-1180-y] [PMID: 18449504]

[18]   Lopez M, Li N, Kataria J, Russell M, Neu J. Live and ultraviolet-inactivated *Lactobacillus rhamnosus* GG decrease flagellin-induced interleukin-8 production in Caco-2 cells. J Nutr 2008; 138(11): 2264-8.
[http://dx.doi.org/10.3945/jn.108.093658] [PMID: 18936229]

[19]   Paolillo R, Romano Carratelli C, Sorrentino S, Mazzola N, Rizzo A. Immunomodulatory effects of *Lactobacillus plantarum* on human colon cancer cells. Int Immunopharmacol 2009; 9(11): 1265-71.
[http://dx.doi.org/10.1016/j.intimp.2009.07.008] [PMID: 19647100]

[20]   Pagnini C, Saeed R, Bamias G, Arseneau KO, Pizarro TT, Cominelli F. Probiotics promote gut health through stimulation of epithelial innate immunity. Proc Natl Acad Sci USA 2010; 107(1): 454-9.
[http://dx.doi.org/10.1073/pnas.0910307107] [PMID: 20018654]

[21]   Ferreira dos Santos T, Alves Melo T, Almeida ME, Passos Rezende R, Romano CC. Immunomodulatory effects of *Lactobacillus plantarum* Lp62 on intestinal epithelial and mononuclear cells. BioMed Res Int 2016; 2016: 1-8.
[http://dx.doi.org/10.1155/2016/8404156] [PMID: 27446958]

[22]   Djaldetti M, Leibovitch CM, Bessler H. Multi-species probiotic modulates cytokine production and the interplay between immune and colon cancer cells. OBM Hepatology and Gastroenterology 2020; 4(4): 1-15.
[http://dx.doi.org/10.21926/obm.hg.2004053]

[23]   Perdigón G, de Moreno de LeBlanc A, Valdez J, Rachid M. Role of yoghurt in the prevention of colon cancer. Eur J Clin Nutr 2002; 56(S3) (Suppl. 3): S65-8.
[http://dx.doi.org/10.1038/sj.ejcn.1601490] [PMID: 12142967]

[24]   Roller M, Femia AP, Caderni G, Rechkemmer G, Watzl B. Intestinal immunity of rats with colon cancer is modulated by oligofructose-enriched inulin combined with *Lactobacillus rhamnosus* and *Bifidobacterium lactis*. Br J Nutr 2004; 92(6): 931-8.
[http://dx.doi.org/10.1079/BJN20041289] [PMID: 15613255]

[25]   Takeda K, Okumura K. Effects of a fermented milk drink containing *Lactobacillus casei* strain *Shirota* on the human NK-cell activity. J Nutr 2007; 137(3) (Suppl. 2): S791-3.
[http://dx.doi.org/10.1093/jn/137.3.791S] [PMID: 17311976]

[26] Gamallat Y, Meyiah A, Kuugbee ED, *et al. Lactobacillus rhamnosus* induced epithelial cell apoptosis, ameliorates inflammation and prevents colon cancer development in an animal model. Biomed Pharmacother 2016; 83: 536-41.
[http://dx.doi.org/10.1016/j.biopha.2016.07.001] [PMID: 27447122]

[27] Casas-Solís J, Huizar-López MR, Irecta-Nájera CA, Pita-López ML, Santerre A. Immunomodulatory effect of *Lactobacillus casei* in a murine model of colon carcinogenesis. Probiotics Antimicrob Proteins 2020; 12(3): 1012-24.
[http://dx.doi.org/10.1007/s12602-019-09611-z] [PMID: 31797281]

[28] Shang F, Jiang X, Wang H, *et al.* The inhibitory effects of probiotics on colon cancer cells: *in vitro* and *in vivo* studies. J Gastrointest Oncol 2020; 11(6): 1224-32.
[http://dx.doi.org/10.21037/jgo-20-573] [PMID: 33456995]

[29] Eslami M, Yousefi B, Kokhaei P, *et al.* Importance of probiotics in the prevention and treatment of colorectal cancer. J Cell Physiol 2019; 234(10): 17127-43.
[http://dx.doi.org/10.1002/jcp.28473] [PMID: 30912128]

[30] Fong W, Li Q, Yu J. Gut microbiota modulation: a novel strategy for prevention and treatment of colorectal cancer. Oncogene 2020; 39(26): 4925-43.
[http://dx.doi.org/10.1038/s41388-020-1341-1] [PMID: 32514151]

[31] Lim HY, Joo HJ, Choi JH, *et al.* Increased expression of cyclooxygenase-2 protein in human gastric carcinoma. Clin Cancer Res 2000; 6(2): 519-25.
[PMID: 10690533]

[32] Ma EL, Choi YJ, Choi J, Pothoulakis C, Rhee SH, Im E. The anticancer effect of probiotic *Bacillus polyfermenticus* on human colon cancer cells is mediated through ErbB2 and ErbB3 inhibition. Int J Cancer 2010; 127(4): 780-90.
[PMID: 19876926]

[33] Kahouli I, Malhotra M, Alaoui-Jamali M, Prakash S. *In-vitro* characterization of the anti-cancer activity of the probiotic bacterium *Lactobacillus fermentum* NCIMB 5221 and potential against colorectal cancer. J Cancer Sci Ther 2015; 7(7): 224-35.

[34] Han KJ, Lee NK, Park H, Paik HD. Anticancer and anti-inflammatory activity of probiotic *Lactococcus lactis* NK34. J Microbiol Biotechnol 2015; 25(10): 1697-701.
[http://dx.doi.org/10.4014/jmb.1503.03033] [PMID: 26165315]

[35] Dubey V, Ghosh AR, Bishayee K, Khuda-Bukhsh AR. Appraisal of the anti-cancer potential of probiotic *Pediococcus pentosaceus* GS4 against colon cancer: *in vitro* and *in vivo* approaches. J Funct Foods 2016; 23: 66-79.
[http://dx.doi.org/10.1016/j.jff.2016.02.032]

[36] Molska M, Reguła J. Potential mechanisms of probiotics action in the prevention and treatment of colorectal cancer. Nutrients 2019; 11(10): 2453.
[http://dx.doi.org/10.3390/nu11102453] [PMID: 31615096]

[37] Hsieh CY, Osaka T, Moriyama E, Date Y, Kikuchi J, Tsuneda S. Strengthening of the intestinal epithelial tight junction by *Bifidobacterium bifidum*. Physiol Rep 2015; 3(3)e12327
[http://dx.doi.org/10.14814/phy2.12327] [PMID: 25780093]

[38] Blackwood BP, Yuan CY, Wood DR, Nicolas JD, Grothaus JS, Hunter CJ. Probiotic *Lactobacillus* species strengthen intestinal barrier function and tight junction integrity in experimental necrotizing enterocolitis. J Probiotics Health 2017; 5(1): 159.
[http://dx.doi.org/10.4172/2329-8901.1000159] [PMID: 28638850]

[39] Martín R, Chamignon C, Mhedbi-Hajri N, *et al.* The potential probiotic *Lactobacillus rhamnosus* CNCM I-3690 strain protects the intestinal barrier by stimulating both mucus production and cytoprotective response. Sci Rep 2019; 9(1): 5398.
[http://dx.doi.org/10.1038/s41598-019-41738-5] [PMID: 30931953]

[40]   Kruszewska D, Lan J, Lorca G, Yanagisawa N, Marklinder I, Ljungh Å. Selection of lactic acid bacteria as probiotic strains by *in vitro* tests. Microecology and Therapy 2002; 29: 37-49.

[41]   Burnett-Hartman AN, Newcomb PA, Potter JD. Infectious agents and colorectal cancer: a review of *Helicobacter pylori, Streptococcus bovis*, JC virus, and human papillomavirus. Cancer Epidemiol Biomarkers Prev 2008; 17(11): 2970-9.
[http://dx.doi.org/10.1158/1055-9965.EPI-08-0571] [PMID: 18990738]

[42]   Baldwin C, Millette M, Oth D, Ruiz MT, Luquet FM, Lacroix M. Probiotic *Lactobacillus acidophilus* and *L. casei* mix sensitize colorectal tumoral cells to 5-fluorouracil-induced apoptosis. Nutr Cancer 2010; 62(3): 371-8.
[http://dx.doi.org/10.1080/01635580903407197] [PMID: 20358475]

[43]   Borowicki A, Michelmann A, Stein K, *et al.* Fermented wheat aleurone enriched with probiotic strains LGG and Bb12 modulates markers of tumor progression in human colon cells. Nutr Cancer 2011; 63(1): 151-60.
[PMID: 21161821]

[44]   Orlando A, Refolo MG, Messa C, *et al.* Antiproliferative and proapoptotic effects of viable or heat-killed *Lactobacillus paracasei* IMPC2.1 and *Lactobacillus rhamnosus* GG in HGC-27 gastric and DLD-1 colon cell lines. Nutr Cancer 2012; 64(7): 1103-11.
[http://dx.doi.org/10.1080/01635581.2012.717676] [PMID: 23061912]

[45]   Tiptiri-Kourpeti A, Spyridopoulou K, Santarmaki V, *et al. Lactobacillus casei* exerts anti-proliferative effects accompanied by apoptotic cell death and up-regulation of TRAIL in colon carcinoma cells. PLoS One 2016; 11(2)e0147960
[http://dx.doi.org/10.1371/journal.pone.0147960] [PMID: 26849051]

[46]   Han W, Mercenier A, Ait-Belgnaoui A, *et al.* Improvement of an experimental colitis in rats by lactic acid bacteria producing superoxide dismutase. Inflamm Bowel Dis 2006; 12(11): 1044-52.
[http://dx.doi.org/10.1097/01.mib.0000235101.09231.9e] [PMID: 17075345]

[47]   De Moreno de LeBlanc A, LeBlanc JG, Perdigón G, *et al.* Oral administration of a catalase-producing *Lactococcus lactis* can prevent a chemically induced colon cancer in mice. J Med Microbiol 2008; 57(1): 100-5.
[http://dx.doi.org/10.1099/jmm.0.47403-0] [PMID: 18065674]

[48]   Chang JH, Shim YY, Cha SK, Reaney MJT, Chee KM. Effect of *Lactobacillus acidophilus* KFRI342 on the development of chemically induced precancerous growths in the rat colon. J Med Microbiol 2012; 61(3): 361-8.
[http://dx.doi.org/10.1099/jmm.0.035154-0] [PMID: 22034161]

[49]   Zhu J, Zhu C, Ge S, *et al. Lactobacillus salivarius* Ren prevent the early colorectal carcinogenesis in 1, 2-dimethylhydrazine-induced rat model. J Appl Microbiol 2014; 117(1): 208-16.
[http://dx.doi.org/10.1111/jam.12499] [PMID: 24754742]

[50]   Lee HA, Kim H, Lee KW, Park KY. Dead nano-sized *Lactobacillus plantarum* inhibits azoxymethane/dextran sulfate sodium-induced colon cancer in Balb/c mice. J Med Food 2015; 18(12): 1400-5.
[http://dx.doi.org/10.1089/jmf.2015.3577] [PMID: 26595186]

[51]   Zhang M, Fan X, Fang B, Zhu C, Zhu J, Ren F. Effects of *Lactobacillus salivarius* Ren on cancer prevention and intestinal microbiota in 1, 2-dimethylhydrazine-induced rat model. J Microbiol 2015; 53(6): 398-405.
[http://dx.doi.org/10.1007/s12275-015-5046-z] [PMID: 26025172]

[52]   Irecta-Nájera CA, del Rosario Huizar-López M, Casas-Solís J, Castro-Félix P, Santerre A. Protective effect of *Lactobacillus casei* on DMH-induced colon carcinogenesis in mice. Probiotics Antimicrob Proteins 2017; 9(2): 163-71.
[http://dx.doi.org/10.1007/s12602-017-9253-2] [PMID: 28316010]

[53] Horvat M, Krebs B, Potrč S, Ivanecz A, Kompan L. Preoperative synbiotic bowel conditioning for elective colorectal surgery. Wien Klin Wochenschr 2010; 122(S2) (Suppl. 2): 26-30.
[http://dx.doi.org/10.1007/s00508-010-1347-8] [PMID: 20517667]

[54] Lee JY, Chu SH, Jeon JY, *et al.* Effects of 12 weeks of probiotic supplementation on quality of life in colorectal cancer survivors: A double-blind, randomized, placebo-controlled trial. Dig Liver Dis 2014; 46(12): 1126-32.
[http://dx.doi.org/10.1016/j.dld.2014.09.004] [PMID: 25442120]

[55] Kotzampassi K, Stavrou G, Damoraki G, *et al.* A four-probiotics regimen reduces postoperative complications after colorectal surgery: a randomized, double-blind, placebo-controlled study. World J Surg 2015; 39(11): 2776-83.
[http://dx.doi.org/10.1007/s00268-015-3071-z] [PMID: 25894405]

[56] Liu Z, Li C, Huang M, *et al.* Positive regulatory effects of perioperative probiotic treatment on postoperative liver complications after colorectal liver metastases surgery: a double-center and double-blind randomized clinical trial. BMC Gastroenterol 2015; 15(1): 34.
[http://dx.doi.org/10.1186/s12876-015-0260-z] [PMID: 25881090]

[57] Tan CK, Said S, Rajandram R, Wang Z, Roslani AC, Chin KF. Pre-surgical administration of microbial cell preparation in colorectal cancer patients: a randomized controlled trial. World J Surg 2016; 40(8): 1985-92.
[http://dx.doi.org/10.1007/s00268-016-3499-9] [PMID: 27098538]

[58] Flesch AT, Tonial ST, Contu PDC, Damin DC. Perioperative synbiotics administration decreases postoperative infections in patients with colorectal cancer: a randomized, double-blind clinical trial. Rev Col Bras Cir 2017; 44(6): 567-73.
[http://dx.doi.org/10.1590/0100-69912017006004] [PMID: 29267553]

[59] Hibberd AA, Lyra A, Ouwehand AC, *et al.* Intestinal microbiota is altered in patients with colon cancer and modified by probiotic intervention. BMJ Open Gastroenterol 2017; 4(1)e000145
[http://dx.doi.org/10.1136/bmjgast-2017-000145] [PMID: 28944067]

[60] Polakowski CB, Kato M, Preti VB, Schieferdecker MEM, Ligocki Campos AC. Impact of the preoperative use of synbiotics in colorectal cancer patients: A prospective, randomized, double-blind, placebo-controlled study. Nutrition 2019; 58: 40-6.
[http://dx.doi.org/10.1016/j.nut.2018.06.004] [PMID: 30278428]

CHAPTER 5

Probiotics Based Anticancer Immunity in Colorectal Cancer

Prashant Shankar Giri[1] and **Mitesh Kumar Dwivedi**[1,*]

[1] *C. G. Bhakta Institute of Biotechnology, Faculty of Science, Uka Tarsadia University, Bardoli, Surat, Gujarat, India*

Abstract: Colorectal cancer (CRC) is the third most common cancer, originating in the colon and rectal region, leading to abnormal growth in the colon or rectal region. The gut microbiota plays a critical role in the maintenance of gut homeostasis, and dysbiosis in the gut microbiota has been associated with CRC pathogenesis. Probiotics can manipulate the gut microbiota, which can be effective in CRC treatment. Additionally, probiotics, through the modulation of host immune response, inhibition of tumor growth, reduction of microbial infection, inhibition of cancerogenic compounds, and regulation of apoptosis, can become a novel therapeutic option for the prevention and treatment of CRC. Therefore, this chapter mainly focuses on the mechanisms of probiotics-based anticancer immunity in CRC, so the existing knowledge could help in developing a safe and effective treatment for CRC.

Keywords: Apoptosis, *B. bifidum*, Colorectal cancer (CRC), Dysbiosis, Gut microbiota, *L. rhamnosus*, *L. acidophilus*, Probiotics, Short chain fatty acids (SCFAs), Tyrosine kinase.

1. INTRODUCTION

Colorectal cancer (CRC) originates in the colon or rectal region, leading to abnormal growth [1]. CRC emerges in the large intestine, where the heightened replication of the epithelial cells gives rise to benign adenoma, which can metastasize and result in carcinoma [1]. CRC is preventable, if there is early detection of growth or polyps in the colon, which can develop into cancer cells [2]. Symptoms include abdominal pain, weight loss, weakness, fatigue, diarrhoea, constipation, blood in stools, bleeding in rectum, changes in consistency of stool, *etc* [3]. The risk factors for CRC include family history, age, diabetes, smoking, alcohol, inflammatory bowel disease, lifestyle, *etc* [4]. It is one of the most

[*] **Corresponding author Mitesh Kumar Dwivedi:** C. G. Bhakta Institute of Biotechnology, Faculty of Science, Uka Tarsadia University, Bardoli, Surat, Gujarat; India; E-mail: mitesh_dwivedi@yahoo.com

Mitesh Kumar Dwivedi, Alwarappan Sankaranarayanan & Sanjay Tiwari (Eds.)

diagnosed cancers worldwide, and its prevalence is rising in developing countries [3]. In 2020, there were approximately 1.9 million new cases of CRC, which are estimated to be responsible for 93,500 cancer deaths [3]. A higher incidence of CRC is found in males compared to females, and approximately 4.4% of males and 4.1% of females are estimated to be affected by CRC in their lifetime [5].

Currently, surgeries and chemotherapy are the first choice of treatment for CRC. Chemotherapy includes single agent and multiple agent regimens, but limitations include systemic toxicity, unsatisfying response rate, and low specificity. Additionally, surgeries are difficult for patients in advanced stages of CRC [6]. Moreover, for patients with unresectable lesions or who are intolerant to surgery radiotherapy and chemotherapy, treatments which can lead to maximum shrinkage of tumor are the only options [6]. Therefore, there is a need to develop novel approaches for treatment of CRC.

Probiotics are live microorganisms residing in the gastrointestinal tract (GIT) that confer health benefits to the host [7]. Probiotics organisms have specific characteristics, including gastric acid, bile salt stability and the ability to adhere and colonize the intestinal mucosa [7]. Additionally, probiotics provide essential nutrients to the host and help in metabolizing indigestible compounds in the host gut [8]. Additionally, probiotics provide immunity and maintain homeostasis *via* production of short chain fatty acids (SCFAs) such as acetate butyrate, *etc* [8].

In the case of CRC, the intestine is characterized by high proportion of bacteria that cause inflammation in the GI tract [9]. Probiotics can reduce the bacteria from the intestine that contribute to CRC [10]. Moreover, probiotics through the modulation of host immune response, inhibition of tumor growth, reduction of microbial infection, inhibition of cancerogenic compounds, and regulation of apoptosis, can serve a novel therapeutic option for CRC [10]. Multiple strategies including probiotics, prebiotics, synbiotics and fecal microbiota transplantation (FMT) can be used to treat CRC [11]. Therefore, this chapter discusses the mechanisms of probiotics based anticancer immunity in CRC, provides animal and human clinical trials evidences for these probiotics use in CRC treatment and prevention, in addition to the role of gut microbiota in CRC development.

2. PATHOGENESIS OF COLORECTAL CANCER

The pathogenesis of CRC is complex; multiple factors, including smoking, diabetes, inflammatory bowel disease, eating habits, obesity, alcohol consumption, and genetics are involved in the progression of CRC [4]. CRC can be sporadic, inherited, or arise from inflammatory bowel disease (IBD) [12].

Chromosome instability pathway, microsatellite instability pathway, and CpG Island Methylator Phenotype (CIMP) pathway are mainly responsible for sporadic CRC cases [12]. The chromosomal instability arises from either gain or loss of chromosomes, which leads to activation of oncogenes such as KRAS and BRAF, inhibiting tumor suppressor genes and resulting in CRC tumorigenesis [12, 13]. Microsatellite instability (MSI) pathway is another mechanism of sporadic CRC development [12]. It refers to the biochemical detection of frame shifted microsatellite sequences from genomic DNA. This MSI leads to frameshift mutations in the coding region of tumor suppressor genes or oncogenes contributing to carcinogenesis [12]. For the CIMP pathway, epigenetic instability in CRC has been demonstrated, and global hypomethylation was associated with genetic instability and chromosomal aberrations [12]. Moreover, hypermethylation of the promoter region of tumor suppressor genes can lead to cancer initiation. Additionally, the altered methylation patterns affect cell cycle regulation, transcription, cell-cell adhesion, invasion, and metastasis [14].

The hereditary CRC is most inherited in autosomal dominant pattern; however *MUTYH*-associated polyposis and NTHL1 are also inherited in autosomal recessive patterns [15]. Evidence of hereditary CRC comes from the family history of CRC, presence of multiple other cancers in patients, and early age diagnosis of CRC [15]. Hereditary CRC is mainly of two types: i) polyposis, which includes familial adenomatous polyposis (FAP) and attenuated FAP (genetic variation in *APC* gene) and *MUTYH* associated polyposis (genetic variation in *MUTYH* gene) [16], and ii) lynch syndrome caused by genetic variation in the *MMR* genes (*MLH1, MSH2, MSH6,* and *PMS2)* and *EPCAM* genes [17].

Patients with IBD have a 60% higher risk of developing CRC. Chronic mucosal inflammation is the primary cause of CRC carcinogenesis in IBD patients [18]. The factors that are responsible for increased risk of CRC in IBD patients are active inflammation, primary sclerosing cholangitis, family history of CRC, extent and duration of severe inflammatory conditions, cytokine secretion, and shortened tubular colon and vascularization, significantly increased the risk of CRC in IBD patients [18]. However, folic acid use, ursodeoxycholic acid, 5-ASA treatment, colectomy, and compliance with CRC surveillance guidelines can prevent CRC development in IBD patients [6].

3. CORRELATION BETWEEN THE GUT MICROBIOTA AND COLO-RECTAL CANCER

Dysbiosis in the gut microbiota and infections with bacteria can lead to the occurrence of CRC [19]. The dysbiosis of gut microbiota, infections, and infiltration of commensal bacteria or their products lead to inflammation which can further activate tumor-associated myeloid cells [19]. The microbial communities can induce tumorigenesis through IL-6 and STAT3 activation. Additionally, these infectious bacteria and viruses adhere to intestinal epithelial cells, and the toxins produced by such bacteria can lead to DNA damage, which triggers CRC development [20]. Moreover, chronic inflammation post infections, inflammatory cells, microbial metabolites, and bile acids can lead to the generation of reactive oxygen species (ROS), which can further lead to DNA damage and initiate CRC development [19, 21]. The alpha bug hypothesis and the driver-passenger model explain the relationship between microbiota and CRC [22, 23].

Sears and Pardoll [22] proposed the alpha bug hypothesis. It suggests that the single intestinal bacterium and gut microbiota can initiate carcinogenesis [22]. The hypothesis was based on cancer induced by *Enterotoxigenic Bacteroides fragilis* (ETBF) mediated carcinogenesis in Apc$^{+/-}$ mice. The ETBF secretion of *B. fragilis toxin* (BFT) binds to colonic epithelial cells and stimulates the cleavage of tumor suppressor protein E-cadherin. This cleavage of E-cadherin activates cell signalling *via* β-catenin/Wnt pathway, which is constitutively activated in CRC. Additionally, BFT activates the nuclear factor-kappa B (NF-κB) pathway, which promotes pro-inflammatory cytokine secretion, and further contributes to CRC [22]. Moreover, the alpha bugs not only initiate tumors but also shape the gut microbiota in such a manner that promotes the mucosal immune response and alteration in intestinal epithelial cells leading to the carcinogenesis. The potential alpha bugs include ETBF, *S. bovis, E. fecalis* and *E. coli* [22].

Tjalsma *et al.* [23] proposed the driver-passenger model for CRC development. The model suggests that the "drivers" (bacterial infections) cause damage in the epithelial cells initiating CRC, which allows the "passenger" (commensal bacteria) or their by-products to mediate tumorigenesis. The CRC-associated microbes such as ETBF, *S. bovis, E. fecalis, E. coli, S. gallalyticus* and *F. nucleatum* persistently adhere to epithelial cells and increase epithelial cell permeability and the DNA damage initiates CRC [23]. This epithelial alteration by the drivers' further favours passenger growth and proliferation, such as *Fusobacterium* spp., which further mediates colorectal tumorigenesis [23].

3.1. Dysbiosis of Gut Microbiota in Colorectal Cancer

The gut microbiota maintains intestinal homeostasis by regulating the mucosal immune system, mucosal barrier integrity and metabolic processes [24]. Previous studies suggest that gut microbiota is crucial in maintaining human health [7]. Dysbiosis in the gut microbiota has been found to be associated with various diseases such as rheumatoid arthritis (RA), diabetes, vitiligo, IBD, cystic fibrosis [7]. The complex relationship between tumor cells, immune cells and the gut microbiota is responsible for the development of carcinoma [25]. Studies have highlighted that the gut microbiota can govern the development of carcinoma by activating tumor-associated genes and suppressing tumor suppressor genes [25]. Gut microbiota can be shaped through healthy food, lifestyle, and probiotics; thus, gut microbiota modulation can be a potent therapeutic target for CRC [26].

It is challenging to define gut dysbiosis as the gut microbiota can be affected by factors such as age, sex, lifestyle, food, medication, smoking, alcoholism, *etc* [27]. Nevertheless, previous studies have suggested that bacterial species such as *Fusobacterium nucleatum, E. coli, Bacteroides fragilis* play a significant role in CRC development [28]. *F. nucleatum* is associated with various inflammatory diseases. In CRC, *F. nucleatum* has been found from the rectum to the cecum [28]. Additionally, studies have suggested that *F. nucleatum* causes CRC through microsatellite instability [29]. Sequence-based analysis in CRC patients suggested a significant increase in *Parvimonas micra, Streptococcus anginosus, Parabacteroides distasonis, Proteobacteria* and *Fusobacterimn* species [30]. The butyrate producing *Faecalibacterium prausnitzii* has been inversely associated with CRC [31]. The bacterium is reduced in CRC patients [31]. Similarly, *Bifidobacterium* species suppressed the CRC development [32]. They can suppress carcinoma by preventing the growth of infectious bacteria and producing bile acids [32].

Previous studies suggest dysbiosis in the gut microbiota of CRC patients [20]. Dysbiosis in the gut microbiome can disrupt the mucosal membrane and immune system, resulting in increased epithelial barrier integrity [7]. The disrupted epithelial barrier results in increased inflammation and production of IL-6, tumor necrosis factor-beta (TNF-β), which promote the growth and survival of tumor cells [33]. Moreover, bacterial film formation and DNA damage mediated by bacteria result in malignant transformation, further contributing to CRC pathogenesis [34]. Therefore, future studies must examine the microbial heterogeneity of CRC patients, which could lead to better diagnosis and screening of CRC. Moreover, the probiotics-based treatment approaches could lead to novel therapeutics for CRC.

4. ROLE OF PROBIOTICS IN COLORECTAL CANCER

The gut microbiota comprises infectious microbes which produce toxins that can lead to carcinogenesis [31]. However, the butyric acid (SCFA)-producing probiotics can suppress such microbes and modify the gut microbiota reducing dysbiosis and CRC pathogenesis [10]. Probiotics can act through various mechanisms such as the modulation of gut microbiota, inhibition of cancerogenic compounds, modulation of host immune response, inhibition of tumor growth, and regulation of apoptosis, and may serve a novel therapeutic option for CRC [10]. Moreover, personalized microbiome therapy can be developed for the treatment of CRC [11]. Table. 1 enlists such *in vitro* and *in vivo* studies involving the effect of such probiotics in suppression of CRC.

Table 1. *In vitro* and *in vivo* studies of probiotics treatment for colorectal cancer.

Bacteria	Function	Mechanism	Reference
Faecalibacterium prausnitzii	Suppresses CRC development	Butyrate producing *Faecalibacterium prausnitzii* prevents the growth of infectious bacteria and produces bile acids	[31]
Bifidobacterium species	Suppresses CRC development	Prevents the growth of infectious bacteria increases epithelial barrier integrity and produces bile acids.	[32]
Lactobacillus species	Suppresses carcinoma cell line proliferation	By modulating the WNt/- β-catenin, which plays a critical role in CRC development. It detoxes N-nitrosodimethylamine and suppressing cancer development.	[35]
L. acidophilus CICC 6074 S-layer	Suppression of colon cancer	Causes G1 phase arrest by upregulating tumor suppressor proteins.	[11]
L. acidophilus fermented brown rice	Suppresses CRC development	Suppresses TNF-α, IL-6, and IL-1 levels and increases pro-apoptotic cleaved caspase-3 and Bax.	[36]
Long-term dietary supplementation of *L. rhamnosus*	Protects against CRC in rats	Maintains the gut microbiome.	[11, 37]
L. casei	Suppresses carcinoma cells	Upregulates TNF-related apoptosis-inducing ligand (TRAIL).	[38]
Bifidobacterium cocktail	Suppresses CRC development	Decreases *Mucispirillum*, *Desulfovibrio,* and *Odoribacter* species.	[39]
B. bifidum	Tumor suppression in mice	Induces apoptosis of adenocarcinoma cells and increases anti-tumor response.	[39]
L. acidophilus, L. rhamnosus, and *B. bifidum* probiotic mixture	Suppresses CRC development	Suppress tumor size and number in mice.	[40]

(Table 1) cont.....

Bacteria	Function	Mechanism	Reference
L. plantarum	Suppresses CRC development	Decreases carcinoma cell line proliferation; it reduces cholesterol levels, TNF-α, and bacterial pro-carcinogenic fecal enzymes.	[41]
Lactobacillus reuteri	Suppresses CRC development	Suppresses tumor progression, decreases inflammation, and prevents metastasis.	[42]
Bacillus licheniformis	Suppresses CRC cell line	Exerts anti-cancerous activity in carcinoma cell line.	[43]
E. coli probiotics	Suppresses CRC development	Upregulate phosphatase, tensin homolog and Bax and downregulate AKT serine/threonine kinase 1 and *Bcl-xL* genes.	[44]
E. faecalis strains	Tumor suppression in CRC	Suppress the growth of carcinoma cell lines.	[45]
Streptomycetes	Cancer suppression	Production of compounds: tacrolimus and rapamycin.	[46, 47]
Propionibacterium freudenreichii	CRC suppression	Through SCFAs production suppresses the proliferation of CRC cells and increases cancer cell death.	[48]
Probiotic yeasts *Kluyveromyces marxianus* and *Pichia kudriavzevii* from dairy products	CRC suppression	Inhibit AKT-1, and Janus Kinase 1 pathways and induce apoptosis in different human colon cancer cell lines.	[49]
Lactobacillus and *Bifidobacterium species*	Anti-cancerous activity	Through antioxidants, it reduce reactive oxygen species, regulates cell cycle, activate caspases leading to the death of cancerous cells, and activate pro-apoptotic Bax protein.	[11]
A randomized phase III clinical trial probiotic supplementation of *L. rhamnosus* with FU-based chemotherapy	Relives CRC symptoms	Reduces abdominal pain and diarrhoea frequency.	[50]
E. faecalis, *L. acidophilus* and *B. longum*	CRC suppression	Reduces *Fusobacterium* species.	[51]
Dietary synbiotic (*L. rhamnosus* GG, *B. lactis* Bb12, and oligofructose-enriched insulin)	CRC suppression	Improves the epithelial barrier and reduces tumor cell proliferation.	[52]
A randomized clinical trial dietary fibre with *L. casei*	Reduces colorectal tumors	Reduces tumor cell proliferation.	[53]

(Table 1) cont.....

Bacteria	Function	Mechanism	Reference
Mixture of probiotic strains: *B. longum, B. bifidum, B. infanis, L. casei, L. acidophilus* and *L. lacis* with ω-3 fatty acid	Improves the health of CRC patients	Reduces inflammation.	[52]
A placebo-controlled clinical trial mixture of probiotic, prebiotic and symbiotic	Improves CRC patients' health	Improves gut microbiota, DNA methylation and CRC biomarkers.	[54]
Lactobacillus strains	Improves CRC patients' health	Reduces inflammation after surgery.	[55 - 58]
B. longum and *L. johnsonii* probiotics	Improves CRC patients' health	Reduces serum zonulin level, infections, and post-surgery compilations.	[59]
L. acidophilus	Reduces tumor in colitis-associated CRC models and alleviation of gut inflammation	Activation of immune response; Cytotoxic effect on tumor cells; Decreases the expression of the inflammation-associated genes.	[60 - 63]
L. acidophilus and *L. bulgaricus*	Protection against *H. Pylori*	Inhibition of *H. pylori* adherence by production of acetic acid and other bactericidal substances.	[64]
L. acidophilus, and *B. animalis subsp. Lactis*	Suppression of crypt foci and CRC	Inhibition of pre-neoplastic lesions Suppression of antioxidant enzymes (SOD) and apoptosis-related proteins (caspase-3 and Bcl-2).	[65]
L. acidophilus CL1285, *L. casei* LBC80R and *L. rhamnosus* CLR2	Inhibition of colon cancer (HT-29) cell proliferation	Protection against toxic and reactive chemical species and stimulation of quinone reductase activity.	[66]
L. plantarum and *L. salivarius*	Prevention of CRC development	Upregulation of IL-18 production.	[67]
B. longum	Inhibition of CRC growth	Enhancement of SCFAs production and reducing the amount of *Bacteroides fragilis* enterotoxin	[68]
VSL#3	Reduction of pre-neoplastic lesions in colitis-associated cancer models	Regulation of the intestinal barrier integrity and endogenous antioxidant defense system.	[69]
P. pentosaceus FP3, *L. salivarius* FP35 and FP25, *E. faecium* FP51	Inhibition of colon cancer cell proliferation	Production of SCFAs like propionic and butyric acid.	[70]

4.1. Animal Model Studies

Studies suggested that the administration of *Lactobacillus* species probiotics can suppress carcinoma cell line proliferation by modulating the WNt/- β-catenin, which plays a critical role in CRC development [35] (Table. **1**). The *Lactobacillus* species can detox N-nitrosodimethylamine, and suppress the cancer development [35]. The *L. acidophilus* CICC 6074 S-layer exhibits G1 phase arrest by upregulating tumor suppressor proteins resulting in the suppression of colon cancer [11]. *L. acidophilus* fermented brown rice has been shown to suppress TNF-α, IL-6, and IL-1 levels and increased the pro-apoptotic cleaved caspase-3 and Bax, which resulted in the suppression of CRC [36].

Furthermore, the long-term dietary supplementation of *L. rhamnosus* maintained the gut microbiome [11]. Additionally, *L. rhamnosus* protected against CRC in rats [37]. *L. casei,* through upregulation of TNF-related apoptosis-inducing ligand (TRAIL) was shown to suppress carcinoma cells [38]. The oral administration of *Bifidobacterium* cocktail decreased *Mucispirillum, Desulfovibrio,* and *Odoribacter* species, thereby suppressing the cancer development. It was suggested that *Bifidobacterium* induces apoptosis of adenocarcinoma cells and increases anti-tumor response resulting in the tumor suppression in mice [39]. A combined mixture of *L. acidophilus, L. rhamnosus,* and *B. bifidum* probiotics also suppressed the tumor size and number in mice [40].

In vitro studies involving *L. plantarum* showed decreased carcinoma cell line proliferation, reduction in cholesterol levels, TNF-α, and bacterial pro-carcinogenic fecal enzymes, suggesting it to be suitable for CRC treatment [41]. In another study, *Lactobacillus reuteri* suppressed the tumor progression, decreased inflammation, and prevented metastasis [42]. Moreover, secretory molecules such as SCFAs, polysaccharides, nucleic acids, or proteins can be used to treat CRC and reduce metastasis [71]. *Bacillus licheniformis* has been shown to have anti-cancerous activity in carcinoma cell line [43]. *E. coli* probiotics upregulate phosphatase, tensin homolog and Bax and downregulate AKT serine/threonine kinase 1 and Bcl-xL genes, thereby suppressing the CRC development [44]. Additionally, *E. faecalis* strains suppressed the growth of carcinoma cell lines [45]. Interestingly, the compounds tacrolimus and rapamycin isolated from *Streptomycetes* have been shown to contribute in the cancer suppression [46, 47]. SCFAs produced by *Propionibacterium freudenreichii* suppressed the proliferation of CRC cells and increased the cancer cell death [48]. The probiotic yeasts *Kluyveromyces marxianus* and *Pichia kudriavzevii* from dairy products have been demonstrated to inhibit AKT-1, and Janus Kinase 1 pathways and to induce apoptosis in different human colon cancer cell lines [49]. Furthermore, both the *Lactobacillus* and *Bifidobacterium* spp. suppressed CRC by increasing antioxidant capacity. The *Lactobacillus* and *Bifidobacterium* species can produce antioxidants, reduce ROS, regulate cell cycle, activate caspases leading to the death of cancerous cells, and activate pro-apoptotic Bax protein, thereby contributing to anti-cancerous activity [11].

4.2. Human Clinical Trials

A randomized phase III clinical trial suggested probiotic supplementation of *L. rhamnosus* with FU-based chemotherapy substantially reduced abdominal pain and diarrhoea frequency [50] (Table. 1). Additionally, gut microbiota density and frequency of *Fusobacterium* species were also found to be decreased after treatment with *E. faecalis, L. acidophilus* and *B. longum* [51]. Dietary synbiotic (*L. rhamnosus* GG, *B. lactis* Bb12, and oligofructose-enriched insulin) was shown to improve epithelial barrier and to reduce tumor cell proliferation [52]. A randomized clinical trial suggested that dietary fibre with *L. casei* reduces the colorectal tumors [53]. Moreover, a mixture of probiotic strains *B. longum, B. bifidum, B. infanis, L. casei, L. acidophilus* and *L. lacis* along with ω-3 fatty acid reduced the inflammation and improved the health of CRC patients [72]. Supplementation with *L. rhamnosus* and *L. acidophilus* also improved CRC patients' health [73]. Interestingly, A placebo-controlled clinical trial suggested that a mixture of probiotic, prebiotic and symbiotic improves gut microbiota, DNA methylation and CRC biomarkers [54].

Furthermore, meta-analysis of randomized controlled trials suggested that *Lactobacillus* strains reduce inflammation after surgery, post-operative complications, improves intestinal mucosal barrier function and improves CRC patients' health [55 - 58]. Additionally, *L. rhamnosus* and *L. acidophilus* supplementation significantly improved CRC patients' health. Moreover, a combination of *B. lactis, L. acidophilus, L. plantarum,* and *Saccharomyces boulardii* improves quality of life of CRC patients after surgery [74]. Studies also suggested that *Enterococcus faecalis, Clostridium butyricum, Bacillus mesentericus, L. acidophilus, L. casei, L. lactis, B. infantis. B. bifidum,* and *B. longum* before surgery significantly improved post-operational complications [75, 76]. In addition, *B. longum* and *L. johnsonii* probiotics improved CRC patients' health, by reducing serum zonulin level, infections, and post-surgery compilations [59].

5. PROBIOTICS MECHANISMS INVOLVED IN TREATMENT OF COLORECTAL CANCER

Currently, a clear understanding of the anti-cancerous activity of probiotics in the treatment of CRC is lacking. However, recent studies suggest that probiotics can modify the gut microbiota composition, secrete anti-cancer and anti-microbial compounds, improve antioxidant levels, enhance immune response, promote apoptosis of cancerous cells, and inhibit tumor growth, and exert anti-proliferative effects, thereby suppressing the CRC development [10] (Fig. 1).

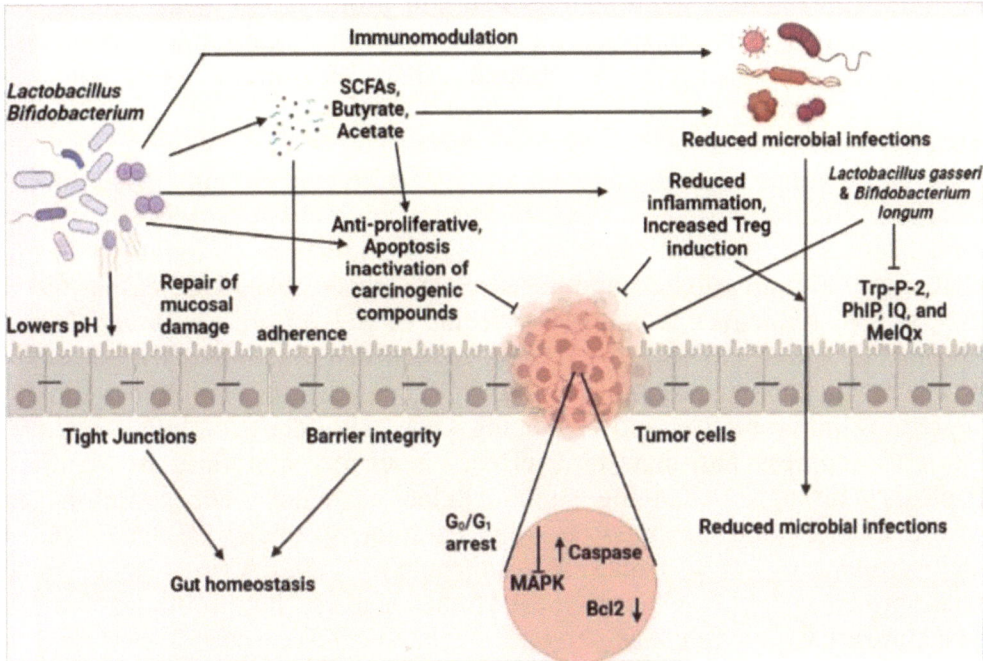

Fig. (1). Mechanism of action of probiotics in the treatment of colorectal cancer.

Probiotic treatment by enhancing host innate and adaptive immune response suppresses the CRC development. Furthermore, probiotics through the production of short chain fatty acids (SCFAs) such as butyrate and acetate, induce anti-proliferative and apoptotic responses in CRC cells. Additionally, probiotics protect the intestinal mucosal layer against invasion and bacterial infection. Probiotics can also inhibit carcinogenic agents by binding or deactivating heterocyclic aromatic amines [HCA] and N-nitroses. Probiotics can exert anti-cancerous effects in CRC by regulating tyrosine kinase signalling pathway. Overall, probiotics suppress CRC development by altering the gut microbiota composition, producing anti-microbial compounds, improving antioxidant levels, enhancing immune response, promoting apoptosis of cancerous cells, and inhibiting the tumor growth.

5.1. Regulation of Apoptosis

In cancerous cells, alteration of cell proliferation and decreased apoptosis is one of the key pathogenic mechanisms [77]. The regulation of apoptosis, cell proliferation, and cell growth can lead to advances in cancer treatment [78]. Probiotics can regulate the apoptosis and cell proliferation of cancerous cells, leading to effective therapeutics for CRC [10]. The oral administration of *L. acidophilus* was shown to have cytotoxic effects on tumor cells by enhancing apoptosis and activating the NF-κB pathway [64]. Additionally, *L. acidophilus* probiotics treatment has been shown to inhibit Bcl-2 [65]. *L. reuteri* can regulate apoptosis *via* enhancing pro-apoptotic mitogen-activated protein kinase [MAPK] signalling [79]. Moreover, *Lactobacillus* EPSs (exopolysaccharides) have shown anti-cancerous effects and prevented CRC by induction of apoptosis through enhancing the expression of apoptosis-related genes caspase-3, caspase-9 and BAX, and by reducing the expression levels of Bcl-2 [80]. Moreover, *L. casei* prevented CRC development by enhancing apoptosis through modulation of IL-22 and increasing the expression of caspase-7 [81]. *L. plantarum* inhibited colitis by suppressing inflammation and enhancing apoptosis [82]. *L. lactis* species was shown to suppress anti-metastatic effects in cancer cell lines by regulating apoptosis through changing intracellular calcium concentration and downregulating the expression of carcinoembryonic antigen (CEA), carcinoembryonic cell adhesion molecule 6 (CEAM6), and matrix metalloproteinases [83]. Overall, these studies suggest that probiotics treatment can suppress CRC by enhancing apoptosis related genes caspase-3, caspase-9 and caspase-7 and regulating calcium concentration, CEA, CEAM6, and matrix metalloproteinases (Fig. **1**).

5.2. Inhibition of Tumor Cell Proliferation

Probiotic species can suppress tumor cells by regulating cell differentiation and proliferation, thereby preventing CRC. *Lactobacillus reuteri* can suppress TNF-induced NF-κB activation [79]. Additionally, *L. reuteri* can regulate cell proliferation by inhibiting IκBα ubiquitination and inducing the expression of the MAPK signalling pathway [79]. The COX-2 expression is generally enhanced in CRC tumors and was suppressed by probiotic mixture VSL#3, leading to the prevention of CRC [84]. Fermented milk containing combination of bacteria: *L. acidophilus, L. helveticus, L. bulgaricus, Bifidobacterium,* and *Streptococcus thermophilus* decreased the number of tumor cells [85]. *Bifidobacterium breve* R0070 + *Lactobacillus lactis* R1058 + *oligoalternan* showed inhibition of tumor cell growth by suppressing intestinal alkaline phosphatase, a biomarker of colic differentiation [85]. Additionally, *B. longum* inhibited ornithine decarboxylase activity, which was involved in colonic tumor cell proliferation and differentiation [86]. Overall, these studies suggest that probiotics can prevent CRC by suppressing tumor cell differentiation and proliferation pathway [10] (Fig. **1**).

5.3. Modulation of Host Immune Response

The immune response plays a crucial role in tumor regulation. Probiotics can modulate the immune response to control the tumor growth [10]. *Lactobacillus* species were shown to have anti-tumor activity *in vivo*. *Lactobacillus casei Shirota* demonstrated to contribute to enhanced host immune response that led to anti-tumor effects in CRC [87]. After the probiotics are ingested into the host, they get phagocytosed by dendritic cells (DCs) and macrophages; then the components are recognized by toll-like receptors in APCs and lead to the production of cytokines such as IFN-γ, TNF-α, IL-1β that stimulate the anti-tumor immune response [10]. Moreover, probiotics can lead to tumor suppression through specific and non-specific mechanisms. The possible mechanism of tumor suppression is through the proliferation and activation of natural killer (NK) cells, which leads to killing of tumor cells [88]. Additionally, probiotic species have been shown to activate Th1 cells, that further induce the tumor specific cellular immunity [89]. Furthermore, *L. acidophilus* SNUL, *L. casei* YIT9029 and *B. longum* HY8001 were shown to suppress the cancer cells by activation of cytotoxic T cells and NK cells [90]. Thus, probiotic treatment by enhancing host innate and adaptive immune response can suppress the CRC development (Fig. **1**).

5.4. Short Chain Fatty Acids (SCFAs)

Probiotics can transform dietary products into SCFAs associated with anti-cancerous properties [91]. The fermentation of indigestible foods can generate SCFAs such as butyrate, acetate, and propionate [92]. This SCFAs are reduce secondary bile salts and provide nutrients and energy for the growth of intestinal mucosa [7]. Additionally, SCFAs reduce the proliferation of tumor cells [93, 94]. Moreover, probiotics regulate immune response and maintain homeostasis *via* the production of acetate butyrate, and other SCFAs [7]. Interestingly, butyrate producing *Faecalibacterium prausnitzii* is inversely associated with CRC [31]. Moreover, acetate and propionate have been found to actively regulate apoptosis in cancerous cells [95, 96]. Synbiotics comprising probiotics and butyrate have also been shown to induce apoptosis leading to CRC treatment [91]. Thus, these studies indicate that probiotics, through the production of SCFAs, can prevent CRC *via* maintaining immune homeostasis and regulating cancer cell proliferation (Fig. **1**).

5.5. Reduction of Microbial Infection

Various bacteria colonize the GIT [10] and play a crucial role in maintaining gut homeostasis [97]. They are essential in the absorption of nutrients, carbohydrates, vitamins, and activation of immune response [10]. However, dysbiosis in the gut microbiota is linked with CRC pathogenesis. The dysbiosis leads to the growth of opportunistic infections in the gut [7]. For example, antibiotic treatments are linked with the development of *Clostridium difficile* colitis [98]. Additionally, there was abundance of *Bacteroides* and *clostridium* spp. in CRC, whereas *Lactobacillus* and *Eubacterium aerofaciens* were found to be protective against CRC [99]. Interestingly, in CRC patients, probiotics alter the gut microbiota, leading to a significant reduction in pathogenic bacteria and a significant increase in protective *Lactobacillus* and *Bifidobacterium* [100, 101]. *L. reuteri* supressed CRC by inhibiting enteropathogenic *E. coli* infection by binding to the mucus layer and providing a strong epithelial barrier [102]. Moreover, the probiotic treatment, *B. longum* inhibited the CRC cells growth by significantly enhancing SCFAs production and reducing *Bacteroides fragilis* enterotoxin [68]. Furthermore, *B. pullicaecorum* reduced the CRC development by suppressing the pathogens in the cecum and ileum [77]. *L. acidophilus* showed protection against *H. pylori* infection by producing acetic acid and other bactericidal substances [64]. Additionally, probiotics VSL#3 treatment has been shown to reduce the size and number of pre-neoplastic lesions by regulating intestinal microbiota composition [69]. Although the exact mechanisms are unknown, the probiotic treatment generally improves the intestinal barrier integrity, and reduces the pathogenic bacterial infection. Moreover, it also adheres to the enterocytes, lowers pH, and enhances the antioxidant system and SCFAs production. Importantly, the probiotic species modulate the immune response in such way that pathogenic bacteria get eliminated [10]. Thus, probiotics maintain gut homeostasis by reducing pathogenic bacteria, which may efficiently counteract the CRC development (Fig. **1**).

5.6. Inactivation of Carcinogenic Compounds

The GIT is a habitat to countless microbes which can activate carcinogenic compounds [103, 104]. The carcinogenic bacteria can cause cancerous mutations in the colon [104]. Probiotic species can be used to treat CRC as they are capable of binding or degrading such carcinogenic compounds [105 - 107]. Interestingly, studies have suggested that commensal bacteria and *Lactobacillus* bind to and metabolize carcinogenic compounds such as heterocyclic amine (HCA) and N-nitroso compounds, thereby reducing mutagenicity. The probiotic species can also bind to mutagens such as Trp-P-2, PhIP, IQ, and MeIQx [10, 106]. For example, *Lactobacillus gasseri* and *Bifidobacterium longum* bind efficiently to Trp-P-1 and Trp-P-2 36. *L. acidophilus* and *Bifidobacterium* spp. bind to Trp-P-1 and by binding to such compounds *Lactobacillus casei* decreases the concentration of IQ, MelQx and PhIP [108]. Furthermore, *B. longum* and lactulose administration in rat increased the activity of glutathione-S-transferase, which is responsible for detoxification [109]. Thus, probiotic species by reducing the mutagenic compounds and increasing the enzymes responsible for detoxification can be useful for prevention and treatment of CRC (Fig. **1**).

5.7. Regulation of Tyrosine Kinase Pathway

The binding of ligands to receptors or the cellular proteins with tyrosine kinase activity activates signalling pathway [110]. The tyrosine kinase pathway plays a crucial role in cancer cell growth and development [10]. *Saccharomyces boulardii* used to treat GI disorders can regulate cell proliferation and suppress cancer cell growth by regulating mucosal immunity [111, 112]. It down-regulates the MAPK signalling pathway, and mainly, suppresses cancer cell growth by inhibiting the epidermal growth factor receptor, which plays a crucial role in cancer development [113]. Although detailed studies are lacking, the bacterium has shown to inhibit the cancer cell growth and tumor formation [10]. Thus, probiotics can have anti-cancerous effects in CRC by regulating tyrosine kinase signalling pathways (Fig. **1**).

6. FUTURE PERSPECTIVES

Although recent research has suggested beneficial effects of probiotics in CRC treatment, the detailed mechanism is unknown. Additionally, multiple interactions between the probiotics and host may vary from individual to individual. These interactions may render differential effects of the probiotics for CRC treatment. Therefore, detailed research is required in this field to develop personalized microbiome therapy for CRC treatment. Additionally, research is required to develop novel strategies, including probiotics, prebiotics, synbiotics, and fecal microbiota transplantation for the efficient treatment of CRC. In particular, synergistic effects of probiotics with anti-cancer drugs must be explored for the treatment of CRC. Moreover, it is unknown what could be the effect of multiple probiotic strains on CRC, as it may have a beneficial effect or, on the contrary. In addition, the combination therapies may have limited effectives which would be detrimental to CRC treatment and even cause other side effects. Therefore, a detailed study is required to unearth the probiotic mechanism for safe and effective treatment of CRC.

CONCLUSIONS

Promising research has highlighted the importance of probiotics in the treatment of CRC. However, the distinct mechanisms for using probiotics in treating CRC are still unclear, as different probiotic strains exert different specific mechanisms. Moreover, it is necessary to study probiotic strains' role in managing and preventing CRC in susceptible individuals. Additionally, human clinical trials are required to investigate probiotics' safety and effectiveness in treating CRC. Therefore, detailed *in vitro* and *in vivo* studies are warranted to assess the efficacy of the use of different probiotic strains in the treatment and prevention of CRC.

CONSENT FOR PUBLICATION

Not applicable.

CONFLICT OF INTEREST

The authors declare no conflict of interest, financial or otherwise.

ACKNOWLEDGEMENT

We are grateful to Uka Tarsadia University, Maliba Campus, Tarsadi, Gujarat, India for providing the facilities needed for the preparation of this chapter.

REFERENCES

[1]   Rawla P, Sunkara T, Barsouk A. Epidemiology of colorectal cancer: incidence, mortality, survival, and risk factors. Prz Gastroenterol 2019; 14(2): 89-103.
[http://dx.doi.org/10.5114/pg.2018.81072] [PMID: 31616522]

[2]   Binefa G, Rodríguez-Moranta F, Teule A, Medina-Hayas M. Colorectal cancer: From prevention to personalized medicine. World J Gastroenterol 2014; 20(22): 6786-808.
[http://dx.doi.org/10.3748/wjg.v20.i22.6786] [PMID: 24944469]

[3]   Sawicki T, Ruszkowska M, Danielewicz A, Niedźwiedzka E, Arłukowicz T, Przybyłowicz KE. A Review of Colorectal Cancer in Terms of Epidemiology, Risk Factors, Development, Symptoms and Diagnosis. Cancers (Basel) 2021; 13(9): 2025. Epub ahead of print
[http://dx.doi.org/10.3390/cancers13092025] [PMID: 33922197]

[4]   Johnson CM, Wei C, Ensor JE, *et al.* Meta-analyses of colorectal cancer risk factors. Cancer Causes Control 2013; 24(6): 1207-22.
[http://dx.doi.org/10.1007/s10552-013-0201-5] [PMID: 23563998]

[5]   Siegel RL, Miller KD, Goding Sauer A, *et al.* Colorectal cancer statistics, 2020. CA Cancer J Clin 2020; 70(3): 145-64.
[http://dx.doi.org/10.3322/caac.21601] [PMID: 32133645]

[6]   Xie YH, Chen YX, Fang JY. Comprehensive review of targeted therapy for colorectal cancer. Signal Transduct Target Ther 2020; 5(1): 22.
[http://dx.doi.org/10.1038/s41392-020-0116-z] [PMID: 32296018]

[7]   Giri PS, Shah F, Dwivedi MK. Probiotics and prebiotics in the suppression of autoimmune

diseases.Probiotics in the Prevention and Management of Human Diseases. Academic Press 2022; pp. 161-86.
[http://dx.doi.org/10.1016/B978-0-12-823733-5.00019-2]

[8]   Khalighi A, Behdani R, Kouhestani S. Probiotics: A Comprehensive Review of Their Classification, Mode of Action and Role in Human Nutrition. Probiotics Prebiotics Hum Nutr Heal 2016; 13 Epub ahead of print
[http://dx.doi.org/10.5772/63646]

[9]   Rinninella E, Raoul P, Cintoni M, *et al.* What is the Healthy Gut Microbiota Composition? A Changing Ecosystem across Age, Environment, Diet, and Diseases. Microorganisms 2019; 7(1): 14. Epub ahead of print
[http://dx.doi.org/10.3390/microorganisms7010014] [PMID: 30634578]

[10]   Uccello M, Malaguarnera G, Basile F, *et al.* Potential role of probiotics on colorectal cancer prevention. BMC Surg 2012; 12(S1) (Suppl. 1): S35.
[http://dx.doi.org/10.1186/1471-2482-12-S1-S35] [PMID: 23173670]

[11]   Jampílek J, Kráľová K, Bella V. Probiotics and prebiotics in the prevention and management of human cancers (colon cancer, stomach cancer, breast cancer, and cervix cancer.Probiotics in the Prevention and Management of Human Diseases Chapter 13. 187-212.

[12]   Malki A, ElRuz RA, Gupta I, Allouch A, Vranic S, Al Moustafa AE. Molecular Mechanisms of Colon Cancer Progression and Metastasis: Recent Insights and Advancements. Int J Mol Sci 2020; 22(1): 130. Epub ahead of print
[http://dx.doi.org/10.3390/ijms22010130] [PMID: 33374459]

[13]   Pino MS, Chung DC. The chromosomal instability pathway in colon cancer. Gastroenterology 2010; 138(6): 2059-72.
[http://dx.doi.org/10.1053/j.gastro.2009.12.065] [PMID: 20420946]

[14]   Cohen Y, Merhavi-Shoham E, Avraham RB, Frenkel S, Pe'er J, Goldenberg-Cohen N. Hypermethylation of CpG island loci of multiple tumor suppressor genes in retinoblastoma. Exp Eye Res 2008; 86(2): 201-6.
[http://dx.doi.org/10.1016/j.exer.2007.10.010] [PMID: 18068703]

[15]   Board PCGE. https://www.ncbi.nlm.nih.gov/books/NBK126744/2022.

[16]   Leoz ML, Carballal S, Moreira L, Ocaña T, Balaguer F. The genetic basis of familial adenomatous polyposis and its implications for clinical practice and risk management. Appl Clin Genet 2015; 8: 95-107.
[PMID: 25931827]

[17]   Jasperson KW, Tuohy TM, Neklason DW, Burt RW. Hereditary and familial colon cancer. Gastroenterology 2010; 138(6): 2044-58.
[http://dx.doi.org/10.1053/j.gastro.2010.01.054] [PMID: 20420945]

[18]   Kim ER, Chang DK. Colorectal cancer in inflammatory bowel disease: The risk, pathogenesis, prevention and diagnosis. World J Gastroenterol 2014; 20(29): 9872-81.
[http://dx.doi.org/10.3748/wjg.v20.i29.9872] [PMID: 25110418]

[19]   Sánchez-Alcoholado L, Ramos-Molina B, Otero Λ, *et al.* The Role of the Gut Microbiome in Colorectal Cancer Development and Therapy Response. Cancers (Basel) 2020; 12(6): 1406. Epub ahead of print
[http://dx.doi.org/10.3390/cancers12061406] [PMID: 32486066]

[20]   Dai Z, Zhang J, Wu Q, *et al.* The role of microbiota in the development of colorectal cancer. Int J Cancer 2019; 145(8): 2032-41.
[http://dx.doi.org/10.1002/ijc.32017] [PMID: 30474116]

[21]   Cheng Y, Ling Z, Li L. The Intestinal Microbiota and Colorectal Cancer. Front Immunol 2020; 11: 615056.

[http://dx.doi.org/10.3389/fimmu.2020.615056] [PMID: 33329610]

[22]   Sears CL, Pardoll DM. Perspective: alpha-bugs, their microbial partners, and the link to colon cancer. J Infect Dis 2011; 203(3): 306-11.
[http://dx.doi.org/10.1093/jinfdis/jiq061] [PMID: 21208921]

[23]   Tjalsma H, Boleij A, Marchesi JR, Dutilh BE. A bacterial driver–passenger model for colorectal cancer: beyond the usual suspects. Nat Rev Microbiol 2012; 10(8): 575-82.
[http://dx.doi.org/10.1038/nrmicro2819] [PMID: 22728587]

[24]   Wu HJ, Wu E. The role of gut microbiota in immune homeostasis and autoimmunity. Gut Microbes 2012; 3(1): 4-14.
[http://dx.doi.org/10.4161/gmic.19320] [PMID: 22356853]

[25]   Vivarelli S, Salemi R, Candido S, *et al.* Gut Microbiota and Cancer: From Pathogenesis to Therapy. Cancers (Basel) 2019; 11(1): 38. Epub ahead of print
[http://dx.doi.org/10.3390/cancers11010038] [PMID: 30609850]

[26]   Conlon M, Bird A. The impact of diet and lifestyle on gut microbiota and human health. Nutrients 2014; 7(1): 17-44.
[http://dx.doi.org/10.3390/nu7010017] [PMID: 25545101]

[27]   Redondo-Useros N, Nova E, González-Zancada N, Díaz LE, Gómez-Martínez S, Marcos A. Microbiota and Lifestyle: A Special Focus on Diet. Nutrients 2020; 12(6): 1776. Epub ahead of print
[http://dx.doi.org/10.3390/nu12061776] [PMID: 32549225]

[28]   Rye MS, Garrett KL, Holt RA, Platell CF, McCoy MJ. *Fusobacterium nucleatum* and *Bacteroides fragilis* detection in colorectal tumours: Optimal target site and correlation with total bacterial load. PLoS One 2022; 17(1): e0262416.
[http://dx.doi.org/10.1371/journal.pone.0262416] [PMID: 34995318]

[29]   Sun CH, Li BB, Wang B, *et al.* The role of *Fusobacterium nucleatum* in colorectal cancer: from carcinogenesis to clinical management. Chronic Dis Transl Med 2019; 5(3): 178-87.
[http://dx.doi.org/10.1016/j.cdtm.2019.09.001] [PMID: 31891129]

[30]   Shah MS, DeSantis TZ, Weinmaier T, *et al.* Leveraging sequence-based faecal microbial community survey data to identify a composite biomarker for colorectal cancer. Gut 2018; 67(5): 882-91.
[http://dx.doi.org/10.1136/gutjnl-2016-313189] [PMID: 28341746]

[31]   Gao R, Gao Z, Huang L, Qin H. Gut microbiota and colorectal cancer. Eur J Clin Microbiol Infect Dis 2017; 36(5): 757-69.
[http://dx.doi.org/10.1007/s10096-016-2881-8] [PMID: 28063002]

[32]   Ding S, Hu C, Fang J, Liu G. The Protective Role of Probiotics against Colorectal Cancer. Oxid Med Cell Longev 2020; 2020: 1-10.
[http://dx.doi.org/10.1155/2020/8884583] [PMID: 33488940]

[33]   Michalaki V, Syrigos K, Charles P, Waxman J. Serum levels of IL-6 and TNF-α correlate with clinicopathological features and patient survival in patients with prostate cancer. Br J Cancer 2004; 90(12): 2312-6.
[http://dx.doi.org/10.1038/sj.bjc.6601814] [PMID: 15150588]

[34]   Avril M, DePaolo RW. "Driver-passenger" bacteria and their metabolites in the pathogenesis of colorectal cancer. Gut Microbes 2021; 13(1): 1941710.
[http://dx.doi.org/10.1080/19490976.2021.1941710] [PMID: 34225577]

[35]   Ghanavati R, Akbari A, Mohammadi F, *et al. Lactobacillus* species inhibitory effect on colorectal cancer progression through modulating the Wnt/β-catenin signaling pathway. Mol Cell Biochem 2020; 470(1-2): 1-13.
[http://dx.doi.org/10.1007/s11010-020-03740-8] [PMID: 32419125]

[36]   Lin PY, Li SC, Lin HP, Shih CK. Germinated brown rice combined with *Lactobacillus acidophilus* and *Bifidobacterium animalis* subsp. *lactis* inhibits colorectal carcinogenesis in rats. Food Sci Nutr

2019; 7(1): 216-24.
[http://dx.doi.org/10.1002/fsn3.864] [PMID: 30680175]

[37]   Huang J, Wang D, Zhang A, Zhong Q, Huang Q. *Lactobacillus rhamnosus* confers protection against colorectal cancer in rats. Trop J Pharm Res 2021; 18(7): 1449-54.
[http://dx.doi.org/10.4314/tjpr.v18i7.12]

[38]   Tiptiri-Kourpeti A, Spyridopoulou K, Santarmaki V, *et al. Lactobacillus casei* Exerts Anti-Proliferative Effects Accompanied by Apoptotic Cell Death and Up-Regulation of TRAIL in Colon Carcinoma Cells. PLoS One 2016; 11(2): e0147960.
[http://dx.doi.org/10.1371/journal.pone.0147960] [PMID: 26849051]

[39]   Parisa A, Roya G, Mahdi R, Shabnam R, Maryam E, Malihe T. Anti-cancer effects of *Bifidobacterium* species in colon cancer cells and a mouse model of carcinogenesis. PLoS One 2020; 15(5): e0232930.
[http://dx.doi.org/10.1371/journal.pone.0232930] [PMID: 32401801]

[40]   Mendes MCS, Paulino DSM, Brambilla SR, Camargo JA, Persinoti GF, Carvalheira JBC. Microbiota modification by probiotic supplementation reduces colitis associated colon cancer in mice. World J Gastroenterol 2018; 24(18): 1995-2008.
[http://dx.doi.org/10.3748/wjg.v24.i18.1995] [PMID: 29760543]

[41]   Chundakkattumalayil HC, Kumar S, Narayanan R, Thalakattil Raghavan K. Role of *L. plantarum* KX519413 as Probiotic and Acacia Gum as Prebiotic in Gastrointestinal Tract Strengthening. Microorganisms 2019; 7(12): 659. Epub ahead of print
[http://dx.doi.org/10.3390/microorganisms7120659]

[42]   Bistas KG, Bistas E, Nyamwaya ME. *Lactobacillus reuteri's* role in the prevention of colorectal cancer: a review of literature. Univ Toronto Med J 2020; 97: 29-36.

[43]   Mahajan RV, Kumar V, Rajendran V, Saran S, Ghosh PC, Saxena RK. Purification and characterization of a novel and robust L-asparaginase having low-glutaminase activity from *Bacillus licheniformis*: *in vitro* evaluation of anti-cancerous properties. PLoS One 2014; 9(6): e99037.
[http://dx.doi.org/10.1371/journal.pone.0099037] [PMID: 24905227]

[44]   Alizadeh S, Esmaeili A, Omidi Y. Anti-cancer properties of *Escherichia coli* Nissle 1917 against HT-29 colon cancer cells through regulation of Bax/Bcl-xL and AKT/PTEN signaling pathways. Iran J Basic Med Sci 2020; 23(7): 886-93.
[PMID: 32774810]

[45]   Williamson AJ, Jacobson R, van Praagh JB, *et al. Enterococcus faecalis* promotes a migratory and invasive phenotype in colon cancer cells. Neoplasia 2022; 27: 100787.
[http://dx.doi.org/10.1016/j.neo.2022.100787] [PMID: 35366466]

[46]   Bolourian A, Mojtahedi Z. Immunosuppressants produced by *Streptomyces* : evolution, hygiene hypothesis, tumour rapalog resistance and probiotics. Environ Microbiol Rep 2018; 10(2): 123-6.
[http://dx.doi.org/10.1111/1758-2229.12617] [PMID: 29377607]

[47]   Bolourian A, Mojtahedi Z. Streptomyces, shared microbiome member of soil and gut, as 'old friends' against colon cancer. FEMS Microbiol Ecol 2018; 94(8): fiy120.
[http://dx.doi.org/10.1093/femsec/fiy120] [PMID: 29912397]

[48]   Casanova MR, Azevedo-Silva J, Rodrigues LR, Preto A. Colorectal Cancer Cells Increase the Production of Short Chain Fatty Acids by *Propionibacterium freudenreichii* Impacting on Cancer Cells Survival. Front Nutr 2018; 5: 44.
[http://dx.doi.org/10.3389/fnut.2018.00044] [PMID: 29881727]

[49]   Rahbar Saadat Y, Yari Khosroushahi A, Movassaghpour AA, Talebi M, Pourghassem Gargari B. Modulatory role of exopolysaccharides of *Kluyveromyces marxianus* and *Pichia kudriavzevii* as probiotic yeasts from dairy products in human colon cancer cells. J Funct Foods 2020; 64: 103675.
[http://dx.doi.org/10.1016/j.jff.2019.103675]

[50]   Österlund P, Ruotsalainen T, Korpela R, *et al. Lactobacillus* supplementation for diarrhoea related to

chemotherapy of colorectal cancer: a randomised study. Br J Cancer 2007; 97(8): 1028-34.
[http://dx.doi.org/10.1038/sj.bjc.6603990] [PMID: 17895895]

[51]   Gao Z, Guo B, Gao R, Zhu Q, Wu W, Qin H. Probiotics modify human intestinal mucosa-associated
       microbiota in patients with colorectal cancer. Mol Med Rep 2015; 12(4): 6119-27.
       [http://dx.doi.org/10.3892/mmr.2015.4124] [PMID: 26238090]

[52]   Rafter J, Bennett M, Caderni G, *et al.* Dietary synbiotics reduce cancer risk factors in polypectomized
       and colon cancer patients. Am J Clin Nutr 2007; 85(2): 488-96.
       [http://dx.doi.org/10.1093/ajcn/85.2.488] [PMID: 17284748]

[53]   Sivamaruthi BS, Kesika P, Chaiyasut C. The Role of Probiotics in Colorectal Cancer Management
       Evid Based Complement Alternat Med 2020. Epub ahead of print 2020
       [http://dx.doi.org/10.1155/2020/3535982]

[54]   Worthley DL, Le Leu RK, Whitehall VL, *et al.* A human, double-blind, placebo-controlled, crossover
       trial of prebiotic, probiotic, and synbiotic supplementation: effects on luminal, inflammatory,
       epigenetic, and epithelial biomarkers of colorectal cancer. Am J Clin Nutr 2009; 90(3): 578-86.
       [http://dx.doi.org/10.3945/ajcn.2009.28106] [PMID: 19640954]

[55]   He D, Wang HY, Feng JY, Zhang MM, Zhou Y, Wu XT. Use of pro-/synbiotics as prophylaxis in
       patients undergoing colorectal resection for cancer: A meta-analysis of randomized controlled trials.
       Clin Res Hepatol Gastroenterol 2013; 37(4): 406-15.
       [http://dx.doi.org/10.1016/j.clinre.2012.10.007] [PMID: 23182673]

[56]   De Andrade Calaça PR, Bezerra RP, Albuquerque WWC, Porto ALF, Cavalcanti MTH. Probiotics as
       a preventive strategy for surgical infection in colorectal cancer patients: a systematic review and meta-
       analysis of randomized trials. Transl Gastroenterol Hepatol 2017; 2(8): 67. Epub ahead of print
       [http://dx.doi.org/10.21037/tgh.2017.08.01] [PMID: 28905008]

[57]   Ouyang X, Li Q, Shi M, *et al.* Probiotics for preventing postoperative infection in colorectal cancer
       patients: a systematic review and meta-analysis. Int J Colorectal Dis 2019; 34(3): 459-69.
       [http://dx.doi.org/10.1007/s00384-018-3214-4] [PMID: 30539265]

[58]   Liu D, Jiang XY, Zhou LS, Song JH, Zhang X. Effects of Probiotics on Intestinal Mucosa Barrier in
       Patients With Colorectal Cancer after Operation. Medicine (Baltimore) 2016; 95(15): e3342. Epub
       ahead of print
       [http://dx.doi.org/10.1097/MD.0000000000003342] [PMID: 27082589]

[59]   Liu ZH, Huang MJ, Zhang XW, *et al.* The effects of perioperative probiotic treatment on serum
       zonulin concentration and subsequent postoperative infectious complications after colorectal cancer
       surgery: a double-center and double-blind randomized clinical trial. Am J Clin Nutr 2013; 97(1): 117-
       26.
       [http://dx.doi.org/10.3945/ajcn.112.040949] [PMID: 23235200]

[60]   Lau S. Bacterial lysates in food allergy prevention. Curr Opin Allergy Clin Immunol 2013; 13(3): 293-
       5.
       [http://dx.doi.org/10.1097/ACI.0b013e328360ede9] [PMID: 23842540]

[61]   Zhuo Q, Yu B, Zhou J etal. *et al.* Lysates of *Lactobacillus acidophilus* combined with CTLA-
       -blocking antibodies enhance antitumor immunity in a mouse colon cancer model. Sci Reports 2019
       91 2019; 9: 1-12.

[62]   Deol PK, Khare P, Bishnoi M, Kondepudi KK, Kaur IP. Coadministration of ginger extract-
       Lactobacillus acidophilus (cobiotic) reduces gut inflammation and oxidative stress *via* downregulation
       of *COX-2*, *i-NOS*, and *c-Myc*. Phytother Res 2018; 32(10): 1950-6.
       [http://dx.doi.org/10.1002/ptr.6121] [PMID: 29876980]

[63]   El-Deeb NM, Yassin AM, Al-Madboly LA, El-Hawiet A. A novel purified *Lactobacillus acidophilus*
       20079 exopolysaccharide, LA-EPS-20079, molecularly regulates both apoptotic and NF-κB
       inflammatory pathways in human colon cancer. Microb Cell Fact 2018; 17(1): 29. Epub ahead of print
       [http://dx.doi.org/10.1186/s12934-018-0877-z] [PMID: 29466981]

[64]   Song H, Zhou L, Liu D, Ge L, Li Y. Probiotic effect on *Helicobacter☐pylori* attachment and inhibition of inflammation in human gastric epithelial cells. Exp Ther Med 2019; 18(3): 1551-62. Epub ahead of print
[http://dx.doi.org/10.3892/etm.2019.7742] [PMID: 31410109]

[65]   Lin PY, Li SC, Lin HP, Shih CK. Germinated brown rice combined with *Lactobacillus acidophilus* and *Bifidobacterium animalis* subsp. *lactis* inhibits colorectal carcinogenesis in rats. Food Sci Nutr 2019; 7(1): 216-24.
[http://dx.doi.org/10.1002/fsn3.864] [PMID: 30680175]

[66]   Desrouillères K, Millette M, Bagheri L, Maherani B, Jamshidian M, Lacroix M. The synergistic effect of cell wall extracted from probiotic biomass containing *Lactobacillus acidophilus* CL1285, *L. casei* LBC80R, and *L. rhamnosus* CLR2 on the anticancer activity of cranberry juice—HPLC fractions. J Food Biochem 2020; 44(5): e13195.
[http://dx.doi.org/10.1111/jfbc.13195] [PMID: 32185816]

[67]   Hradicka P, Beal J, Kassayova M, Foey A, Demeckova V. A Novel Lactic Acid Bacteria Mixture: Macrophage-Targeted Prophylactic Intervention in Colorectal Cancer Management. Microorg 2020; Vol 8: Page 387. 2020; 8: 387.

[68]   Ohara T, Suzutani T. Intake of *Bifidobacterium longum* and Fructo-oligosaccharides prevents Colorectal Carcinogenesis Euroasian J hepato-gastroenterology. 2018; 8: 11-7.

[69]   Cruz BCS, Conceição LL, Mendes TAO, Ferreira CLLF, Gonçalves RV, Peluzio MCG. Use of the synbiotic VSL#3 and yacon-based concentrate attenuates intestinal damage and reduces the abundance of Candidatus Saccharimonas in a colitis-associated carcinogenesis model. Food Res Int 2020; 137: 109721.
[http://dx.doi.org/10.1016/j.foodres.2020.109721] [PMID: 33233290]

[70]   Thirabunyanon M, Hongwittayakorn P. Potential Probiotic Lactic Acid Bacteria of Human Origin Induce Antiproliferation of Colon Cancer Cells *via* Synergic Actions in Adhesion to Cancer Cells and Short-Chain Fatty Acid Bioproduction. Appl Biochem Biotechnol 2012 1692. 2012; 169: 511-25.

[71]   Mahdavi M, Laforest-Lapointe I, Massé E. Preventing Colorectal Cancer through Prebiotics. Microorganisms 2021; 9(6): 1325. Epub ahead of print
[http://dx.doi.org/10.3390/microorganisms9061325] [PMID: 34207094]

[72]   Golkhalkhali B, Rajandram R, Paliany AS, *et al.* Strain-specific probiotic (microbial cell preparation) and omega-3 fatty acid in modulating quality of life and inflammatory markers in colorectal cancer patients: a randomized controlled trial. Asia Pac J Clin Oncol 2018; 14(3): 179-91.
[http://dx.doi.org/10.1111/ajco.12758] [PMID: 28857425]

[73]   Lee JY, Chu SH, Jeon JY, *et al.* Effects of 12 weeks of probiotic supplementation on quality of life in colorectal cancer survivors: A double-blind, randomized, placebo-controlled trial. Dig Liver Dis 2014; 46(12): 1126-32.
[http://dx.doi.org/10.1016/j.dld.2014.09.004] [PMID: 25442120]

[74]   Kotzampassi K, Stavrou G, Damoraki G, *et al.* A Four-Probiotics Regimen Reduces Postoperative Complications After Colorectal Surgery: A Randomized, Double-Blind, Placebo-Controlled Study. World J Surg 2015; 39(11): 2776-83.
[http://dx.doi.org/10.1007/s00268-015-3071-z] [PMID: 25894405]

[75]   Aisu N, Tanimura S, Yamashita Y, *et al.* Impact of perioperative probiotic treatment for surgical site infections in patients with colorectal cancer. Exp Ther Med 2015; 10(3): 966-72.
[http://dx.doi.org/10.3892/etm.2015.2640] [PMID: 26622423]

[76]   Tan CK, Said S, Rajandram R, Wang Z, Roslani AC, Chin KF. Pre-surgical Administration of Microbial Cell Preparation in Colorectal Cancer Patients: A Randomized Controlled Trial. World J Surg 2016; 40(8): 1985-92.
[http://dx.doi.org/10.1007/s00268-016-3499-9] [PMID: 27098538]

[77]   Torres-Maravilla E, Boucard AS, Mohseni AH, Taghinezhad-S S, Cortes-Perez NG, Bermúdez-Humarán LG. Role of Gut Microbiota and Probiotics in Colorectal Cancer: Onset and Progression. Microorganisms 2021; 9(5): 1021. Epub ahead of print
[http://dx.doi.org/10.3390/microorganisms9051021] [PMID: 34068653]

[78]   Fesik SW. Promoting apoptosis as a strategy for cancer drug discovery. Nat Rev Cancer 2005; 5(11): 876-85.
[http://dx.doi.org/10.1038/nrc1736] [PMID: 16239906]

[79]   Otte JM, Mahjurian-Namari R, Brand S, Werner I, Schmidt W, Schmitz F. Probiotics regulate the expression of COX-2 in intestinal epithelial cells. Nutr Cancer 2009; 61(1): 103-13.
[http://dx.doi.org/10.1080/01635580802372625] [PMID: 19116880]

[80]   Tukenmez U, Aktas B, Aslim B, Yavuz S. The relationship between the structural characteristics of lactobacilli-EPS and its ability to induce apoptosis in colon cancer cells *in vitro*. Sci Reports 2019 91 2019; 9: 1-14.

[81]   Jacouton E, Chain F, Sokol H, Langella P, Bermúdez-Humarán LG. Probiotic Strain *Lactobacillus casei* BL23 Prevents Colitis-Associated Colorectal Cancer. Front Immunol 2017; 8: 1553. Epub ahead of print
[http://dx.doi.org/10.3389/fimmu.2017.01553] [PMID: 29209314]

[82]   Lee HA, Kim H, Lee KW, Park KY. Dead Nano-Sized Lactobacillus plantarum Inhibits Azoxymethane/Dextran Sulfate Sodium-Induced Colon Cancer in Balb/c Mice. https://home.liebertpub.com/jmf 2015; 18: 1400–1405.

[83]   Norouzi Z, Salimi A, Halabian R, Fahimi H. Nisin, a potent bacteriocin and anti-bacterial peptide, attenuates expression of metastatic genes in colorectal cancer cell lines. Microb Pathog 2018; 123: 183-9.
[http://dx.doi.org/10.1016/j.micpath.2018.07.006] [PMID: 30017942]

[84]   Sano H, Kawahito Y, Wilder RL, *et al*. Expression of cyclooxygenase-1 and -2 in human colorectal cancer. Cancer Res 1995; 55(17): 3785-9.
[PMID: 7641194]

[85]   Grimoud J, Durand H, de Souza S, *et al. In vitro* screening of probiotics and synbiotics according to anti-inflammatory and anti-proliferative effects. Int J Food Microbiol 2010; 144(1): 42-50.
[http://dx.doi.org/10.1016/j.ijfoodmicro.2010.09.007] [PMID: 20951454]

[86]   Moorehead RJ, Hoper M, McKelvey STD. Assessment of ornithine decarboxylase activity in rectal mucosa as a marker for colorectal adenomas and carcinomas. Br J Surg 2005; 74(5): 364-5.
[http://dx.doi.org/10.1002/bjs.1800740513] [PMID: 3594125]

[87]   Kato I, Kobayashi S, Yokokura T, Mutai M. Antitumor activity of *Lactobacillus casei* in mice. Gann 1981; 72(4): 517-23.
[PMID: 6796451]

[88]   Takagi A, Matsuzaki T, Sato M, Nomoto K, Morotomi M, Yokokura T. Enhancement of natural killer cytotoxicity delayed murine carcinogenesis by a probiotic microorganism. Carcinogenesis 2001; 22(4): 599-605.
[http://dx.doi.org/10.1093/carcin/22.4.599] [PMID: 11285195]

[89]   Yasui H, Shida K, Matsuzaki T, Yokokura T. Immunomodulatory function of lactic acid bacteria. Antonie van Leeuwenhoek 1999; 76(1/4): 383-9.
[http://dx.doi.org/10.1023/A:1002041616085] [PMID: 10532394]

[90]   Lee JW, Shin JG, Kim EH, *et al*. Immunomodulatory and antitumor effects *in vivo* by the cytoplasmic fraction of *Lactobacillus casei* and *Bifidobacterium longum*. J Vet Sci 2004; 5(1): 41-8.
[http://dx.doi.org/10.4142/jvs.2004.5.1.41] [PMID: 15028884]

[91]   Mirzaei R, Afaghi A, Babakhani S, *et al*. Role of microbiota-derived short-chain fatty acids in cancer development and prevention. Biomed Pharmacother 2021; 139: 111619.

[http://dx.doi.org/10.1016/j.biopha.2021.111619] [PMID: 33906079]

[92]   Mai V. Dietary modification of the intestinal microbiota. Nutr Rev 2004; 62(6): 235-42.
[http://dx.doi.org/10.1111/j.1753-4887.2004.tb00045.x] [PMID: 15291396]

[93]   Topping DL, Clifton PM. Short-chain fatty acids and human colonic function: roles of resistant starch and nonstarch polysaccharides. Physiol Rev 2001; 81(3): 1031-64.
[http://dx.doi.org/10.1152/physrev.2001.81.3.1031] [PMID: 11427691]

[94]   Whitehead RH, Young GP, Bhathal PS. Effects of short chain fatty acids on a new human colon carcinoma cell line (LIM1215). Gut 1986; 27(12): 1457-63.
[http://dx.doi.org/10.1136/gut.27.12.1457] [PMID: 3804021]

[95]   Lan A, Lagadic-Gossmann D, Lemaire C, Brenner C, Jan G. Acidic extracellular pH shifts colorectal cancer cell death from apoptosis to necrosis upon exposure to propionate and acetate, major end-products of the human probiotic *propionibacteria*. Apoptosis 2007; 12(3): 573-91.
[http://dx.doi.org/10.1007/s10495-006-0010-3] [PMID: 17195096]

[96]   Jan G, Belzacq A-S, Haouzi D, *et al. Propionibacteria* induce apoptosis of colorectal carcinoma cells *via* short-chain fatty acids acting on mitochondria. Cell Death Differ 2002; 9(2): 179-88.
[http://dx.doi.org/10.1038/sj.cdd.4400935] [PMID: 11840168]

[97]   Manning TS, Gibson GR. Prebiotics. Best Pract Res Clin Gastroenterol 2004; 18(2): 287-98.
[http://dx.doi.org/10.1016/j.bpg.2003.10.008] [PMID: 15123070]

[98]   Mullish BH, Williams HRT. *Clostridium difficile* infection and antibiotic-associated diarrhoea. Clin Med (Lond) 2018; 18(3): 237-41.
[http://dx.doi.org/10.7861/clinmedicine.18-3-237] [PMID: 29858434]

[99]   Wang T, Cai G, Qiu Y. Structural segregation of gut microbiota between colorectal cancer patients and healthy volunteers *et al.* Structural segregation of gut microbiota between colorectal cancer patients and healthy volunteers. ISME J 2012 62. 2011; 6: 320-9.

[100] O'Mahony L, Feeney M, O'Halloran S, *et al.* Probiotic impact on microbial flora, inflammation and tumour development in IL-10 knockout mice. Aliment Pharmacol Ther 2001; 15(8): 1219-25.
[http://dx.doi.org/10.1046/j.1365-2036.2001.01027.x] [PMID: 11472326]

[101] Berretta M, Lleshi A, Fisichella R. *et al.* The role of nutrition in the development of esophageal cancer: What do we know? Front Biosci - Elit 2012; 4E: 351-7.

[102] Walsham ADS, MacKenzie DA, Cook V, *et al. Lactobacillus reuteri* Inhibition of Enteropathogenic *Escherichia coli* Adherence to Human Intestinal Epithelium. Front Microbiol 2016; 7: 244.
[http://dx.doi.org/10.3389/fmicb.2016.00244] [PMID: 26973622]

[103] Van Tassell RL, Kingston DGI, Wilkins TD. Metabolism of dietary genotoxins by the human colonic microflora; the fecapentaenes and heterocyclic amines. Mutat Res Rev Genet Toxicol 1990; 238(3): 209-21.
[http://dx.doi.org/10.1016/0165-1110(90)90013-2] [PMID: 2160606]

[104] Wakabayashi K, Nagao M, Esumi H, Sugimura T. Food-derived mutagens and carcinogens. Cancer Res 1992; 52(7) (Suppl.): 2092s-8s.
[PMID: 1544146]

[105] Kumar M, Kumar A, Nagpal R, *et al.* Cancer-preventing attributes of probiotics: an update. Int J Food Sci Nutr 2010; 61(5): 473-96.
[http://dx.doi.org/10.3109/09637480903455971] [PMID: 20187714]

[106] Orrhage K, Sillerström E, Gustafsson JÅ, Nord CE, Rafter J. Binding of mutagenic heterocyclic amines by intestinal and lactic acid bacteria. Mutat Res 1994; 311(2): 239-48.
[http://dx.doi.org/10.1016/0027-5107(94)90182-1] [PMID: 7526189]

[107] Ragusa M, Statello L, Maugeri M, *et al.* Specific alterations of the microRNA transcriptome and global network structure in colorectal cancer after treatment with MAPK/ERK inhibitors. J Mol Med

(Berl) 2012; 90(12): 1421-38.
[http://dx.doi.org/10.1007/s00109-012-0918-8] [PMID: 22660396]

[108]   Ohta Y, Ohta Y. Antimutagenicity of cell fractions of microorganisms on potent mutagenic pyrolysates. Mutat Res Genet Toxicol Test 1993; 298(4): 247-53.
[http://dx.doi.org/10.1016/0165-1218(93)90003-V] [PMID: 7678160]

[109]   Nowak A, Libudzisz Z. Ability of probiotic *Lactobacillus casei* DN 114001 to bind or/and metabolise heterocyclic aromatic amines *in vitro*. Eur J Nutr 2009; 48(7): 419-27.
[http://dx.doi.org/10.1007/s00394-009-0030-1] [PMID: 19448966]

[110]   Lemmon MA, Schlessinger J. Cell signaling by receptor tyrosine kinases. Cell 2010; 141(7): 1117-34.
[http://dx.doi.org/10.1016/j.cell.2010.06.011] [PMID: 20602996]

[111]   Sullivan Å, Nord CE. The place of probiotics in human intestinal infections. Int J Antimicrob Agents 2002; 20(5): 313-9.
[http://dx.doi.org/10.1016/S0924-8579(02)00199-1] [PMID: 12431865]

[112]   Guslandi M, Mezzi G, Sorghi M, Testoni PA. *Saccharomyces boulardii* in maintenance treatment of Crohn's disease. Dig Dis Sci 2000; 45(7): 1462-4.
[http://dx.doi.org/10.1023/A:1005588911207] [PMID: 10961730]

[113]   Czerucka D, Dahan S, Mograbi B, Rossi B, Rampal P. *Saccharomyces boulardii* preserves the barrier function and modulates the signal transduction pathway induced in enteropathogenic *Escherichia coli*-infected T84 cells. Infect Immun 2000; 68(10): 5998-6004.
[http://dx.doi.org/10.1128/IAI.68.10.5998-6004.2000] [PMID: 10992512]

CHAPTER 6

Probiotics-based Anticancer Immunity in Breast Cancer

Nosheen Masood[1,*] and **Saima Shakil Malik**[2,*]

[1] *Department of Biotechnology, Fatima Jinnah Women University, The Mall, Rawalpindi, Pakistan*

[2] *Department of Genetics, Research Division, The University of Alabama at Birmingham, AL, USA*

Abstract: A growing number of evidence is available in support of the advantageous role of a balanced intestinal microbiota in the progression and manifestation of malignant tumors, not only in the gastrointestinal tract but in other distant tissues as well, with the most potential role in breast carcinoma. Breast cancer involves a complex interplay of several factors, such as familial history, use of hormonal replacement therapy, dietary habits, lifestyle, environment, clinical features, genetics and epigenetics. Recently, a positive correlation between a patient's breast microbiome and cancer has beocme a novel potential risk factor. In the present chapter, we tried to discuss the role of microbiome as a potential breast cancer risk factor and tried to investigate the literature focussing on the proposed mechanisms behind the interaction of microbiome, human genetic makeup involved in the onset of breast carcinogenesis and determining the effect of transformed breast, milk and gut microbiome on the physiological status of both normal and malignant breast. We also tried to shed light on the resistance to chemotherapeutic treatment among individuals with altered microbiomes with an emphasis on the role of the microbiome in developing and maintaining inflammation, epigenetic alterations and estrogen metabolism. Interestingly, bacterial species are indispensable modulatory agents of widely used chemotherapeutic/ immunotherapeutic regiments. But the exact role of commensal bacteria in immunity, formation of neoplasia and response to treatment needs much more research because most of the available knowledge is based on animal model studies and needs its translation to humans which requires great precision and has various hurdles too. Therefore, we tried to give a comprehensive overview of current knowledge in terms of breast cancer therapeutics and suggest integrating probiotic bacteria and/or modulation of the intestinal microbiota to be used as immune adjuvants, targeting to enhance the effectiveness of conventional anti-tumor treatments and cancer immunotherapies as well.

Keywords: Breast microbiome, Breast cancer, Cancer therapeutics, Immunotherapies, Probiotic bacteria.

[*] **Corresponding authors Nosheen Masood and Saima Shakil Malik:** Department of Biotechnology, Fatima Jinnah Women University, The Mall, Rawalpindi, Pakistan; and Department of Genetics, Research Division, The University of Alabama at Birmingham, AL, USA; E-mails: dr.nosheen@fjwu.edu.pk and saimamalik25@yahoo.com

[#] These authors have contributed equally to this chapter

Mitesh Kumar Dwivedi, Alwarappan Sankaranarayanan & Sanjay Tiwari (Eds.)
All rights reserved-© 2023 Bentham Science Publishers

1. INTRODUCTION

Breast cancer is the 2nd most commonly occurring cancer and is the main cause of cancer-related deaths worldwide [1]. There are several factors that influence the initiation and aggressiveness of tumor, including genetic and environmental. A comparatively new agent responsible for cancer is probiotics (the beneficial microorganisms, *e.g.*, bacteria). Once cancer appears, the body responds by activating the immune cells of the body. Immune cells and epithelial cells of mucosal surface bidirectionally interact with the bacterial population present in the gastro-intestinal tract (GIT) of humans [2]. The bacterial population in GIT are dynamic, and they can perform multiple functions of metabolizing bile salts, synthesizing vitamin B and K, and regulating cytokine production for fighting against pathogenic organisms. The population of probiotics is easily altered by numerous factors like pharmaceutical use, infections, travelling to international destinations, diet, race, ethnicity and age. Changes in the GIT bacterial population is an ongoing process, therefore this means that they tend to change throughout the lifetime of an individual [3]. Various diseases like asthma, arthritis, diabetes and obesity are also linked with a change in the bacterial flora. It has been found in many studies that the excessive use of antibiotics leads to tumor development which means these bacteria have a role in carcinogenesis as well [4].

Keeping in mind the overall importance of bacteria for human health, the term probiotic was first coined by Elie Metchnikoff 100 years back. Later probiotics were defined by WHO (World Health Organization) and FAO (Food and Agricultural Organization) as 'live microorganisms which, when administered in adequate amounts (in food or as a dietary supplement) confer a health benefit on the host'. Some of the most commonly used strains of bacteria for the purpose of probiotics are summarised in Fig. (**1**). A number of probiotics stay in the GIT, and they vary from person to person and are known to reduce carcinogen exposure by restricting their absorption [5]. In the case of colon cancer, they are known to alter physio-chemical conditions, produce anti-mutagenic components, degrade carcinogens, alter the activity of metabolic micro-flora and enhance the immune response of the host [6]. In this chapter, detailed information is provided regarding how these probiotics affect breast tissue and their effects on the treatment of breast cancer patients.

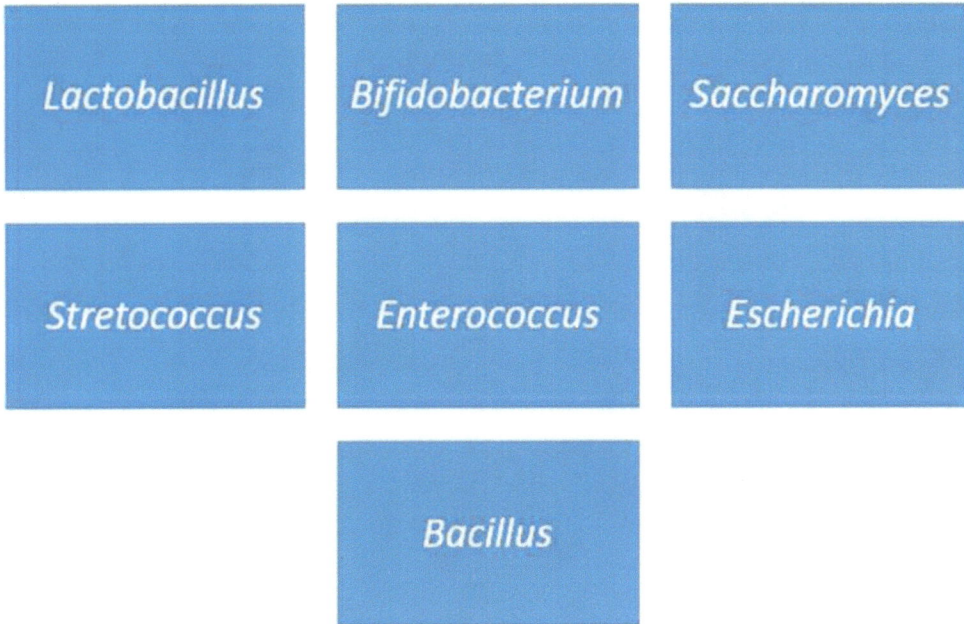

Fig. (1). Most commonly used bacteria as probiotics.

Most cancer therapies are immune-based, but unluckily, breast cancer does not respond to these immune checkpoints. Breast cancer patients are mostly kept on antibiotics that destroy the microbiota irrespective of harmful or beneficial bacteria and give rise to resistant strains that kill people all over the world; additionally, not all breast cancer patients respond well to antibiotics [7]. In order to overcome these problems, it is important to understand what the normal microbiota looks like and which bacteria are the probiotics, and which drugs can be administered to these patients (personalized treatment). Another observation is that whatever applies to breast cancer may not be applicable to all cancers and *vice versa* [8].

2. GUT MICROBIOME

Numerous viruses and microorganisms are present in the human body that usually exceed the number of human cells [9]. These microorganisms are collectively known as microbiota. It consists of different communities of archaea, viruses, eukaryotes, and bacteria and affects our health by cross-talking with one another [10]. Ideally, this should be an organ of our body that is forgotten and is mostly present in the GIT. It is estimated that most (35%) of cancers are due to diet, and one of the most prominent among them is breast cancer (50%) [11]. If the diet is a factor for breast cancer, this means there is an abnormality of GI tract probiotics (Fig. **2**).

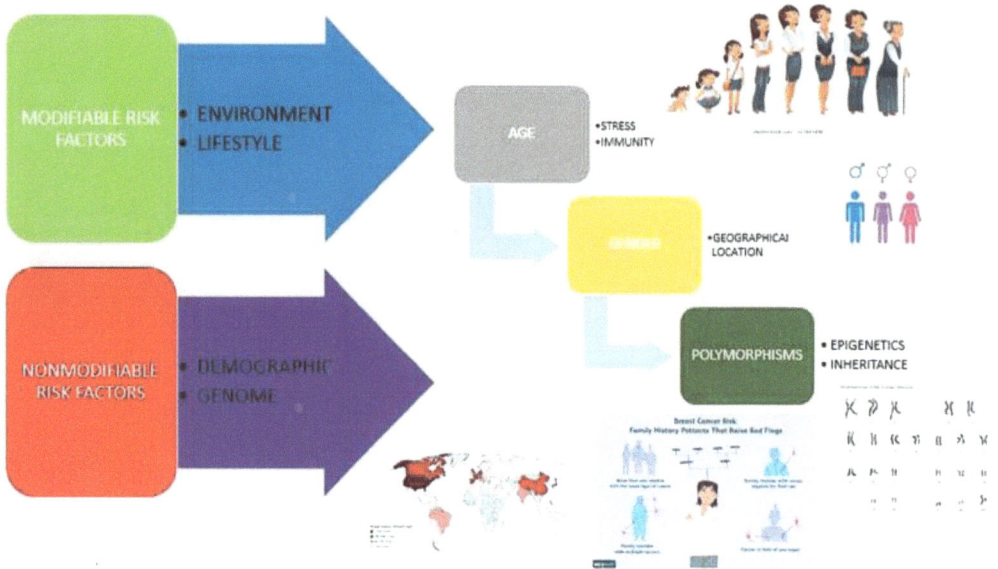

Fig. (2). Modifiable risk factors like lifestyle (junk food, lack of physical activities, *etc*.), environment (air pollution, use of antibiotics, hormonal drugs exposure, *etc*.) and detailed non-modifiable risk factors may influence the microbiota of human body and ultimately lead to breast cancer.

During cancer therapy, the synergistic effect of microbiome and diet has been found, specifically linking the Mediterranean diet with breast cancer. In a study on *Macaca fasciculus* monkey, the Western diet was compared with the Mediterranean diet, and it was reported that the population of *Lactobacillus* was comparatively higher in the former diet pattern because of high saturated fats and sucrose intake compared with fibre intake in this diet [12]. Bioactive compounds that are released by bacteria were higher in Mediterranean diet individuals. The breast tissue of such monkeys was rich in bile acid metabolites, conferring a protective role against breast cancer [13]. Particularly how gastrointestinal bacteria affect breast bacteria is still unknown. However, it was found that in mice, estrogen exposure for a long time affects the gut microbiome as well as estrogen metabolism and inflammation [14]. Therefore, from this information, it may be concluded that probiotics are directly associated with estrogen exposure.

Probiotics play a role in breast cancer as they reduce the number of β-glucuronidase expressing bacteria. These bacteria are responsible for the conversion of pre-carcinogens to active ones [15]. Probiotics play an important role in modulating estrogens circulating in humans as they secrete β-glucuronidase enzyme, which is responsible for the deconjugation of estrogen, leading to its uptake by tissue due to its conversion into the biologically free and active form. This free and active estrogen available for uptake is associated with many cancers that are hormone associated, like breast cancer. β-glucuronidase was also extracted from a breast cancer survivor's nipple aspiration [16].

The term microbiome and microbiota are nowadays used interchangeably. But both refer to the microbiota genome collectively and refer to the functions or traits expressed by microorganisms in that particular habitat [17]. Another terminology frequently used in conjunction with the microbiome is dysbiosis, which means that a part of the body or the whole body has abnormal microbiota. Although the composition of microbiota varies throughout the body, it is specific in an individual and can be used as a prognostic for disease identification and aggressiveness of the disease, specifically cancers [18]. The majority of these microorganisms are present in the gut, but recent studies have shown them to be associated with sporadic breast cancer [19]. Researchers are working to identify the changes and particular habitats of different microbiota in breast cancer patients as compared to normal individuals to identify the exact role. They have worked using shotgun-sequencing for metagenomics studies and NGS (next-generation sequencing) for 16S-rRNA for a targeted approach for identifying the qualitative and quantitative changes in the microbiota of the gut in breast cancer and healthy people, but conclusive results are still lacking [20]. Gut microbiota dysbiosis occurs through estrogen-independent as well as estrogen-dependant pathways that lead to breast cancer [21].

Most of the microorganisms present in gut microbiota belong to phyla of *Lentisphaerae, Tenericutes, Verrucomicrobia, Fusobacteria, Proteobacteria, Actinobacteria, Bacteriodetes* and *Firmicutes* [22]. The genera most commonly found in gut microbiota are *Bifidobacterium, Streptomyces, Streptococcus, Lactobacillus, Peptostreptococcus, Peptococcus, Ruminococcus, Eubacterium, Faecalibacterium, Clostridium* and *Bacteroides* [19]. Normally these organisms are present in homeostasis, known as normobiosis. However, if harmful bacteria outnumber the beneficial ones, dysbiosis leads to breast cancer. Several factors such as radiation, chemotherapy, use of antibiotic, smoking, alcohol, hygiene, stress, probiotics, prebiotics, diet, hormones, ethnicity, age and other factors change the microbiota of gut.

3. BREAST MICROBIOME

Breast tissue is mainly fatty in nature and is rich in lymphatic vessels serving as an ideal place for the growth of bacteria. Bacteria are translocated from GIT to breast tissue, which may change the breast microbiota. Other factors like sexual activity, diet, medication, disease and breastfeeding, along with genetic changes, also alter the microbiome ecology. The microbiome plays an important role in tumor microenvironment (TME) regulation and may affect the immune system leading to carcinogenesis. In 2019, Chen *et al.* reported that microorganisms in GIT of breast cancer patients differ from normal controls [23]. The variations in microbiota at immunologic and metabolic levels are comparatively less in cancer patients depicting a protective role of microorganisms in cancer. The presence of an increased number of bacteria that are not in normal breast tissue but in malignant tissue showed that they can cause double-stranded DNA breaks leading to cancer [24]. DNA sequencing analysis also confirmed a changed microbiota in cancer patients [25]. Malignant breast cancer patients had higher levels of bacteria that belong to phylum *Proteobacteria*, genus *Propionicimonas* and families *Methylobacteriaceae, Nocordioidaceae, Rhodobacteraceae, Caulobacteraceae* and *Micrococcaceae* as compared to benign breast tissue [26]. Heiken *et al.* reported that ER$^+$ breast cancer tissue had microbiota mostly belonging to genera *Lactobaccilus, Gluconacetobacter, Hydrogenophaga, Fusobacterium,* and *Atopobium* in invasive carcinoma as compared to that of benign [27].

Various studies, both *in vitro* as well as *in vivo* have been done to evaluate the role of probiotics in breast cancer. Animal studies have shown the health benefits of probiotics in the case of breast cancer [28]. It was shown that anti-inflammatory cytokines (IL-4 & IL-10) inhibition and overexpression of pro-inflammatory cytokines (IFN-γ) resulted in higher survival time in a group that was given *L acidophilus*. The group was orally administered 0.5 ml of *Lactobacillis acidophilus* (2.78108 CFU/ml) two weeks before the cancer transplant and 30 days afterwards with an interval of 3 days [29]. Researchers used the same suspension in mice before transplanting breast cancer and the suspension was administered for two consecutive weeks before the surgery and continued in a similar manner after surgery with 3 days intervals. All the studies showed the antitumor activity in mice with bacteria and prolonged survival [15]. Another study concluded that oral administration of *L. casei* can affect stimulation of the Th1 cytokine production in mouse spleen cell culture and NK cell cytotoxicity [30].

Breast cancer is a hormone-dependent disease, and free circulating estrogen leads to carcinogenesis. Microbiota of breast tissue is responsible for the conjugation and deconjugation of estrogen, and the assessment of microbiota may be used as prognostic factors for ER-positive breast cancer. Another important role of these microorganisms is to modulate the immune system. Probiotics give signals to immune cells in case of pathogenic attack, but dysbiosis can send false signals to the immune system, leading to inflammation and tissue damage, thereby providing a ground for tumorigenesis. Thus, this may lead to an immune-compromised situation with higher inflammation that leads to tumor promotion [31].

4. MILK MICROBIOME

When a baby is born, he is blessed with microbiota inherited from the mother in the uterine cavity as well as the vagina that provides an initial shield against pathogens. Later, due to feeding, gut microbiota develops further, which helps the infant strengthen the immune system. The microbiota of a human develops in 3 stages during childhood. The developmental is the first stage in which the diversity and composition of microbiota are defined. If a child is fed on mother milk, then most of the *Bacteroides* species will be present. The second stage is the transition phase, when the child is 1 year old and is exposed to different environments in the house (*e.g.*, pets, siblings, hygiene, medicinal uses, *etc.*), and the third stage is the stable one that remains in the human till adulthood and is modified by the lifestyle. At the age of 65 years, dysbiosis is observed mostly and is the most stable microbiota period [32]. It was found that the microbiota of breast tissue was similar to the microbiota of breast milk [33]. During the breastfeed process, the maternal skin interacts with the mouth of the infant and develops GI tract microflora through which it enters the mammary pathway [34]. The microbiota of mammary milk is influenced by a number of factors like postpartum duration, childbirth, pregnancy, use of antibiotics, diet quality as well as geographical location [35]. Researchers demonstrated that Spanish, Chinese, South African and Finnish women's milk mostly contains microorganisms of phyla *Actinobacteria* and *Bacteroidetes* and bacterial strains *of Staphylococcus, Serratia* and *Corynebacterium* [36]. In another study using metagenomics analysis, it was revealed that 34% of microbiota belongs to *Firmicutes* phyla and 65% are *Proteobacteria*, whereas 0.5% were *Streptococcus*, 33.4% were *Staphylococcus* and 61.1% belonged to the genera *Pseudomonas* [24].

Joice *et al.* claimed that there is still a 50% unidentified genome that constitutes microbiota that may be used as treatment option, prognosis or even diagnoses [37]. How do cancer occurrence and recurrence take place? How does the microbiota modulate breast cancer? These questions are still open, and there are a lot of missing pieces of information regarding the physiological functions of metabolites and proteins that are released by microorganisms.

5. MECHANISMS OF MICROBIAL MODULATION IN ANTI-TUMOR IMMUNE RESPONSES BY PROBIOTICS

The interface between the immune system and commensal bacteria was known to have positive effects on the progress of anticancer responses [38] *via* any one of the three mechanisms discussed below. In one of the mechanisms, T-cell responses induced by microorganisms, cross-react with tumor antigens or aid in anticancer immune responses' generation. In the second, pattern recognition receptors (PRRs) regulate anti-inflammatory and immune system activities through microbial induction, whereas, in the last one, systemic effects are modulated by metabolite's secretion [39 - 41].

Several T cell receptors get triggered when they encounter variable bacterial structures, leading to the circulation and expansion of a wide range of T helper lymphocytes [42]. These T lymphocytes can invade the tumors, possibly due to the production of chemokines in the TME. Once settled in the TME, they start assisting cytotoxic T cells through either co-stimulatory signal's induction or the production of cytokines [43]. On the other hand, researchers have also reported that their cross-reactivity might support T cells in antigen recognition on the surface of tumor cells [44 - 46].

Commensal bacteria not only absolutely influence T cells activation but also activate innate immunity cells by interacting with PRRs, and thus prompt the exposed dendritic cells (DCs) to lead to the promotion of potential anti-tumor CD8$^+$ and Th1 T cell responses [47]. *Lactobacillus*-treated human myeloid DCs showed increased levels of various maturation and activation markers on their surface, including CD86, CD83, CD80, CD40 and MHCII. Research has shown that the treated DCs also produce IFN-γ, IL18 and IL-12, thereby tilting the CD4$^+$ and CD8$^+$ T cells towards polarization of Tc1 and Th1 cells. Additionally, these dendritic cells have no role in the secretion of IL-13, IL-4 or IL-10 cytokines. IFN-γ - a cytokine, secreted by Th1 T cells, meditates several anti-tumor effects like antigen presentation, cytotoxicity and inhibition of angiogenesis [48].

Furthermore, they straightforwardly participate in CD8$^+$ cytotoxic T cell priming, which are the most energetic predators of tumor cells installed by the immune system. Even after *E. coli*-derived lipopolysaccharide's stimulation, IL-10 suppression and elevated production of IL-12 maintain their status [49, 50]. It has been shown that *Lactobacillus kefiri* formulation augmented the maturation and co-stimulation biomarkers' expression on DCs along with IFN-γ production and the efficacy of CD8$^+$ T cell stimulation [51, 52]. Researchers have reported the related effects through co-culture of other *Lactobacilli* species, in human DCs priming to Th1 polarization by IL-12 facilitation and IFN-γ secretion [53, 54]. *Lactococcus lactis* subsp. *Cremoris* FC activates IL-18 and IL-12-induced (combined) production of IFN-γ in mice DCs [55]. A group of scientists have used a mixture of three different probiotics, including *Clostridium butyricum, Bacillus mesentericus* and *Enterococcus faecalis* (bio-three) and found increased IL-12 production, elevated expression of activation markers and antigen presentation on DCs. Additionally, they have detected an accumulation of IFN-γ in CD4+ T cells supernatants and probiotic-initiated DCs [56, 57]. In conclusion, all these findings indicate that some specific probiotic species can elicit *in vitro* DCs' facilitated polarization of anti-tumor human T lymphocytes. Consequently, the aforementioned and other related strains are potent aspirants as natural adjuvants targeting the immune responses of DCs.

Direct bacterial and immune system interactions are not the only mechanisms that regulate immunity. A plethora of metabolites of microbial origin also employs immunomodulatory effects [58]. Gut microorganisms are the chief supplier of polyamines [59, 60], responsible for autophagy induction [61, 62]. Immune cells detect SCFAs *via* G protein-coupled receptors [63] and butyrate with the help of DCs, thereby regulating the antigen presentation and successive T-cell differentiation [64]. It has been observed that butyrate, by using its histone deacetylase (HDAC) inhibitory action, can restrain the growth of lymphoma by causing cancer cells' apoptosis [65]. Gut microbes produce Vitamin B6, which had a synergetic effect in combination with cisplatin to treat non-small cell lung cancer (NSCLC), but only in immune-competent mice, revealing the signs of immunogenic cell death and calreticulin exposure on the surface of these lung cancer cells [66]. Furthermore, histamine is found to be implicated in maintaining DCs reactions to bacterial ligands, causing increased antigen-presenting capability [58, 67].

6. MICROBIOME EFFECTS AND APPLICATIONS IN BREAST CANCER

Associations among breast cancer and human microbiome open novel perspectives for cancer treatment and prognosis and have gathered scientists' attention towards the therapeutic application of microbiome, as illustrated in Fig. (3). Various studies explored the probiotics' effects on breast cancer, such as: cell proliferation inhibition, and apoptosis induction along with cell cycle arrest [68]. The researchers studied two mice groups; one of the groups was fed the western style diet comprising of high sugar and fat, low vitamin C, D3 and fiber for developing mammary tumors, whereas the other group was directed for the development of human breast tumors. Both groups were given oral intake of probiotic lactic acid microbes. They found that probiotic *Lactobacillus reuteri* administration resulted in the inhibition of early-stage carcinogenesis and increased breast cell sensitivity to apoptosis [69].

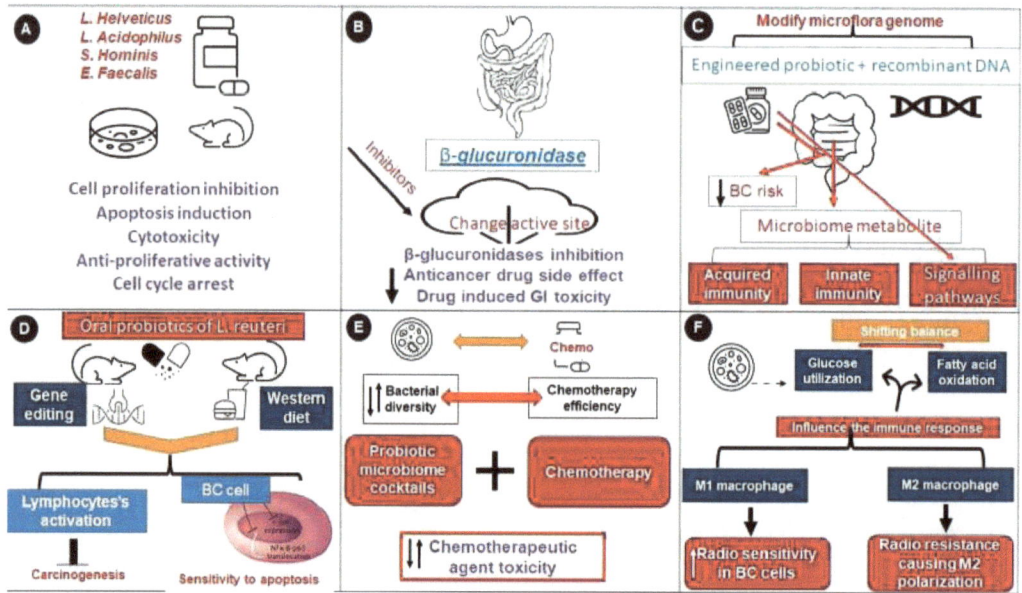

Fig. (3). Effects of the microbiome and its applications in breast carcinoma. A: use of probiotics to affect tumor progression by the induction of apoptosis and cell proliferation inhibition, B: Various catalytic activities & β-glucuronidase's conformational changes accompanied with genetic engineering might be helpful in decreasing the anti-cancerous drug-induced toxicity, C: use of potential tailored recombinant probiotic which can target and modify gut microbiome leading to decreased breast cancer (BC) risk, D: Genetic manipulation of mice to develop human BC (shown in center side) and fed by westernized diet for the development of mammary tumors (shown in the right side). Both were fed with *L. reuteri* and showed lymphocyte activation (CD4$^+$ & CD25$^+$), early-stage BC inhibition and increased breast cell sensitivity to apoptosis *via* NKK-B-P65 translocation, E: Chemotherapy's reciprocal communication with bacterial diversity – probiotics and chemotherapy combinations represented no effect with reduced or amplified (in some cases) chemotherapy agent toxicity, and F: the microbiome indirectly affects the immune system by shifting fatty acid oxidation and glucose utilization balance.

Furthermore, researchers established that the *L. acidophilus* oral administration signifies anticancer activity among mice producing breast tumors [70]. Mendoza *et al.* compiled the results from various sources and represented the anti-cancerous effects of probiotics on cell lines, such as apoptosis, anti-proliferative activity, cell cycle arrest and cytotoxicity [15]. Even though the aforementioned studies presented the testimony of probiotics displaying activity against breast cancer, there are even fundamental inquiries on probiotics' use in breast cancer. Probiotics dosage, strains and regimen need to be established on the basis of breast carcinoma related clinical feature and interaction of probiotics with the conventional treatment. Some of the clinical trials related to breast cancer and probiotics' role are in progress. Two *Lactobacillus* species have been reported to treat mastitis, and the study suggested that probiotics might be potential alternatives to antibiotics during breastfeeding for the treatment of breast infections [71].

7. BENEFICIAL MODULATION OF ANTI-TUMOR IMMUNE RESPO-NSES BY PROBIOTIC BACTERIA

It is obvious that GIT-related cancers are the most studied malignancies with respect to the administration of probiotics, but microbial identification with immunomodulatory properties encouraged researchers to expand their knowledge in other cancers as well, most possibly breast cancer due to many reasons, including greater disease incidence and role of breast microbiome in therapeutics [72, 73]. A group of investigators emphasized the defensive mechanism of *Lactobacillus reuteri* ATCC-PTA-6475 facilitated by regulatory T cells' (Tregs) accumulation, early-stage transformation of malignancy and inhibition of inflammatory diseases in mouse models encompassing mammary tumor [69]. Another study with rats explored *Lactobacillus plantarum* LS/07 effects in N-nitroso-N-methyl urea mammary carcinoma. Although they have been unable to observe any decrease in the tumor growth or development, but reduced ratio between low/high grade tumor along with decreased Ki67 expression, a proliferation marker was observed [74]. Furthermore, enhanced infiltration of CD4$^+$ and CD8$^+$ T cells in tumor serves as motivation towards the exploration of probiotic approaches in breast cancer diagnostics and therapeutics [29, 75].

A group of researchers in their two different studies have shown significant inhibition of tumor growth with selenium nanoparticles enriched *Lactobacillus brevis* and *Lactobacillus plantarum,* when injected in mice with 4T1 cells. Both cases showed increased cytotoxicity and production of NK cells and IFN-γ, respectively. They also observed increased TNF-α [29] and IL-2 production with the administration of *L. plantarum,* which leads to reduced liver metastasis and IL-17 up-regulation [75]. Intriguingly, *Lactobacillus casei* CRL 431 fermented milk was found to be diminutive of tumor growth in breast cancer models with reduced serum IL-6 levels and elevated ratio of CD8$^+$/CD4$^+$ T lymphocytes [76]. Dietary supplementation of *Lactobacillus acidophilus* among animal models injected with 4T1 cells promoted secretion of IFN-γ and reduced the tumor volume in spleen cultured cells intensified with tumor antigens, whereas it led to significantly decreased TGF-β production [77].

Additionally, scientists have reported a positive association of other extra-intestinal cancers with probiotic consumption as well. One of the groups discovered *Bifidobacterium* species as imperative to produce the finest immune responses against bladder cancer and melanoma. To confirm this, researchers used mice models and administered them with a mixture of *Bifidobacterium* species. They observed an immense level of change or betterment in the tumor control which was comparable to anti-PD-L1 treatment. Moreover, their combination remarkably eradicated the overgrowth of tumor [78].

Table 1. Anti-cancerous effects of probiotics in breast cancer cells.

Probiotic Stain	Duration & Treatment	Cell Lines used	Findings	Reference
Kefir grains water 50mg/mL (mixture of Lactobacillus acidophilus, L. casei & L. lactis	MTT assay	4T1	IC50 value at 48hrs = 12.5 IC50 value at 72hrs = 8.3	[79]
Lactobacillus acidophilus & Lactobacillus crispatus		MDA-MB-231	*Lactobacilli* were capable of decreasing transcriptional activity of 4 different cancer-testis antigens; Antiproliferative activity	[80]
Lactobacillus plantarum	Several concentrations		NFκB pathway downregulation mediated the apoptosis	[81]
Staphylococcus hominis & Enterococcus faecalis	Bacterial live, heat killed cells or cytoplasmic fractions were of 25µg/mL, 50µg/mL, 100µg/mL & 200µg/mL and were incubated for 24hrs / 48hrs / 72 hrs	MCF-7	Exerted cell cycle arrest, cellular proliferation inhibition, & induction of apoptosis	[68]
Lactobacillus rhamnosus & Lactobacillus crispatus	Supernatant & incubation of several concentrations		Cytotoxicity along with hypoxia-inducible factor (HIF)-1 suppression	[82]
Lactococcus lactis KC24	Inoculation of 105 or 106CFU/well of bacteria incubation for 48 hrs		Exerted significant toxicity in cancerous cells	[83]
Enterecoccus lactis NK34	Inoculation of 10^5 or 10^6 CFU/well of bacteria incubation for 44 hrs		59% cytotoxicity at 10^5 CFU/well 98% cytotoxicity at 10^6 CFU/well	[84]
Lactoccocus lactis IW5	Incubation (24 hrs) with EL metabolites		30% cell inhibition	[85]

Enterococcus hirae 13144 was found to improve the cyclophosphamide-induced effects upon oral administration against sarcoma and increased the Th1-mediated immune responses, such as the intra-tumoral ratio of cytotoxic cells to Tregs. They also observed the outcomes of *Barnesiella intestinihominis* administration, which resulted in the promotion of IFN-γ production followed by infiltration of γδ-T cells in the tumor [86]. All these findings encouraged the researchers to explore the beneficial modulation of anti-tumor immune responses by probiotic bacteria in different cancers leading to better therapeutic and health outcomes. Some of the *in vitro* studies are shown in Table **1**, representing probiotics' anti-cancerous effects in breast cancer cells.

CONCLUSION

A number of studies have explored the impact of intestinal microflora and emphasized probiotics consumption for the development of effective anticancer immune responses. Commensal microorganisms come forward as a practical approach either at earlier stages of cancer development or during the treatment with conventional methods to modify an individual's potential to fight against cancer. Immune function regulation through immunomodulatory activity of probiotic species and gut microbiota is coming up with fascinating interpretations. The systemic disposition of these endeavours suggests that they can impact not only the GIT but also other malignancies and distant tissues as well. Remarkably, probiotic microorganisms modulate and affect different stages of the cancer-immunity relationship. Here, an important thing to consider is that most of the research is conducted in animal models, so it is a big challenge to translate them in humans. Perceptibly, all the microorganisms identified as potential probiotics for cancer therapeutics in animals are not present in the humans or able to exist in human hosts. Therefore, it is mandatory to identify the common strains in both the environments and hosts or at least capable of performing their activity equally. This will basically narrow down the potential targets and need more precise research. Nonetheless, considering the outcomes of completed clinical trials or ongoing ones, we can foresee an alternative and potential strategy worth of consideration in cancer treatment/therapeutics on the basis of functional foods or probiotic formulations as immune adjuvants in traditional treatment and immunotherapies.

CONSENT FOR PUBLICATION

Not applicable.

CONFLICT OF INTEREST

The authors declare no conflict of interest, financial or otherwise.

ACKNOWLEDGEMENTS

Declared none.

REFERENCES

[1]   Fahad Ullah M. Breast cancer: current perspectives on the disease status. Adv Exp Med Biol 2019; 1152. 51-64.
       [http://dx.doi.org/10.1007/978-3-030-20301-6_4] [PMID: 31456179]

[2]   Olaimat AN, Aolymat I, Al-Holy M. *et al.* The potential application of probiotics and prebiotics for the prevention and treatment of COVID-19. npj Science of Food 2020; 4(1): 1-7.

[3]   Frost I, Van Boeckel TP, Pires J, Craig J, Laxminarayan R. Global geographic trends in antimicrobial resistance: the role of international travel. J Travel Med 2019; 26(8): taz036.
       [http://dx.doi.org/10.1093/jtm/taz036] [PMID: 31115466]

[4]   Fong W, Li Q, Yu J. Gut microbiota modulation: a novel strategy for prevention and treatment of colorectal cancer. Oncogene 2020; 39(26): 4925-43.
       [http://dx.doi.org/10.1038/s41388-020-1341-1] [PMID: 32514151]

[5]   Arun KB, Madhavan A, Sindhu R, *et al.* Probiotics and gut microbiome – Prospects and challenges in remediating heavy metal toxicity. J Hazard Mater 2021; 420: 126676.
       [http://dx.doi.org/10.1016/j.jhazmat.2021.126676] [PMID: 34329091]

[6]   Joseph SK, Sabitha M, Nair SC. Stimuli-responsive polymeric nanosystem for colon specific drug delivery. Adv Pharm Bull 2019; 10(1): 1-12.
       [http://dx.doi.org/10.15171/apb.2020.001] [PMID: 32002356]

[7]   Cabaluna ND, Uy GB, Galicia RM, Cortez SC, Yray MDS, Buckley BS. A randomized, double-blinded placebo-controlled clinical trial of the routine use of preoperative antibiotic prophylaxis in modified radical mastectomy. World J Surg 2013; 37(1): 59-66.
       [http://dx.doi.org/10.1007/s00268-012-1816-5] [PMID: 23052809]

[8]   McKee AM, Hall LJ, Robinson SD. The microbiota, antibiotics and breast cancer. Breast Cancer Manag 2019; 8(3): BMT29.
       [http://dx.doi.org/10.2217/bmt-2019-0015] [PMID: 31857826]

[9]   Liang G, Bushman FD. The human virome: assembly, composition and host interactions. Nat Rev Microbiol 2021; 19(8): 514-27.
       [http://dx.doi.org/10.1038/s41579-021-00536-5] [PMID: 33785903]

[10]   Matijašić M, Meštrović T, Čipčić Paljetak H, Perić M, Barešić A, Verbanac D. Gut microbiota beyond bacteria—Mycobiome, virome, archaeome, and eukaryotic parasites in IBD. Int J Mol Sci 2020; 21(8): 2668.
       [http://dx.doi.org/10.3390/ijms21082668] [PMID: 32290414]

[11]   Lavalette C, Adjibade M, Srour B, *et al.* Cancer-specific and general nutritional scores and cancer risk: results from the prospective NutriNet-Sante cohort. Cancer Res 2018; 78(15): 4427-35.
       [http://dx.doi.org/10.1158/0008-5472.CAN-18-0155] [PMID: 30049821]

[12]   Thames A, Sade Spencer LE, McClintock S, Nurmi E. ACNP 59th annual meeting: panels, mini-panels and study groups. Neuropsychopharmacology 2020; 45(S1) (Suppl. 1): 1-67.
       [http://dx.doi.org/10.1038/s41386-020-00889-0] [PMID: 33279933]

[13]   Sipe LM, Chaib M, Pingili AK, Pierre JF, Makowski L. Microbiome, bile acids, and obesity: How microbially modified metabolites shape anti-tumor immunity. Immunol Rev 2020; 295(1): 220-39.
       [http://dx.doi.org/10.1111/imr.12856] [PMID: 32320071]

[14]   Kaliannan K, Robertson RC, Murphy K, *et al.* Estrogen-mediated gut microbiome alterations influence sexual dimorphism in metabolic syndrome in mice. Microbiome 2018; 6(1): 205.
       [http://dx.doi.org/10.1186/s40168-018-0587-0] [PMID: 30424806]

[15]   Mendoza L. Potential effect of probiotics in the treatment of breast cancer. Oncol Rev 2019; 13(2): 422.
       [http://dx.doi.org/10.4081/oncol.2019.422] [PMID: 31583054]

[16]   Chan AA, Bashir M, Rivas MN, *et al.* Characterization of the microbiome of nipple aspirate fluid of breast cancer survivors. Sci Rep 2016; 6(1): 28061.
[http://dx.doi.org/10.1038/srep28061] [PMID: 27324944]

[17]   Boon E, Meehan CJ, Whidden C, Wong DHJ, Langille MGI, Beiko RG. Interactions in the microbiome: communities of organisms and communities of genes. FEMS Microbiol Rev 2014; 38(1): 90-118.
[http://dx.doi.org/10.1111/1574-6976.12035] [PMID: 23909933]

[18]   Wei MY, Shi S, Liang C, *et al.* The microbiota and microbiome in pancreatic cancer: more influential than expected. Mol Cancer 2019; 18(1): 97.
[http://dx.doi.org/10.1186/s12943-019-1008-0] [PMID: 31109338]

[19]   Fernández M, Reina-Pérez I, Astorga J, Rodríguez-Carrillo A, Plaza-Díaz J, Fontana L. Breast cancer and its relationship with the microbiota. Int J Environ Res Public Health 2018; 15(8): 1747.
[http://dx.doi.org/10.3390/ijerph15081747] [PMID: 30110974]

[20]   Palacios A. Concepts and techniques in the study of the gut microbiota

[21]   Buchta Rosean C, Bostic RR, Ferey JCM, *et al.* Preexisting commensal dysbiosis is a host-intrinsic regulator of tissue inflammation and tumor cell dissemination in hormone receptor–positive breast cancer. Cancer Res 2019; 79(14): 3662-75.
[http://dx.doi.org/10.1158/0008-5472.CAN-18-3464] [PMID: 31064848]

[22]   Fujio-Vejar S, Vasquez Y, Morales P, *et al.* The gut microbiota of healthy chilean subjects reveals a high abundance of the phylum *verrucomicrobia*. Front Microbiol 2017; 8: 1221.
[http://dx.doi.org/10.3389/fmicb.2017.01221] [PMID: 28713349]

[23]   Chen J, Douglass J, Prasath V, *et al.* The microbiome and breast cancer: a review. Breast Cancer Res Treat 2019; 178(3): 493-6.
[http://dx.doi.org/10.1007/s10549-019-05407-5] [PMID: 31456069]

[24]   Eslami-S Z, Majidzadeh-A K, Halvaei S, Babapirali F, Esmaeili R. Microbiome and breast cancer: new role for an ancient population. Front Oncol 2020; 10: 120.
[http://dx.doi.org/10.3389/fonc.2020.00120] [PMID: 32117767]

[25]   Xuan C, Shamonki JM, Chung A, *et al.* Microbial dysbiosis is associated with human breast cancer. PLoS One 2014; 9(1): e83744.
[http://dx.doi.org/10.1371/journal.pone.0083744] [PMID: 24421902]

[26]   Meng S, Chen B, Yang J, *et al.* Study of microbiomes in aseptically collected samples of human breast tissue using needle biopsy and the potential role of *in situ* tissue microbiomes for promoting malignancy. Front Oncol 2018; 8: 318.
[http://dx.doi.org/10.3389/fonc.2018.00318] [PMID: 30175072]

[27]   Hieken TJ, Chen J, Hoskin TL, *et al.* The microbiome of aseptically collected human breast tissue in benign and malignant disease. Sci Rep 2016; 6(1): 30751.
[http://dx.doi.org/10.1038/srep30751] [PMID: 27485780]

[28]   Imani Fooladi AA, Yazdi MH, Pourmand MR, *et al.* Th1 cytokine production induced by *Lactobacillus acidophilus* in BALB/c mice bearing transplanted breast tumor. Jundishapur J Microbiol 2015; 8(4): e17354.
[http://dx.doi.org/10.5812/jjm.8(4)2015.17354] [PMID: 26034546]

[29]   Yazdi M, Mahdavi M, Kheradmand E, Shahverdi A. The preventive oral supplementation of a selenium nanoparticle-enriched probiotic increases the immune response and lifespan of 4T1 breast cancer bearing mice. Arzneimittelforschung 2012; 62(11): 525-31.
[http://dx.doi.org/10.1055/s-0032-1323700] [PMID: 22945771]

[30]   Soltan Dallal MM, Yazdi MH, Holakuyee M, Hassan ZM, Abolhassani M, Mahdavi M. *Lactobacillus casei* ssp.casei induced Th1 cytokine profile and natural killer cells activity in invasive ductal carcinoma bearing mice. Iran J Allergy Asthma Immunol 2012; 11(2): 183-9.

[PMID: 22761192]

[31]   Dzutsev A, Goldszmid RS, Viaud S, Zitvogel L, Trinchieri G. The role of the microbiota in inflammation, carcinogenesis, and cancer therapy. Eur J Immunol 2015; 45(1): 17-31.
[http://dx.doi.org/10.1002/eji.201444972] [PMID: 25328099]

[32]   Maynard C, Weinkove D. The gut microbiota and ageing. Biochemistry and Cell Biology of Ageing. Subcell Biochem 2018; 90: 351-71.
[http://dx.doi.org/10.1007/978-981-13-2835-0_12] [PMID: 30779015]

[33]   Ojo-Okunola A, Nicol M, du Toit E. Human breast milk bacteriome in health and disease. Nutrients 2018; 10(11): 1643.
[http://dx.doi.org/10.3390/nu10111643] [PMID: 30400268]

[34]   Lyons KE, Ryan CA, Dempsey EM, Ross RP, Stanton C. Breast milk, a source of beneficial microbes and associated benefits for infant health. Nutrients 2020; 12(4): 1039.
[http://dx.doi.org/10.3390/nu12041039] [PMID: 32283875]

[35]   Vandenplas Y, Carnielli VP, Ksiazyk J, et al. Factors affecting early-life intestinal microbiota development. Nutrition 2020; 78: 110812.
[http://dx.doi.org/10.1016/j.nut.2020.110812] [PMID: 32464473]

[36]   Demmelmair H, Jiménez E, Collado MC, Salminen S, McGuire MK. Maternal and perinatal factors associated with the human milk microbiome. Curr Dev Nutr 2020; 4(4): 4004011.
[http://dx.doi.org/10.1093/cdn/nzaa027] [PMID: 32270132]

[37]   Joice R, Yasuda K, Shafquat A, Morgan XC, Huttenhower C. Determining microbial products and identifying molecular targets in the human microbiome. Cell Metab 2014; 20(5): 731-41.
[http://dx.doi.org/10.1016/j.cmet.2014.10.003] [PMID: 25440055]

[38]   Malik SS, Saeed A, Baig M, Asif N, Masood N, Yasmin A. Anticarcinogenecity of microbiota and probiotics in breast cancer. Int J Food Prop 2018; 21(1): 655-66.
[http://dx.doi.org/10.1080/10942912.2018.1448994]

[39]   Erdman SE, Poutahidis T. Gut microbiota modulate host immune cells in cancer development and growth. Free Radic Biol Med 2017; 105: 28-34.
[http://dx.doi.org/10.1016/j.freeradbiomed.2016.11.013] [PMID: 27840315]

[40]   Goubet A-G, Daillère R, Routy B, Derosa L, M Roberti P, Zitvogel L. The impact of the intestinal microbiota in therapeutic responses against cancer. C R Biol 2018; 341(5): 284-9.
[http://dx.doi.org/10.1016/j.crvi.2018.03.004] [PMID: 29631891]

[41]   Bonvalet M, Daillère R, Roberti MP, et al. The impact of the intestinal microbiota in therapeutic responses against cancer Oncoimmunol. Springer 2018; pp. 447-62.

[42]   Pabst O, Slack E. IgA and the intestinal microbiota: the importance of being specific. Mucosal Immunol 2020; 13(1): 12-21.
[http://dx.doi.org/10.1038/s41385-019-0227-4] [PMID: 31740744]

[43]   Zitvogel L, Ma Y, Raoult D, Kroemer G, Gajewski TF. The microbiome in cancer immunotherapy: Diagnostic tools and therapeutic strategies. Science 2018; 359(6382): 1366-70.
[http://dx.doi.org/10.1126/science.aar6918] [PMID: 29567708]

[44]   Balachandran VP, Łuksza M, Zhao JN, et al. Identification of unique neoantigen qualities in long-term survivors of pancreatic cancer. Nature 2017; 551(7681): 512-6.
[http://dx.doi.org/10.1038/nature24462] [PMID: 29132146]

[45]   Nanjundappa RH, Ronchi F, Wang J. et al. A gut microbial mimic that hijacks diabetogenic autoreactivity to suppress colitis. Cell. 2017; 171(3): 655-7. e17

[46]   Leng Q, Tarbe M, Long Q, Wang F. Pre-existing heterologous T-cell immunity and neoantigen immunogenicity. Clin Transl Immunology 2020; 9(3): e01111.
[http://dx.doi.org/10.1002/cti2.1111] [PMID: 32211191]

[47]   Malik SS, Masood N, Fatima I, *et al.* Microbial-Based Cancer Therapy: Diagnostic Tools and Therapeutic Strategies Microbial Technology for the Welfare of Society. Springer 2019; pp. 53-82.

[48]   Iwasaki A, Medzhitov R. Toll-like receptor control of the adaptive immune responses. Nat Immunol 2004; 5(10): 987-95.
[http://dx.doi.org/10.1038/ni1112] [PMID: 15454922]

[49]   Mohamadzadeh M, Olson S, Kalina WV, *et al.* Lactobacilli activate human dendritic cells that skew T cells toward T helper 1 polarization. Proc Natl Acad Sci USA 2005; 102(8): 2880-5.
[http://dx.doi.org/10.1073/pnas.0500098102] [PMID: 15710900]

[50]   Lawania S, Singh N, Behera D, Sharma S. XPC Polymorphism and Risk for Lung Cancer in North Indian Patients Treated with Platinum Based Chemotherapy and Its Association with Clinical Outcomes. Pathol Oncol Res 2018; 24(2): 353-66.
[http://dx.doi.org/10.1007/s12253-017-0252-0] [PMID: 28540485]

[51]   Ghoneum M, Felo N, Agrawal S, Agrawal A. A novel kefir product (PFT) activates dendritic cells to induce CD4+T and CD8+T cell responses *in vitro*. Int J Immunopathol Pharmacol 2015; 28(4): 488-96.
[http://dx.doi.org/10.1177/0394632015599447] [PMID: 26384392]

[52]   Lee KA, Luong MK, Shaw H, Nathan P, Bataille V, Spector TD. The gut microbiome: what the oncologist ought to know. Br J Cancer 2021; 125(9): 1197-209.
[http://dx.doi.org/10.1038/s41416-021-01467-x] [PMID: 34262150]

[53]   Mohamadzadeh M, Klaenhammer TR. Specific *Lactobacillus* species differentially activate Toll-like receptors and downstream signals in dendritic cells. Expert Rev Vaccines 2008; 7(8): 1155-64.
[http://dx.doi.org/10.1586/14760584.7.8.1155] [PMID: 18844590]

[54]   Ashraf R, Vasiljevic T, Day SL, Smith SC, Donkor ON. Lactic acid bacteria and probiotic organisms induce different cytokine profile and regulatory T cells mechanisms. J Funct Foods 2014; 6: 395-409.
[http://dx.doi.org/10.1016/j.jff.2013.11.006]

[55]   Kosaka A, Yan H, Ohashi S, *et al. Lactococcus lactis* subsp. cremoris FC triggers IFN-γ production from NK and T cells *via* IL-12 and IL-18. Int Immunopharmacol 2012; 14(4): 729-33.
[http://dx.doi.org/10.1016/j.intimp.2012.10.007] [PMID: 23102661]

[56]   Hua MC, Lin T-Y, Lai M-W, Kong MS, Chang HJ, Chen CC. Probiotic Bio-Three induces Th1 and anti-inflammatory effects in PBMC and dendritic cells. World J Gastroenterol 2010; 16(28): 3529-40.
[http://dx.doi.org/10.3748/wjg.v16.i28.3529] [PMID: 20653061]

[57]   Zeng W, Shen J, Bo T. *et al.* Cutting edge: probiotics and fecal microbiota transplantation in immunomodulation. J Immunol Res 2019 2019.

[58]   Wang G, Huang S, Wang Y, *et al.* Bridging intestinal immunity and gut microbiota by metabolites. Cell Mol Life Sci 2019; 76(20): 3917-37.
[http://dx.doi.org/10.1007/s00018-019-03190-6] [PMID: 31250035]

[59]   Tofalo R, Cocchi S, Suzzi G. Polyamines and gut microbiota. Front Nutr 2019; 6: 16.
[http://dx.doi.org/10.3389/fnut.2019.00016] [PMID: 30859104]

[60]   Linsalata M, Russo F, Berloco P, *et al.* Effects of probiotic bacteria (VSL#3) on the polyamine biosynthesis and cell proliferation of normal colonic mucosa of rats. *In vivo* 2005; 19(6): 989-95.
[PMID: 16277012]

[61]   Sobieszczuk-Nowicka E, Paluch-Lubawa E, Mattoo AK, Arasimowicz-Jelonek M, Gregersen PL, Pacak A. Polyamines–A new metabolic switch: Crosstalk with networks involving senescence, crop improvement, and mammalian cancer therapy. Front Plant Sci 2019; 10: 859.
[http://dx.doi.org/10.3389/fpls.2019.00859] [PMID: 31354753]

[62]   Pietrocola F, Pol J, Vacchelli E, *et al.* Caloric restriction mimetics enhance anticancer immunosurveillance. Cancer Cell 2016; 30(1): 147-60.

[http://dx.doi.org/10.1016/j.ccell.2016.05.016] [PMID: 27411589]

[63] Joglekar P, Segre JA. Building a translational microbiome toolbox. Cell 2017; 169(3): 378-80.
[http://dx.doi.org/10.1016/j.cell.2017.04.009] [PMID: 28431240]

[64] Berndt BE, Zhang M, Owyang SY, *et al.* Butyrate increases IL-23 production by stimulated dendritic cells. Am J Physiol Gastrointest Liver Physiol 2012; 303(12): G1384-92.
[http://dx.doi.org/10.1152/ajpgi.00540.2011] [PMID: 23086919]

[65] Wei W, Sun W, Yu S, Yang Y, Ai L. Butyrate production from high-fiber diet protects against lymphoma tumor. Leuk Lymphoma 2016; 57(10): 2401-8.
[http://dx.doi.org/10.3109/10428194.2016.1144879] [PMID: 26885564]

[66] Aranda F, Bloy N, Pesquet J, *et al.* Immune-dependent antineoplastic effects of cisplatin plus pyridoxine in non-small-cell lung cancer. Oncogene 2015; 34(23): 3053-62.
[http://dx.doi.org/10.1038/onc.2014.234] [PMID: 25065595]

[67] Sarasola MP, Táquez Delgado MA, Nicoud MB, Medina VA. Histamine in cancer immunology and immunotherapy. Current status and new perspectives. Pharmacol Res Perspect 2021; 9(5): e00778.
[http://dx.doi.org/10.1002/prp2.778] [PMID: 34609067]

[68] Hassan Z, Mustafa S, Rahim RA, Isa NM. Anti-breast cancer effects of live, heat-killed and cytoplasmic fractions of *Enterococcus faecalis* and *Staphylococcus hominis* isolated from human breast milk. *In vitro* Cell Dev Biol Anim 2016; 52(3): 337-48.
[http://dx.doi.org/10.1007/s11626-015-9978-8] [PMID: 26659392]

[69] Lakritz JR, Poutahidis T, Levkovich T, *et al.* Beneficial bacteria stimulate host immune cells to counteract dietary and genetic predisposition to mammary cancer in mice. Int J Cancer 2014; 135(3): 529-40.
[http://dx.doi.org/10.1002/ijc.28702] [PMID: 24382758]

[70] Yazdi MH, Soltan Dallal MM, Hassan ZM, *et al.* Oral administration of *Lactobacillus acidophilus* induces IL-12 production in spleen cell culture of BALB/c mice bearing transplanted breast tumour. Br J Nutr 2010; 104(2): 227-32.
[http://dx.doi.org/10.1017/S0007114510000516] [PMID: 20193099]

[71] Arroyo R, Martín V, Maldonado A, Jiménez E, Fernández L, Rodríguez JM. Treatment of infectious mastitis during lactation: antibiotics versus oral administration of Lactobacilli isolated from breast milk. Clin Infect Dis 2010; 50(12): 1551-8.
[http://dx.doi.org/10.1086/652763] [PMID: 20455694]

[72] Sehrawat N, Yadav M, Singh M, Kumar V, Sharma VR, Sharma AK, Eds. Probiotics in microbiome ecological balance providing a therapeutic window against cancer Seminars in cancer biology. Elsevier 2021.

[73] Torres-Maravilla E, Boucard AS, Mohseni AH, Taghinezhad-S S, Cortes-Perez NG, Bermúdez-Humarán LG. Role of gut microbiota and probiotics in colorectal cancer: onset and progression. Microorganisms 2021; 9(5): 1021.
[http://dx.doi.org/10.3390/microorganisms9051021] [PMID: 34068653]

[74] Kassayová M, Bobrov N, Strojný L, *et al.* Anticancer and immunomodulatory effects of *Lactobacillus plantarum* LS/07, inulin and melatonin in NMU-induced rat model of breast cancer. Anticancer Res 2016; 36(6): 2719-28.
[PMID: 27272781]

[75] Yazdi MH, Mahdavi M, Setayesh N, Esfandyar M, Shahverdi AR. Selenium nanoparticle-enriched *Lactobacillus brevis* causes more efficient immune responses *in vivo* and reduces the liver metastasis in metastatic form of mouse breast cancer. Daru 2013; 21(1): 33.
[http://dx.doi.org/10.1186/2008-2231-21-33] [PMID: 23631392]

[76] Aragón F, Carino S, Perdigón G, de Moreno de LeBlanc A. The administration of milk fermented by the probiotic *Lactobacillus casei* CRL 431 exerts an immunomodulatory effect against a breast tumour

in a mouse model. Immunobiology 2014; 219(6): 457-64.
[http://dx.doi.org/10.1016/j.imbio.2014.02.005] [PMID: 24646876]

[77]   Maroof H, Hassan ZM, Mobarez AM, Mohamadabadi MA. *Lactobacillus acidophilus* could modulate
       the immune response against breast cancer in murine model. J Clin Immunol 2012; 32(6): 1353-9.
       [http://dx.doi.org/10.1007/s10875-012-9708-x] [PMID: 22711009]

[78]   Sivan A, Corrales L, Hubert N, *et al.* Commensal *Bifidobacterium* promotes antitumor immunity and
       facilitates anti–PD-L1 efficacy. Science 2015; 350(6264): 1084-9.
       [http://dx.doi.org/10.1126/science.aac4255] [PMID: 26541606]

[79]   Zamberi NR, Abu N, Mohamed NE, *et al.* The antimetastatic and antiangiogenesis effects of kefir
       water on murine breast cancer cells. Integr Cancer Ther 2016; 15(4): NP53-66.
       [http://dx.doi.org/10.1177/1534735416642862] [PMID: 27230756]

[80]   Azam R, Ghafouri-Fard S, Tabrizi M, *et al.* *Lactobacillus acidophilus* and *Lactobacillus crispatus*
       culture supernatants downregulate expression of cancer-testis genes in the MDA-MB-231 cell line.
       Asian Pac J Cancer Prev 2014; 15(10): 4255-9.
       [http://dx.doi.org/10.7314/APJCP.2014.15.10.4255] [PMID: 24935380]

[81]   Kadirareddy RH, Vemuri SG, Palempalli UMD. Probiotic Conjugated Linoleic Acid Mediated
       Apoptosis in Breast Cancer Cells by Downregulation of NFκB. Asian Pac J Cancer Prev 2016; 17(7):
       3395-403.
       [PMID: 27509982]

[82]   Bharti V, Mehta A, Singh S, *et al.* Cytotoxicity of live whole cell, heat killed cell and cell free extract
       of *lactobacillus* strain in u-87 human glioblastoma cell line and mcf-7 breast cancer cell line. Int J
       Probio Prebio 2015; 10(4): 153-8.

[83]   Lee NK, Han KJ, Son SH, Eom SJ, Lee S-K, Paik H-D. Multifunctional effect of probiotic
       Lactococcus lactis KC24 isolated from kimchi. Lebensm Wiss Technol 2015; 64(2): 1036-41.
       [http://dx.doi.org/10.1016/j.lwt.2015.07.019]

[84]   Han KJ, Lee NK, Park H, Paik HD. Anticancer and anti-inflammatory activity of probiotic
       Lactococcus lactis NK34. J Microbiol Biotechnol 2015; 25(10): 1697-701.
       [http://dx.doi.org/10.4014/jmb.1503.03033] [PMID: 26165315]

[85]   Nami Y, Haghshenas B, Haghshenas M, Abdullah N, Yari Khosroushahi A. The prophylactic effect of
       probiotic *Enterococcus lactis* IW5 against different human cancer cells. Front Microbiol 2015; 6:
       1317.
       [http://dx.doi.org/10.3389/fmicb.2015.01317] [PMID: 26635778]

[86]   Daillère R, Vétizou M, Waldschmitt N, *et al.* *Enterococcus hirae* and *Barnesiella intestinihominis*
       facilitate cyclophosphamide-induced therapeutic immunomodulatory effects. Immunity 2016; 45(4):
       931-43.
       [http://dx.doi.org/10.1016/j.immuni.2016.09.009] [PMID: 27717798]

CHAPTER 7

Probiotics Based Anticancer Immunity In Stomach Cancer

Shilpi Singh[1], Bindu Kumari[2], Sonal Sinha[3], Gireesh Kumar Singh[2], Suaib Lqman[1,*] and Dhananjay Kumar Singh[2,*]

[1] *Molecular Bioprospection Department, CSIR- Central Institute of Medicinal and Aromatic Plants, Lucknow, U.P., India*

[2] *Department of Pharmacy, Central University of South Bihar, Gaya, Bihar, India*

[3] *Pragya College of Pharmaceutical Sciences, Gaya, Bihar, India*

Abstract: Stomach cancer is a global health challenge due to its increasing prevalence. The intestinal microbiota of humans plays a vital role in producing short-chain fatty acids, developing resistance towards pathogenic microbes, nutrient absorption, modulation in immunological response, metabolism, synthesis of vitamins, and gut immune system development. Many diseases or disorders, including cancers, obesity, psychiatric illnesses, rheumatoid arthritis, and inflammatory bowel syndrome, are associated with an imbalance of microbiotas. Earlier reports suggest that probiotics *via* the oral route act as a functional food and suppress cancer development. Further, some probiotics are clinically effective in reducing post-operative inflammation in cancer patients. Probiotics primarily display inhibitory effects against *H. pylori* infections in the digestive tract. The combination of probiotics with antibiotics has effectively eradicated *H. pylori* infections. Besides, probiotics reduce the pro-carcinogens metabolism, they also diminish the growth of pathogens and improve the consistency of the intestinal barrier. Moreover, compounds produced by the microorganisms are reported to interact unswervingly with cancer cells and affect their survival. The therapeutic efficacy and adverse side-effects of the strategies used for stomach cancer prevention could be improved by using probiotics either as adjuvant or neo-adjuvant as the safety concern of the commercially used strains has been verified. The underlying mechanism describing microbiota's effect on oncogenic activation, carcinogenic metabolite production, DNA damage, inhibition of tumour immunity, and chronic inflammation induction still needs a more detailed investigation. In addition, double-blind, placebo-controlled, randomized, and well-designed clinical studies are required to understand the efficacy and mode of action to reduce the death rate and stomach cancer burden. In depth studies are essential to set probiotics as an eccentric strategy for stomach cancer prevention and treatment.

* **Corresponding authors Dhananjay Kumar Singh and Suaib Lqman:** Department of Pharmacy, Central University of South Bihar, Gaya, Bihar, India; and Molecular Bioprospection Department, CSIR- Central Institute of Medicinal and Aromatic Plants, Lucknow-226015, U.P., India; E-mails: dhananjay@cusb.ac.in and s.luqman@cimap.res.in
\# These authors contributed equally.

Mitesh Kumar Dwivedi, Alwarappan Sankaranarayanan & Sanjay Tiwari (Eds.)

Keywords: Gut immune system, *H. pylori*, Immune system, Inflammation, Intestinal microbiota, Probiotics, Stomach cancer, Tumour immunity.

1. INTRODUCTION

Inflammation influences several biological processes involved in the progression and development of a tumour and acts as an intrinsic tumour characteristic. Non-immune cells, neoplastic and immune cells coexist in tumours, but tumour growth is compromised when an appropriate microenvironment is unavailable [1, 2]. The heterotypic signalling in non-neoplastic and neoplastic cells reshaped the tumour niche. The emergence currently saw a change in the treatment paradigm of the therapies centered on tumour microenvironment [3, 4]. Among the most widely used immunotherapeutics, immune-checkpoint blockers (ICBs) are the principal approaches in cancer [5 - 7]. Despite some significant results in a few cancer types, only a particular type of population gets the beneficial effects. The major challenge is identifying the accurate and precise biomarkers in the clinical setup and personalising an immune treatment [8].

In stomach cancer, chronic inflammation and infection are essential for stomach cancer pathogenesis. The *H. pylori* infection is linked to the intestinal and stomach cancers that trigger persistent and chronic inflammation in gastric mucosa, inflammatory cell infiltration, and diverse inflammatory mediators [9]. Epstein-Barr virus (EBV) is also linked to 10% of total stomach cancer, and CD8$^+$ T cells infiltration is the characteristic feature of EBV-positive stomach cancer [10]. Genetic and environmental determinants play an essential role in the genesis of stomach malignancy; thus, at the molecular level, the ecological and genetic factors make it a complex and heterogeneous disease that increases the clinical complexity. FDA approves the use of pembrolizumab, a programmed cell death protein 1 inhibitor for the recurrent and advanced PD-L1 expressing stomach cancer [11]. Earlier studies indicate that the alliance of PD-1 and PDL-1 expression correlates with the clinical parameters and the survival of patients with stomach cancer [12 - 15]. Besides, few studies suggest inducing PD-L1 expression by *H. pylori* [16 - 19].

Moreover, several other parameters have now been accepted as biomarkers due to the significant clinical relevance for predicting the response against ICBs studied in stomach cancer. Hence this book chapter summarises epidemiology, histology and immune contexture concerning stomach cancer. Further, we discuss the significance of predictive markers concerning the immune microenvironment. Moreover, we include the probiotics, their impact on stomach cancer management, and the probiotics' clinical trials. In addition, we shed light on the significant current gaps in the treatment, diagnosis, prognosis, and prevention of stomach cancer and the challenges that need to be addressed.

2. EPIDEMIOLOGY OF STOMACH CANCER DEVELOPMENT, SYMPTOMS AND RISK FACTORS

Stomach cancer is developed from the stomach lining and is also known as gastric cancer. It is the fifth-leading cancer among the other cancer types, with 7% cases and a 9% death rate; it is the third most common cancer type with the leading cause of death [20]. The stomach lining comprises glands and columnar epithelial cells sensitive to inflammation, especially gastritis, leading to gastric ulcers and gastric cancer [21]. According to the American Institute of Cancer Research (2022), approximately 26,380 new cases and 11,090 deaths were recorded in the United States. It is the fourth most common cancer type among men, while it is the seventh most common cancer type in females in India [22]. According to the statistical analysis, South Korea showed the highest stomach cancer rates, followed by Mongolia in 2018. The order among countries from the highest to the lowest stomach cancer incidence rates was as follows: South Korea > Mongolia > Japan > China > Bhutan > Kyrgyzstan > Chile > Belarus > Peru > Vietnam.

2.1. Incidence and Mortality

Stomach cancer is a more prevalent cancer type in males than females, with 2.2 times in developed countries while the ratio is 1.83 in developing countries. It is the most frequently diagnosed type of cancer [23]. The highest incidences were recorded in Latin America and Central and Eastern Asia. The highest incidence of 60/100000 has been reported in the Republic of Korea [24]. Approximately 783,000 deaths were recorded each year, making it the third most deadly type of cancer in males. It is attributed to about 8.3% of total cancer deaths, and the cumulative death risk is 0.57% in females and 1.36% in males from birth to the age of 74 years [20].

2.2. Geographical Variability and Trends

In the United States, the 5-year survival rate is 31%, indicating that most of the cases were diagnosed at the metastatic stage. Approx 67% of the survival rates were observed for pre-metastatic stomach cancer diagnosis. In Asia, the 5-years survival rate is 12% higher due to early diagnosis by lymph nodes examination, while 19% and 15% survival rate is reported in the United Kingdom for 5-years and 10-years survival, respectively. Europe shows a 26% survival rate, higher than the United Kingdom but less than the United States [25 - 27].

2.3. Symptoms

In the early stages of stomach cancer, there are non-specific symptoms due to small tumour size and expansion of the stomach. No apparent signs can be seen in the early stages, but the symptoms have been observed in advanced settings due to the metastatic stage diagnosis, and the stomach cancer has a poor prognosis. (Fig. **1**) describes the symptoms of stomach cancer, including a feeling of abdominal discomfort and pain at the early stages. Still, when cancer reaches an advanced stage, the pain lasts longer and gets stronger. Besides, the patients also face the problem of indigestion and appetite loss.

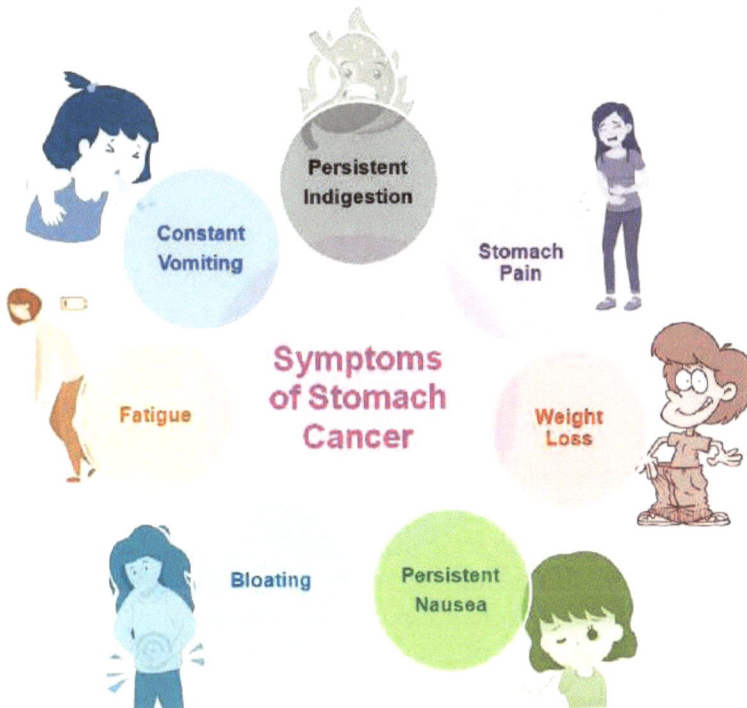

Fig. (1). Symptoms of the early and advanced stages of stomach cancer.

2.4. Risk Factors

Various risk factors have been observed to significantly increase the risk of stomach cancer, including smoking, diet, family history, and infection of *Helicobacter pylori* and Epstein-Bar viruses (EBV), which are recapitulated in (Fig. **2**). Family history is a crucial risk factor because 10% of stomach cancer shows familial aggregation, and >3% of all stomach carcinoma is inherited by following the pattern of Mendelian inheritance [28, 29].

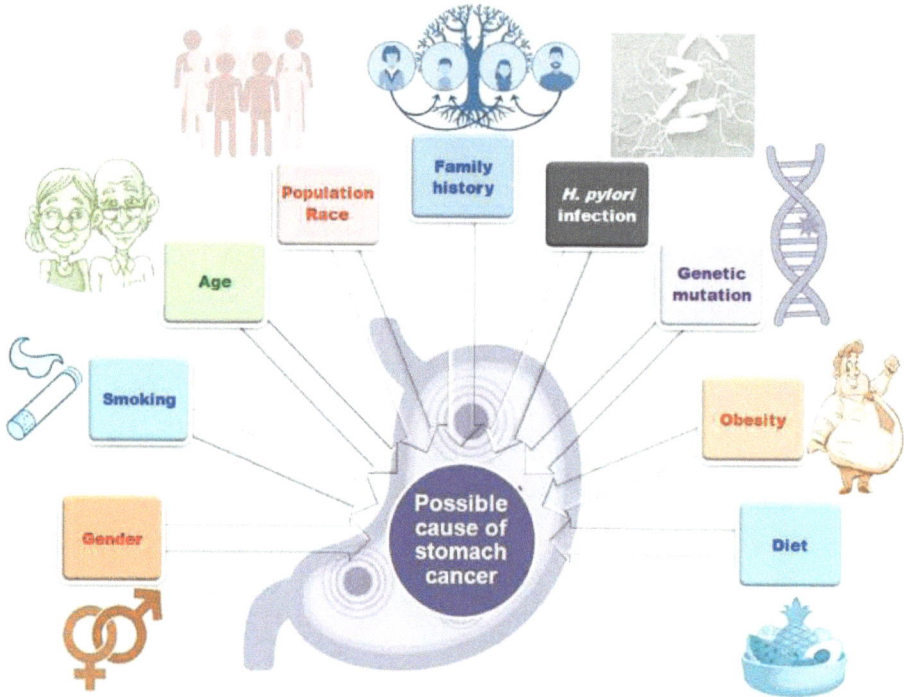

Fig. (2). Risk factors associated with stomach cancer development.

Earlier evidence indicates that vegetables and fruits protect against stomach cancer development, but the smoked foods, salt-preserved foods, and charbroiled and broiled meat increase stomach cancer progression [30 - 32]. About 80% of stomach cancer risk was increased in smokers and heavy drinkers [33, 34]. The gram-negative bacteria *Helicobacter pylori* affect the process of oncogenesis and act as an oncogene for the development of stomach cancer [35 - 40]. Limited reports have been available to describe the role of EBV in the development of stomach cancer, and about 10% of stomach cancer is EBV-positive [41 - 43].

2.5. Diagnosis, Prevention and Treatment

Endoscopy and contrast radiography is generally used to screen and diagnose stomach cancer. Besides this, non-invasive methods such as serum trefoil factor3, pepsinogen level in serum and serology of *H. pylori* are used. Serological detection of *H. pylori* was done by helicon test and Urea breath test. The visual examination of gastric mucosa was done by endoscopy, histological analysis and biopsy [20]. Fig. (**3**) depicts the most commonly used diagnosis and treatment methods for stomach cancer. There are preventive approaches which have been applied to overcome the challenges detailed below.

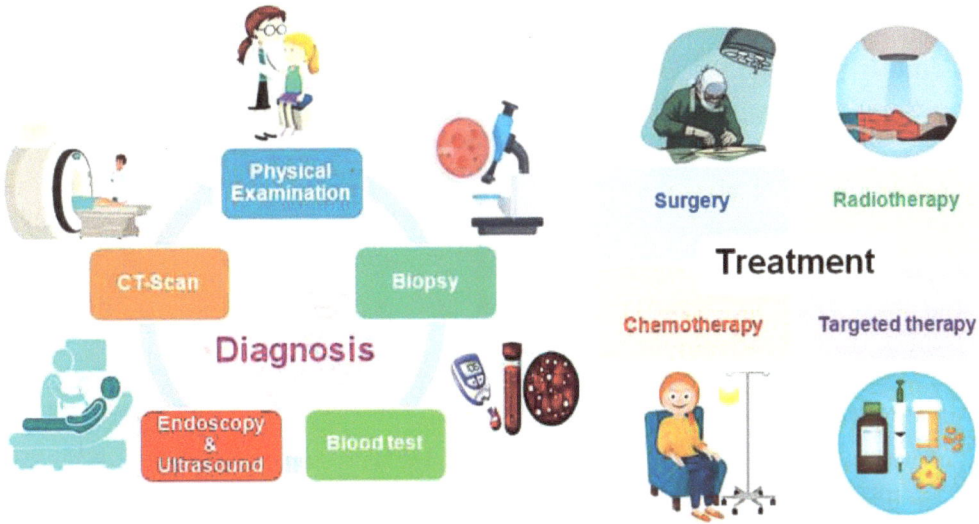

Fig. (3). Commonly used diagnosis and treatment modalities for stomach cancer.

2.5.1. Eradication of H. Pylori Infection

The primary goal of gastric cancer prevention is eradicating infection of *H.pylori* in the developing world because the condition is associated with the non-cardiac type of gastric cancer. The eradication reduced the incidence of gastric cancer in asymptomatic Asian individuals by a meta-analysis [44]. The prevalence of gastric lesions was decreased after administering antibiotics for two weeks in the Shandong Intervention Trial [45]. The development of metachronous stomach carcinoma was prevented by prophylactic eradication of *H. pylori* [46].

2.5.2. Diet Improvement

The prevention might be possible by reducing the consumption of salt-preserved foods and reducing salt consumption. Besides, the intake of fresh fruits and vegetables might be helpful because they contain vitamin C, phytochemicals, folate and carotenoids *etc.*, which have been reported to reduce carcinogenesis. Moreover, lifestyle modification, including limited smoking and increased physical activities, could also reduce the risk of stomach cancer [47 - 49].

2.5.3. Early Detection

The specificity and sensitivity of photofluorography are 80-90% and 70-90%, respectively. Compared to the symptom-detected patients, the 15-30% better survival was observed in screen-detected patients [50]. Endoscopy has high sensitivity toward stomach cancer in the distant and regional regions compared to the radiographic method [51]. According to Matsumoto *et al*. [52], endoscopic and radiographic examination avoids the development of stomach cancer. The endoscopic screening reduced the mortality by up to 30% compared to the non-examined group [53].

3. HISTOPATHOLOGY OF STOMACH CANCER

Lauren, in 1965 established the stomach cancer classification, which is most frequently acceptable compared to other categories. According to this, two histological subtypes include diffuse intestinal and indeterminate type. The intestinal type is the most common, followed by the diffuse and indeterminate varieties. Visible glands and cohesion between cancer cells are the characteristics of the intestinal carcinoma, while poorly cohesive cells, no gland formation and diffusely infiltrating walls are observed in diffuse subtypes.The intestinal subtype is linked with metaplasia of gastric mucosa and infection with *H. pylori*. The studies indicate that diffuse stomach cancer is higher in younger patients and females than in other types [54, 55]. The classification of stomach cancer is represented in Fig. (**4**).

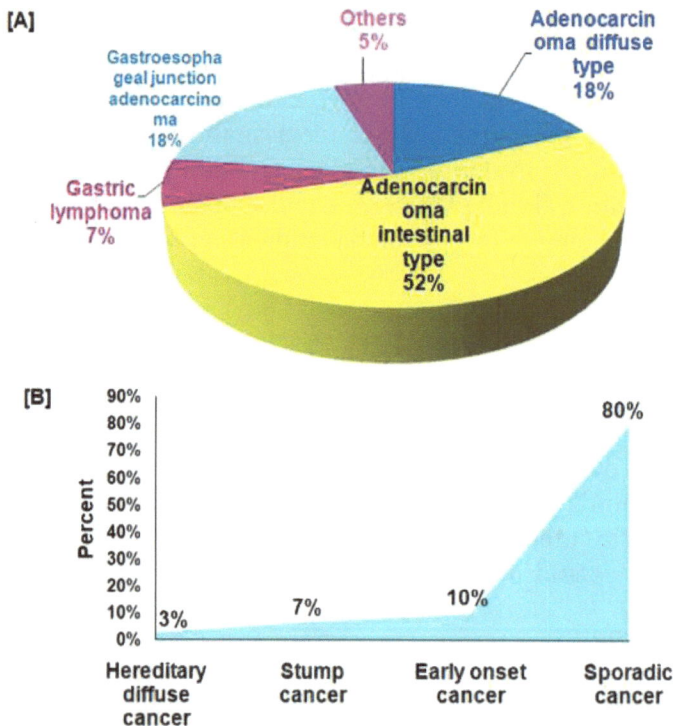

Fig. (**4**). Classification of stomach cancer.

3.1. Sporadic Type

It mainly affects the population over 45 years and is caused by the environmental factors' coincidence. In high-risk countries, males are two times more susceptible than females [56 - 58].

3.2. Early-onset Gastric Cancer

This type of gastric cancer occurs in the population below 45 years, and genetic factors play an essential role in developing this type of cancer. It is diffuse, multifactorial, and due to the hormonal factors mainly observed in females, the pathogenesis remains unclear [59 - 61].

3.3. Gastric Stump Cancer

A type of carcinoma forms after peptic ulcer surgery in gastric remnant. It encompasses about 1-7% of all stomach cancer and majorly affects males compared to females. The primary risk factor is gastrectomy, and after 15 years of gastrectomy, the chance of infection would increase by four to seven folds compared to healthy individuals. The infection of EBV is less prominent in the intact stomach but evident in the gastric remnant and targets the p53 protein. However, the infection of *H. pylori* is less common [61 - 63].

3.4. Hereditary Diffuse Gastric Cancer

It constitutes 1-3% of all gastric cancer types. It is developed from inherited syndromes, especially the germline mutation in the *CDH1* gene that encodes a critical metastasis regulating protein E-cadherin. It is poorly differentiated, infiltrates from the stomach wall, diffuses, and increases the thickening of the wall [58, 61].

The World Health Organization (WHO) also classified stomach cancer based on the origin of cancer from the five layers of the stomach. The classification of stomach cancer is as follows:Adenocarcinoma starts from mucosa and accounts for 90-95% of cancer. Two significant types of adenocarcinoma have been reported, *i.e.* diffuse and intestinal. In intestinal adenocarcinoma, cells have reduced stroma and irregular tubular structures; multiple lume, while in diffuse adenocarcinoma, cells secrete mucus, discohesive, and are poorly differentiated. Besides, about 5% of stomach cancers are lymphomas.

4. TUMOUR-IMMUNE MILIEU IN STOMACH CANCER

The immune system is a remarkable factor in the development of stomach cancer. The immune cells, including neutrophils, several lineages of T-cells, macrophages and dendritic cells (DCs), are important for developing the tumour microenvironment and are involved in various cancer growth and initiation [2, 64]. The immune-suppressive character has been observed in stomach cancer, but variation was noted based on molecular subtype, anatomical location of the lesion, and histology of the tumour [65]. CD4+T-cells, CD68+ macrophages and CD8+ T cells represent about 11%, 13% and 15% of all intra-tumoural cells in stomach cancer respectively. The high infiltration of macrophages, CD4+ and CD8+ cells was observed in EBV-positive tumours, while less infiltration was noted in diffuse-type of stomach cancer. In intestinal subtypes, the presence of infiltrating macrophages was conspicuous and had relatively low T cells. The earlier studies depict that EBV-positive stomach cancer is prominent in filtered tumours, particularly by CD8+ T cells [65 - 69]. Besides, several studies indicate the association between improved survival and the high number of lymphocytes. Stomach cancer cells express a ligand for CD155 and PD-L1 and induce exhaustion of T-cells after interacting with TIGIT and PD-1, respectively, which affects the metabolism of T-cells *via* glycolysis inhibition and suppresses their functions. The downregulation of genes involved in glucose metabolism, the Akt/mTOR pathway and glucose uptake was observed in the TIGIT+ CD8+ T cells obtained from a stomach cancer patient. When the glucose concentration increased, the phenotype of T cell exhaustion was reversed. In the animal model of stomach cancer, the PD-1 inhibition and TIGIT inhibition improve immunity. In stomach cancer, over-expression of inhaled corticosteroids is the reported mechanism for the exhaustion of T-cells. Various reports examined the role of PDL1 and PD-1 in the microenvironment of stomach cancer. Besides, the upregulation of inhaled corticosteroids, including VISTA, CTLA-4, and TIM-3, has been reported [70 - 72].

In 2014, the approval for inhaled corticosteroid inhibitors (nivolumab and pembrolizumab) was initiated for melanoma, leading to the introduction of a new cancer treatment era. Since then, various CTLA-4, PD-1 and PD-L1 inhibitors have been approved against different types of cancer [4]. In 2017, pembrolizumab, a PD-1inhibitor approved for recurrent stomach cancer expressing PD-L1, advanced based on the KEYNOTE-059 phase II clinical trial [14]. The ATTRACTION-2 phase-III trial and ONO-4538 phase-II of nivolumab increased the survival of heavily pretreated stomach cancer patients. After this trial, Japan approved using nivolumab for advanced stages of stomach carcinoma regardless of PD-L1 expression [73]. A combination trial has been conducted to investigate the combined effect of inhaled corticosteroid inhibitors with conventional therapies. The combination of neo-adjuvant short-term-limited local radiotherapy and immune checkpoint blockade therapy was used in the CIRCUIT trial (Clinical trials.gov). The Gal-9 and TIM-3 play an essential role in the exhaustion of T-cells. The overall poor survival is associated with their expression in stomach cancer patients [67]. Recently LAG-3 was found as a therapeutic target that promotes activation of CD8[+] T-cell, increases the survival rate, enhances interferon-γ (IFN-γ) secretion and reduces tumour growth in stomach cancer [74].

5. GUT MICROBIOTA DYSBIOSIS IN STOMACH CANCER

The infection of *H. pylori* alters the microbial habitat, increasing the risk of gastric cancer.Some reports suggest that the reduced microbial diversity was observed in cancer and inflammatory diseases. Some studies indicate that the enrichment of microbial diversity was observed in stomach cancer tissues compared to the healthy tissues [75, 76]. Gantuya *et al*. [77]indicate that the reduced microbiome diversity was observed in stomach cancer, intestinalmetaplasia and gastritis. In the advanced stages of stomach cancer, the microbiome diversity was increased compared to the early stages and *Salinivibrio, Tsukamurella, Burkholderia*, and *Uruburuella* are most abundant in advanced settings. In the case of early stomach cancer the microbiome enriched with *Pseudoxanthomonas, Ralstonia, Anoxybacillus, Novosphingobium*, and *Ochrobactrum* [78]. Liu *et al*. [79]suggested non-significant changes observed in the microbial composition of late and early stages of stomach cancer; however, the richness of microbial diversity was decreased compared to the normal tissues. The study indicates the enrichment of *Streptococcus anginosus, Propionibacterium acnes* and *Prevotella melanogenic,* while the reduced level of *Bacteroides uniformis* and *Prevotella copri* was observed in tumour tissues [79]. The report of Ravegnini *et al*. [80] provides evidence that the high levels of *Acidobacteria* and *Proteobacteria* were observed in adenocarcinoma while in single ring cell carcinoma, high levels of *Patescibacteria, Fusobacteria*, and *Bacteroidetes* were observed.A study in Taiwan suggests that high levels of *Lactobacillus* were observed in stomach cancer patients compared to intestinal metaplasia and gastritis [81];this is supported by others finding [82]. The potential role of lactic acid-producing bacteria in stomach cancer pathogenesis is reported by several groups [76, 83, 84]. The changes in the stomach microbiome were investigated by Park & his group in 2022 in the gastric juice samples collected from 88 patients. The next-generation sequencing and 16S rRNA gene profiling was used to study microbial composition and diversity differences. The findings suggest that the microbial diversity was decreased with the substantial increase in carcinogenesis. The *Veillonella* and *Lactobacillus* enriched genera were observed in cancer groups. Besides, the functional capacity evaluation indicates the delpletion and enrichment of various functional pathways associated with carcinogenesis [85]. Anther report by Coker *et al.* [86], indicates that *Streptococcus anginosus*, *Dialister pneumosintes*, *Parvimonas micra*, *Peptostreptococcus stomatis* and *Slackia exigua* are the major microbes associated with progression of stomach cancer.

6. ROLE OF PROBIOTICS IN STOMACH CANCER MANAGEMENT

Probiotics are a group of microbes (yeast and bacteria) that show health-promoting effects, if consumed appropriately. The administration of probiotics maintains the intestinal microorganisms, restores gut homeostasis, and decreases the gastro-intestinal tract (GIT) pathogenic microorganisms [87–91]. The microorganisms used as probiotics are presented in Table **1**.

Table. (1). List of microorganisms used in human nutrition as probiotics.

Type of Microorganisms	Microorganisms used in Pharmaceutical products	Microorganisms used as Food additives	Both
Lactobacillus	*L. acidophilus* *L. gasseri* *L. helveticus* *L. reuteri*	*L. amylovorus* *L. johnsonii* *L. pentosus* *L. plantarum*	*L. casei* *L. rhamnosus*
Bifidobacterium	*B. adolescentis* *B. animalis* *B. bifidum* *B. infantis* *B. longum*	*B. breve*	-
Lactic Acid Bacteria	*Enterococcus faecium* *Streptococcus thermophiles*	*Lactococcus lactis*	-
Other	*Bacillus clausii* *Escherichia coli Nissle 1917* *Saccharomyces cerevisiae* *(boulardi)*	-	-

6.1. Anticancer Mechanism of Probiotics

Probiotics induce anti-pathogenic ability by promoting gut barrier function, decreasing translocation of bacteria, and modulating microbiota. Besides, it modulates inflammatory response, reducing metastasis and tumour development, thereby promoting gastric cancer prevention and treatment [92 - 94]. Probiotics act as dietary supplements to suppress the development of neoplastic lesions and the tumour's predisposition and trigger immune activity, thereby reducing the development of gastrointestinal cancer [31, 95 - 98]. The previous studies indicate the role of probiotics in oxidative stress markers, inflammation markers and metabolic profiles [99 - 102]. Fig. (**5**) depicts the mechanism adopted by the probiotics for preventing cancer.

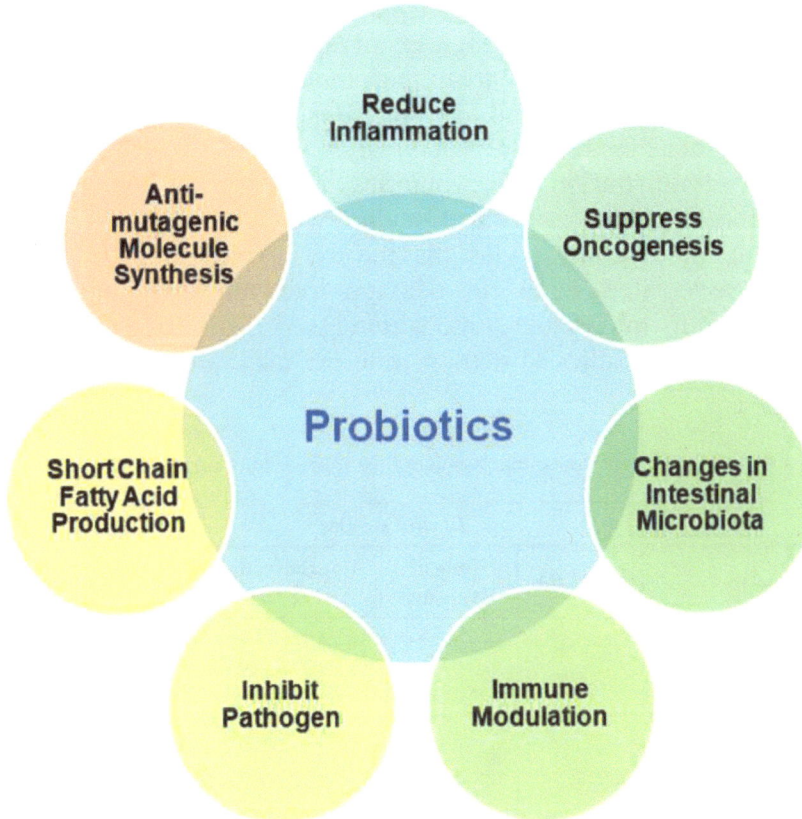

Fig. (5). Targets of probiotics for cancer prevention and treatment.

Majorly the administration of probiotics affects the microbiota in both a quantitative and qualitative manner. Some specific strains, including *Clostridia, Streptococcus bovis, H. pylori*, and *Bacteroides*, produce genotoxic metabolites that bind to surface receptors and affect intracellular signalling, while *B. longum* and *L. acidophilus* inhibit carcinogenic growth. The administration of probiotics increases intestinal barriers' integrity, decreasing the metabolism of pre-carcinogens and suppressing pathogenic growth. The effects are not limited to preventing the carcinogenic agents but also involve the therapeutic effects [93]. The probiotics give therapeutic responses by producing antibiotics and bacteriocins that suppress the growth of undesired microbes. Besides, these products directly interact with tumour cells, thereby suppressing their proliferation, and their competitive nature is due to their ability to adhere to the epithelial cells. Short chain fatty acids' (SCFAs) production is another mode by which probiotics suppress the tumour growth. Probiotics also reduce pro-inflammatory cytokines, including IL-17, thereby showing immunomodu- latory potential in different cancer types [93]. The oral administration of probiotics decreases the side effects of drugs by modulating the intestinal microbiome. Diarrhoea and mucositis are the significant adverse effects caused by anticancer treatments. Among the other treatment modalities, probiotics have various advantages, including safety and low cost. Besides, they reduce respiratory tract infections and diarrhoea due to *Clostridium difficile* and improve antibiotics [103]. The administration of probiotics reestablishes the gut microbiota population both in quantity and functionality, which gets reduced after treatments [104]. Several clinical trials suggest that the consumption of probiotics diminishes the therapy associated with gut damage like mucositis and diarrhoea by maintaining healthy microbiota composition [105]. Table **2** mentions the different *in vitro* and *in vivo* studies to demonstrate the effects of probiotics in stomach cancer.

Table. (2). Effects of probiotics on stomach cancer (*in vitro* & human) studies.

In vitro studies					
Probiotics	**Cell Line**	**Time of Exposure**	**Concentration (CFU/mL)**	**Effect**	**References**
Lactobacillus acidophilus 74-2 *Bifidobacterium lactis 420*	NCI-N87 AGS	-	8.24×10^7 and 2.20×10^8 respectively	Upregulate COX-1 expression	[106]
Lactobacillus rhamnosus GG	HGC-27	24h and 48h	1×10^8	Suppressed proliferation Decreased polyamine content	[107]
Lactobacillus paracasei IMPC2.1 and Lactobacillus rhamnosus GG	HGC-27	24h and 48h	1×10^8	Inhibit growth Induced apoptosis	[108]
Propionibacterium freudenreichii ITG P9	HGT-1	24h, 48h and 72h	9×10^{12}	Increased release of cytochrome c and activate caspase	[109]
Lactobacillus reuteri	AGS	24h, 48h and 72h	1.5×10^8	Reduced proliferation uPAR and uPA	[110]

(Table 2) cont.....

In vitro studies					
Probiotics	**Cell Line**	**Time of Exposure**	**Concentration (CFU/mL)**	**Effect**	**References**
Lactobacillus fermentum UCO979C and Lactobacillus casei Shirota	AGS	0-48 h	1.5×10^9	Inhibited urease activity	[111]
Human Studies					
Probiotics	**Model**	**Duration**	**Sample size**	**Effects**	**Reference**
Bifidobacterium	Gastric cancer patients	4 weeks	112	Reduced small intestine bacterial overgrowth Decreased symptoms of gastric cancer	[112]

The studies by Gianotti *et al.* [113]and Lalla *et al.* [114]suggest that probiotics containing *Lactobacillus* prevent mucositis and diarrhoea in patients who suffered from pelvic malignancy and received pelvic malignancy radiotherapy/ chemotherapy. The evidence indicates that *H. pylori* are involved in gastric cancer initiation; thus, the potential effect of probiotics to suppress the activity of *H. pylori* has been investigated and are presented in Tables **2** and **3** [110, 115 - 118]. The exact anticancer mechanisms of probiotics are still not known. The reports indicate that the gut's microbiota affects various pathways that might be essential for this process. Probiotic microbes maintain the sustainable condition of phytochemicals in the colon by maintaining homeostasis. The reduced pH increases the excessive release of bile acids in the face, leading to the damage of colon epithelium, and showing direct cytotoxicity, thereby promoting colon carcinogenesis. The bacteria, including *B. bifidum* and *L. acidophilus,* modulate the bile acid profile and pH, thus offering cancer-preventive efficiency [119 - 121]. The probiotics balance the microflora's metabolic activity and quantity of natural flora. The gut microbes, including *Clostridium perfringens* and *Escherichia coli* involved in the production of the carcinogenic molecule by utilizing enzymes including nitroreductase, β-glucuronidase and azoreductase [122]. The microbes of probiotics, including *Bifidobacillus* and *Lactobacillus* strains, showed cancer preventive efficacy by degrading carcinogen *via* binding to it. Unhealthy food like fried meat has mutagenic compounds associated with colon cancer risks. Administration of *Lactobacillus* strain decreased the faecal and urine excretion of heterocyclic aromatic amines, thereby alleviating the mutagenic effect of cooked meat [122 - 124]. Gut microbiota metabolized and produced various compounds reported to suppress carcinogenesis and maintain homeostasis. The SCFAs including butyrate, acetate and propionate are created by some specific gut microbiota populations *via* fermentation of fibre rich probiotics. Besides, they act as a high energy source, they also act as signalling molecules that primarily affect proliferation, immune system, production of intestinal hormone and cell death. Moreover, they are also involved in maintaining epithelial integrity [122, 125, 126].

Table. (3). Clinical studies conducted using probiotics with combination therapy for eradication of *H. pylori* infection.

Probiotic Strains	Patients	Sample Size	Exposure Time	Eradication Rate	Side Effects	Adverse Effects	Reference
L. acidophilus L.B.	Dyspeptic adults	120	10 days	Increase	-	-	[127]
L. rhamnosus G.G.	Asymptomatic adults	60	14 days	No effect	Decrease	-	[128]
L. rhamnosus G.G.	Asymptomatic adults	120	14 days	No effect	-	Increase	[129]
L. acidophilus La5 B. lactis Bb12	Dyspeptic adults	160	4 weeks	Increase	-	Decrease	[130]
L. rhamnosus G.G. S. boulardii L. acidophilus La5 B. lactis Bb12	Asymptomatic adults	85	2 weeks	No effect	-	Decrease	[131]
L. caseissp L. casei D.G.	Dyspeptic adults with resistant *H. pylori*	70	10 days	No effect	-	Decrease	[132]
L. casei	Dyspeptic children	86	2 weeks	Increase	-	No effect	[133]
L. reuteri	Dyspeptic children	40	20 days	No effect	-	Decrease	[134]
L. acidophilus La5 B. lactis Bb12	Dyspeptic adults with resistant *H. pylori*	138	4 weeks	Increase	Decrease	-	[130]
B. animalis L. casei	Children	65	-	Increase	-	-	[135]
L. rhamnosus LC P. freudenreichii B. breve	Individuals	118	4 weeks	No effect	-	-	[136]
L. reuteri	Individuals	90	6 weeks	Increase	-	-	[137]

7. CURRENT PROBLEMS AND PROSPECTS

Stomach cancer has been associated with epigenetic and genetic aberrations. Currently, the tumour, node and metastasis(TNM) staging is used for the prognosis of stomach cancer; however, the other factors are also crucial for patients' survival and natural course. Recently used targeted therapy to treat stomach cancer patients has been proven unsuccessful. Thus, the treatment of stomach cancer patients is challenging. Molecular profiling and high-end next-generation sequencing help in improving the understanding of this complex disease. The studies suggest that epigenetic changes, mutations and chromosomal alterations are associated with stomach cancer. The clinical significance of immune-modulatory molecules and their differential expression further needs to be explored. Moreover, few reports are based on the morphological investigation of tumour-infiltrating lymphocytes in stomach cancer; thus, scoring method standardization is still required to quantify lymphocytes in stomach cancer.

Further studies are required to confirm the bonafide stomach cancer driver's clinical and functional levels that could be used as biomarkers and therapeutic targets. Besides, the promising research area is to identify the correlation and mechanism of infectious or environmental agents and the risk of stomach cancer. The studies are also required to explore the impact of risk factors on survival, treatment response and microenvironment, including immune cells, blood cells and stromal cells in stomach cancer patients. Although the advanced diagnostic tools helped to identify and isolate bacterial species involved in cancer pathogenesis, the underlying mechanisms describing the effects of microbiota on oncogenic activation, carcinogenic metabolite production, DNA damage, inhibition of tumour immunity, and chronic inflammation induction are still needed exploration. The improvement in the pathogenesis of stomach cancer might help to improve the survival and prognosis of patients.

The studies revealed that microbiota has an essential role in the treatment and diagnosis of disease.Therefore, microbiota has been considered a promising target for the prevention and treatment of cancer. Earlier evidences indicated that probiotics increased bacteria eradication, reduced toxicities associated with chemotherapy/radiotherapy, and prevented cancer development. The effects of probiotics were mainly observed in colon, breast, hepatocellular carcinoma and lung carcinoma, but limited studies are reported in stomach cancer. Moreover, most of the evidences are based on pre-clinical studies; therefore, further clinical studies will be required to establish their usefulness in the prevention and treatment of stomach cancer. The interplay between microbiota and drug mechanisms needs to be investigated in depth. Some microbes have decreased the efficiency of molecular targeted therapy and chemotherapy. Besides, they also affect conventional drugs' adverse effects and toxicity profiles. Thus, the studies indicate that the microbiota of the GIT is an emerging field with diverse therapeutic applications. Therefore, further studies are needed to explore the combined effect of probiotics and antibiotics with immunotherapy and chemotherapy. The manipulation using intestinal microbiota is a recent strategy by which promising findings have been observed against the infection of *Clostridium difficile*. Thus, the therapeutic implementation against other diseases, including stomach cancer, might help to overcome the challenge of adverse effects. In addition, further studies will be required to find out the potential strains, administration regime and dosage for selective stage and type of cancer to reduce the death rates.

CONCLUSION

Probiotics have been an essential tool in the clinical medicine due to various health-promoting effects. Multiple studies using surfeit experimental models, including human clinical trials, animal models, and *in vitro* studies, have shown that probiotics can help to treat and prevent stomach cancer by activating the immune response, reducing intestinal pH, and suppressing the bacterial conversion of carcinogens from pro-carcinogens, and producing SCFAs. However, probiotics as a bio-therapeutic agent against stomach cancer have not been yet investigated adequately. Besides, the clinical utility of probiotics concerning mortality rates remains unexplored. In addition, the role of probiotics along with immune checkpoint inhibitors needs to be examined. Therefore, further studies and experimental evidences are required to provide information about the significant utility of probiotics and their optimal doses to increase the use of probiotics as a pharmacological tool against stomach cancer.

CONSENT FOR PUBLICATION

Not applicable.

CONFLICT OF INTEREST

The authors declare no conflict of interest, financial or otherwise.

ACKNOWLEDGEMENTS

SS and SL are thankful to CSIR-CIMAP, Lucknow India. DKS and BK acknowledge UGC, New Delhi and Department of Pharmacy, Central University of South Bihar, Gaya, India for their support.

REFERENCES

[1]   Gabrilovich DI, Ostrand-Rosenberg S, Bronte V. Coordinated regulation of myeloid cells by tumours. Nat Rev Immunol 2012; 12(4): 253-68.
[http://dx.doi.org/10.1038/nri3175] [PMID: 22437938]

[2]   Binnewies M, Roberts EW, Kersten K, *et al.* Understanding the tumor immune microenvironment (TIME) for effective therapy. Nat Med 2018; 24(5): 541-50.
[http://dx.doi.org/10.1038/s41591-018-0014-x] [PMID: 29686425]

[3]   Chen DS, Mellman I. Elements of cancer immunity and the cancer–immune set point. Nature 2017; 541(7637): 321-30.
[http://dx.doi.org/10.1038/nature21349] [PMID: 28102259]

[4]   Rotte A, Jin JY, Lemaire V. Mechanistic overview of immune checkpoints to support the rational design of their combinations in cancer immunotherapy. Ann Oncol 2018; 29(1): 71-83.
[http://dx.doi.org/10.1093/annonc/mdx686] [PMID: 29069302]

[5]   Herbst RS, Soria JC, Kowanetz M, *et al.* Predictive correlates of response to the anti-PD-L1 antibody MPDL3280A in cancer patients. Nature 2014; 515(7528): 563-7.
[http://dx.doi.org/10.1038/nature14011] [PMID: 25428504]

[6]   Tumeh PC, Harview CL, Yearley JH, *et al.* PD-1 blockade induces responses by inhibiting adaptive immune resistance. Nature 2014; 515(7528): 568-71.
[http://dx.doi.org/10.1038/nature13954] [PMID: 25428505]

[7]   Wei SC, Levine JH, Cogdill AP, *et al.* Distinct Cellular Mechanisms Underlie Anti-CTLA-4 and Anti-PD-1 Checkpoint Blockade. Cell 2017; 170(6): 1120-1133.e17.
[http://dx.doi.org/10.1016/j.cell.2017.07.024] [PMID: 28803728]

[8]   Samstein RM, Lee CH, Shoushtari AN, *et al.* Tumor mutational load predicts survival after immunotherapy across multiple cancer types. Nat Genet 2019; 51(2): 202-6.
[http://dx.doi.org/10.1038/s41588-018-0312-8] [PMID: 30643254]

[9]   O'Connor A, O'Morain CA, Ford AC. Population screening and treatment of *Helicobacter pylori* infection. Nat Rev Gastroenterol Hepatol 2017; 14(4): 230-40.
[http://dx.doi.org/10.1038/nrgastro.2016.195] [PMID: 28053340]

[10]   Comprehensive molecular characterization of gastric adenocarcinoma. Nature 2014; 513(7517): 202-9.
[http://dx.doi.org/10.1038/nature13480] [PMID: 25079317]

[11]   Joshi SS, Maron SB, Catenacci DV. Pembrolizumab for treatment of advanced gastric and gastroesophageal junction adenocarcinoma. Future Oncol 2018; 14(5): 417-30.
[http://dx.doi.org/10.2217/fon-2017-0436] [PMID: 29094609]

[12]   Cho J, Lee J, Bang H, *et al.* Programmed cell death-ligand 1 expression predicts survival in patients with gastric carcinoma with microsatellite instability. Oncotarget 2017; 8(8): 13320-8.
[http://dx.doi.org/10.18632/oncotarget.14519] [PMID: 28076847]

[13]   Xing X, Guo J, Ding G, *et al.* Analysis of PD1, PDL1, PDL2 expression and T cells infiltration in 1014 gastric cancer patients. OncoImmunology 2018; 7(3)e1356144
[http://dx.doi.org/10.1080/2162402X.2017.1356144] [PMID: 29399387]

[14]   Fuchs CS, Doi T, Jang RW, *et al.* Safety and efficacy of pembrolizumab monotherapy in patients with previously treated advanced gastric and gastroesophageal junction cancer: phase 2 clinical KEYNOTE-059 trial. JAMA Oncol 2018; 4(5): e180013-3.
[http://dx.doi.org/10.1001/jamaoncol.2018.0013] [PMID: 29543932]

[15]   Zhang M, Dong Y, Liu H, *et al.* The clinicopathological and prognostic significance of PD-L1 expression in gastric cancer: a meta-analysis of 10 studies with 1,901 patients. Sci Rep 2016; 6(1): 37933.
[http://dx.doi.org/10.1038/srep37933] [PMID: 27892511]

[16] Das S, Suarez G, Beswick EJ, Sierra JC, Graham DY, Reyes VE. Expression of B7-H1 on gastric epithelial cells: its potential role in regulating T cells during *Helicobacter pylori* infection. J Immunol 2006; 176(5): 3000-9.
[http://dx.doi.org/10.4049/jimmunol.176.5.3000] [PMID: 16493058]

[17] Beswick EJ, Pinchuk IV, Das S, Powell DW, Reyes VE. Expression of the programmed death ligand 1, B7-H1, on gastric epithelial cells after *Helicobacter pylori* exposure promotes development of CD4+ CD25+ FoxP3+ regulatory T cells. Infect Immun 2007; 75(9): 4334-41.
[http://dx.doi.org/10.1128/IAI.00553-07] [PMID: 17562772]

[18] Wu Y-Y, Lin C-W, Cheng K-S, *et al.* Increased programmed death-ligand-1 expression in human gastric epithelial cells in *Helicobacter pylori* infection. Clin Exp Immunol 2010; 161(3): 551-9.
[http://dx.doi.org/10.1111/j.1365-2249.2010.04217.x] [PMID: 20646001]

[19] Lina TT, Alzahrani S, House J, *et al. Helicobacter pylori* cag pathogenicity island's role in B7-H1 induction and immune evasion. PLoS One 2015; 10(3)e0121841
[http://dx.doi.org/10.1371/journal.pone.0121841] [PMID: 25807464]

[20] Rawla P, Barsouk A. Epidemiology of gastric cancer: global trends, risk factors and prevention. Prz Gastroenterol 2019; 14(1): 26-38.
[http://dx.doi.org/10.5114/pg.2018.80001] [PMID: 30944675]

[21] BW S, CP W. World Cancer Report 2014 [Internet]. [cited 2022 Jun 5]. Available from: https://publications.iarc.fr/Non-Series-Publications/World-Cancer-Reports/World-Cancer-Report-2014

[22] Sharma A, Radhakrishnan V. Gastric cancer in India. Indian J Med Paediatr Oncol 2011; 32(1): 12-6.
[http://dx.doi.org/10.4103/0971-5851.81884] [PMID: 21731210]

[23] Bray F, Ferlay J, Soerjomataram I, Siegel RL, Torre LA, Jemal A. Global cancer statistics 2018: GLOBOCAN estimates of incidence and mortality worldwide for 36 cancers in 185 countries. CA Cancer J Clin 2018; 68(6): 394-424.
[http://dx.doi.org/10.3322/caac.21492] [PMID: 30207593]

[24] Balakrishnan M, George R, Sharma A, Graham DY. Changing trends in stomach cancer throughout the world. Curr Gastroenterol Rep 2017; 19(8): 36.
[http://dx.doi.org/10.1007/s11894-017-0575-8] [PMID: 28730504]

[25] Howlader N, Noone A, Krapcho M, Miller D, Bishop K, Kosary CL. Cancer Statistics Review, 1975-2014-SEER Statistics, National Cancer Institute. SEER Cancer Statistics Review 2016; 1975-2014.

[26] Stojanovic MM, Rancic NK, Andjelkovic Apostolovic MR, Ignjatovic AM, Ilic MV. Trends of Stomach Cancer in Central Serbia. Medicina (Kaunas) 2021; 57(7): 665.
[http://dx.doi.org/10.3390/medicina57070665] [PMID: 34203145]

[27] Wang J, Sun Y, Bertagnolli MM. Comparison of gastric cancer survival between Caucasian and Asian patients treated in the United States: results from the Surveillance Epidemiology and End Results (SEER) database. Ann Surg Oncol 2015; 22(9): 2965-71.
[http://dx.doi.org/10.1245/s10434-015-4388-4] [PMID: 25631065]

[28] Yaghoobi M, Bijarchi R, Narod SA. Family history and the risk of gastric cancer. Br J Cancer 2010; 102(2): 237-42.
[http://dx.doi.org/10.1038/sj.bjc.6605380] [PMID: 19888225]

[29] Boland CR, Yurgelun MB. Historical perspective on familial gastric cancer. Cell Mol Gastroenterol Hepatol 2017; 3(2): 192-200.
[http://dx.doi.org/10.1016/j.jcmgh.2016.12.003] [PMID: 28275686]

[30] Kim J, Cho YA, Choi WJ, Jeong SH. Gene-diet interactions in gastric cancer risk: A systematic review. World J Gastroenterol 2014; 20(28): 9600-10.
[http://dx.doi.org/10.3748/wjg.v20.i28.9600] [PMID: 25071358]

[31] Zhang MM, Cheng JQ, Xia L, Lu YR, Wu XT. Monitoring intestinal microbiota profile: A promising

method for the ultraearly detection of colorectal cancer. Med Hypotheses 2011; 76(5): 670-2.
[http://dx.doi.org/10.1016/j.mehy.2011.01.028] [PMID: 21310543]

[32]   Keszei AP, Goldbohm RA, Schouten LJ, Jakszyn P, van den Brandt PA. Dietary N-nitroso
       compounds, endogenous nitrosation, and the risk of esophageal and gastric cancer subtypes in the
       Netherlands Cohort Study. Am J Clin Nutr 2013; 97(1): 135-46.
       [http://dx.doi.org/10.3945/ajcn.112.043885] [PMID: 23193003]

[33]   Moy KA, Fan Y, Wang R, Gao YT, Yu MC, Yuan JM. Alcohol and tobacco use in relation to gastric
       cancer: a prospective study of men in Shanghai, China. Cancer Epidemiol Biomarkers Prev 2010;
       19(9): 2287-97.
       [http://dx.doi.org/10.1158/1055-9965.EPI-10-0362] [PMID: 20699372]

[34]   Duell EJ, Travier N, Lujan-Barroso L, *et al.* Alcohol consumption and gastric cancer risk in the
       European Prospective Investigation into Cancer and Nutrition (EPIC) cohort. Am J Clin Nutr 2014;
       94(5): 1266-75.
       [http://dx.doi.org/10.3945/ajcn.111.012351] [PMID: 21993435]

[35]   Roesler BM, Rabelo-Gonçalves EMA, Zeitune JMR. Virulence Factors of *Helicobacter pylori:* A
       Review. Clin Med Insights Gastroenterol 2014; 7CGast.S13760
       [http://dx.doi.org/10.4137/CGast.S13760] [PMID: 24833944]

[36]   Ishaq S, Nunn L. *Helicobacter pylori* and gastric cancer: a state of the art review. Gastroenterol
       Hepatol Bed Bench 2015; 8 (Suppl. 1): S6-S14.
       [PMID: 26171139]

[37]   Khatoon J, Rai RP, Prasad KN. Role of *Helicobacter pylori* in gastric cancer: Updates. World J
       Gastrointest Oncol 2016; 8(2): 147-58.
       [http://dx.doi.org/10.4251/wjgo.v8.i2.147] [PMID: 26909129]

[38]   Chang WL, Yeh YC, Sheu BS. The impacts of *H. pylori* virulence factors on the development of
       gastroduodenal diseases. J Biomed Sci 2018; 25(1): 68.
       [http://dx.doi.org/10.1186/s12929-018-0466-9] [PMID: 30205817]

[39]   Baj J, Brzozowska K, Forma A, Maani A, Sitarz E, Portincasa P. Immunological aspects of the tumour
       microenvironment and epithelial-mesenchymal transition in gastric carcinogenesis. Int J Mol Sci 2020;
       21(7): 2544.
       [http://dx.doi.org/10.3390/ijms21072544] [PMID: 32268527]

[40]   Baj J, Korona-Głowniak I, Forma A, *et al.* Mechanisms of the epithelial–mesenchymal transition and
       tumour microenvironment in *Helicobacter pylori*-induced gastric cancer. Cells 2020; 9(4): 1055.
       [http://dx.doi.org/10.3390/cells9041055] [PMID: 32340207]

[41]   Fukayama M, Hayashi Y, Iwasaki Y, *et al.* Epstein-Barr virus-associated gastric carcinoma and
       Epstein-Barr virus infection of the stomach. Lab Invest 1994; 71(1): 73-81.
       [PMID: 8041121]

[42]   Camargo MC, Murphy G, Koriyama C, *et al.* Determinants of Epstein-Barr virus-positive gastric
       cancer: an international pooled analysis. Br J Cancer 2011; 105(1): 38-43.
       [http://dx.doi.org/10.1038/bjc.2011.215] [PMID: 21654677]

[43]   Iizasa H, Nanbo A, Nishikawa J, Jinushi M, Yoshiyama H. Epstein-Barr Virus (EBV)-associated
       gastric carcinoma. Viruses 2012; 4(12): 3420-39.
       [http://dx.doi.org/10.3390/v4123420] [PMID: 23342366]

[44]   Ford AC, Forman D, Hunt RH, Yuan Y, Moayyedi P. *Helicobacter pylori* eradication therapy to
       prevent gastric cancer in healthy asymptomatic infected individuals: systematic review and meta-
       analysis of randomised controlled trials. BMJ 2014; 348: g3174.
       [http://dx.doi.org/10.1136/bmj.g3174] [PMID: 24846275]

[45]   Ma JL, Zhang L, Brown LM, *et al.* Fifteen-year effects of *Helicobacter pylori*, garlic, and vitamin
       treatments on gastric cancer incidence and mortality. J Natl Cancer Inst 2012; 104(6): 488-92.

[http://dx.doi.org/10.1093/jnci/djs003] [PMID: 22271764]

[46]   Fukase K, Kato M, Kikuchi S, *et al*. Effect of eradication of *Helicobacter pylori* on incidence of metachronous gastric carcinoma after endoscopic resection of early gastric cancer: an open-label, randomised controlled trial. Lancet 2008; 372(9636): 392-7.
[http://dx.doi.org/10.1016/S0140-6736(08)61159-9] [PMID: 18675689]

[47]   González CA, Pera G, Agudo A, *et al*. Fruit and vegetable intake and the risk of stomach and oesophagus adenocarcinoma in the European Prospective Investigation into Cancer and Nutrition (EPIC–EURGAST). Int J Cancer 2006; 118(10): 2559-66.
[http://dx.doi.org/10.1002/ijc.21678] [PMID: 16380980]

[48]   Elingarami S, Liu M, Fan J, He N. Applications of nanotechnology in gastric cancer: detection and prevention by nutrition. J Nanosci Nanotechnol 2014; 14(1): 932-45.
[http://dx.doi.org/10.1166/jnn.2014.9008] [PMID: 24730310]

[49]   IARC. Fruit and Vegetables [Internet]. [cited 2022 Jun 5]. Available from: https://publications.iarc.fr/Book-And-Report-Series/Iarc-Handbooks-Of--ancer-Prevention/Fruit-And-Vegetables-2003

[50]   Tsubono Y, Hisamichi S. Screening for gastric cancer in Japan. Gastric Cancer 2000; 3(1): 9-18.
[http://dx.doi.org/10.1007/PL00011692] [PMID: 11984703]

[51]   Choi KS, Suh M. Screening for gastric cancer: the usefulness of endoscopy. Clin Endosc 2014; 47(6): 490-6.
[http://dx.doi.org/10.5946/ce.2014.47.6.490] [PMID: 25505713]

[52]   Matsumoto S, Ishikawa S, Yoshida Y. Reduction of gastric cancer mortality by endoscopic and radiographic screening in an isolated island: A retrospective cohort study. Aust J Rural Health 2013; 21(6): 319-24.
[http://dx.doi.org/10.1111/ajr.12064] [PMID: 24299436]

[53]   Hamashima C, Ogoshi K, Okamoto M, Shabana M, Kishimoto T, Fukao A. A community-based, case-control study evaluating mortality reduction from gastric cancer by endoscopic screening in Japan. PLoS One 2013; 8(11)e79088
[http://dx.doi.org/10.1371/journal.pone.0079088] [PMID: 24236091]

[54]   Laurén P. THE TWO HISTOLOGICAL MAIN TYPES OF GASTRIC CARCINOMA: DIFFUSE AND SO-CALLED INTESTINAL-TYPE CARCINOMA. Acta Pathol Microbiol Scand 1965; 64(1): 31-49.
[http://dx.doi.org/10.1111/apm.1965.64.1.31] [PMID: 14320675]

[55]   Hu B, El Hajj N, Sittler S, Lammert N, Barnes R, Meloni-Ehrig A. Gastric cancer: Classification, histology and application of molecular pathology. J Gastrointest Oncol 2012; 3(3): 251-61.
[PMID: 22943016]

[56]   Kikuchi S, Nakajima T, Nishi T, *et al*. Association between family history and gastric carcinoma among young adults. Jpn J Cancer Res 1996; 87(4): 332-6.
[http://dx.doi.org/10.1111/j.1349-7006.1996.tb00226.x] [PMID: 8641962]

[57]   Forman D, Burley VJ. Gastric cancer: global pattern of the disease and an overview of environmental risk factors. Best Pract Res Clin Gastroenterol 2006; 20(4): 633-49.
[http://dx.doi.org/10.1016/j.bpg.2006.04.008] [PMID: 16997150]

[58]   Skierucha M, Milne AN, Offerhaus GJA, Polkowski WP, Maciejewski R, Sitarz R. Molecular alterations in gastric cancer with special reference to the early-onset subtype. World J Gastroenterol 2016; 22(8): 2460-74.
[http://dx.doi.org/10.3748/wjg.v22.i8.2460] [PMID: 26937134]

[59]   Lim S, Lee HS, Kim HS, Kim YI, Kim WH. Alteration of E-cadherin-mediated adhesion protein is common, but microsatellite instability is uncommon in young age gastric cancers. Histopathology 2003; 42(2): 128-36.

[http://dx.doi.org/10.1046/j.1365-2559.2003.01546.x] [PMID: 12558744]

[60]   Ramos-De la Medina A, Salgado-Nesme N, Torres-Villalobos G, Medina-Franco H. Clinicopathologic characteristics of gastric cancer in a young patient population. J Gastrointest Surg 2004; 8(3): 240-4.
         [http://dx.doi.org/10.1016/j.gassur.2003.12.009] [PMID: 15019915]

[61]   Sitarz R, Skierucha M, Mielko J, Offerhaus J, Maciejewski R, Polkowski W. Gastric cancer: epidemiology, prevention, classification, and treatment. Cancer Manag Res 2018; 10: 239-48.
         [http://dx.doi.org/10.2147/CMAR.S149619] [PMID: 29445300]

[62]   Thorban S, Böttcher K, Etter M, Roder JD, Busch R, Siewert JR. Prognostic factors in gastric stump carcinoma. Ann Surg 2000; 231(2): 188-94.
         [http://dx.doi.org/10.1097/00000658-200002000-00006] [PMID: 10674609]

[63]   van Rees BP, Caspers E, zur Hausen A, *et al.* Different pattern of allelic loss in Epstein-Barr virus-positive gastric cancer with emphasis on the p53 tumor suppressor pathway. Am J Pathol 2002; 161(4): 1207-13.
         [http://dx.doi.org/10.1016/S0002-9440(10)64397-0] [PMID: 12368194]

[64]   Hanahan D, Coussens LM. Accessories to the crime: functions of cells recruited to the tumor microenvironment. Cancer Cell 2012; 21(3): 309-22.
         [http://dx.doi.org/10.1016/j.ccr.2012.02.022] [PMID: 22439926]

[65]   Kim TS, da Silva E, Coit DG, Tang LH. Intratumoural immune response to gastric cancer varies by molecular and histologic subtype. Am J Surg Pathol 2019; 43(6): 851-60.
         [http://dx.doi.org/10.1097/PAS.0000000000001253] [PMID: 30969179]

[66]   Zheng X, Song X, Shao Y, *et al.* Prognostic role of tumor-infiltrating lymphocytes in gastric cancer: a meta-analysis. Oncotarget 2017; 8(34): 57386-98.
         [http://dx.doi.org/10.18632/oncotarget.18065] [PMID: 28915679]

[67]   Wang Y, Zhao E, Zhang Z, Zhao G, Cao H. Association between Tim-3 and Gal-9 expression and gastric cancer prognosis. Oncol Rep 2018; 40(4): 2115-26.
         [http://dx.doi.org/10.3892/or.2015.4170] [PMID: 30106451]

[68]   Zhang D, He W, Wu C, *et al.* Scoring System for Tumor-Infiltrating Lymphocytes and Its Prognostic Value for Gastric Cancer. Front Immunol 2019; 10: 71.
         [http://dx.doi.org/10.3389/fimmu.2019.00071] [PMID: 30761139]

[69]   Kulangara K, Zhang N, Corigliano E, *et al.* Clinical utility of the combined positive score for programmed death ligand-1 expression and the approval of pembrolizumab for treatment of gastric cancer. Arch Pathol Lab Med 2019; 143(3): 330-7.
         [http://dx.doi.org/10.5858/arpa.2018-0043-OA] [PMID: 30028179]

[70]   Wherry EJ, Kurachi M. Molecular and cellular insights into T cell exhaustion. Nat Rev Immunol 2015; 15(8): 486-99.
         [http://dx.doi.org/10.1038/nri3862] [PMID: 26205583]

[71]   Pauken KE, Wherry EJ. Overcoming T cell exhaustion in infection and cancer. Trends Immunol 2015; 36(4): 265-76.
         [http://dx.doi.org/10.1016/j.it.2015.02.008] [PMID: 25797516]

[72]   Collin M. Immune checkpoint inhibitors: a patent review (2010-2015). Expert Opin Ther Pat 2016; 26(5): 555-64.
         [http://dx.doi.org/10.1080/13543776.2016.1176150] [PMID: 27054314]

[73]   Kang YK, Boku N, Satoh T, *et al.* Nivolumab in patients with advanced gastric or gastro-oesophageal junction cancer refractory to, or intolerant of, at least two previous chemotherapy regimens (ONO-4538-12, ATTRACTION-2): a randomised, double-blind, placebo-controlled, phase 3 trial. Lancet 2017; 390(10111): 2461-71.
         [http://dx.doi.org/10.1016/S0140-6736(17)31827-5] [PMID: 28993052]

[74]   Li N, Jilisihan B, Wang W, Tang Y, Keyoumu S. Soluble LAG3 acts as a potential prognostic marker

of gastric cancer and its positive correlation with CD8+T cell frequency and secretion of IL-12 and INF-γ in peripheral blood. Cancer Biomark 2018; 23(3): 341-51.
[http://dx.doi.org/10.3233/CBM-181278] [PMID: 30223387]

[75] Castaño-Rodríguez N, Goh KL, Fock KM, Mitchell HM, Kaakoush NO. Dysbiosis of the microbiome in gastric carcinogenesis. Sci Rep 2017; 7(1): 15957.
[http://dx.doi.org/10.1038/s41598-017-16289-2] [PMID: 29162924]

[76] Chen XH, Wang A, Chu AN, Gong YH, Yuan Y. Mucosa-associated microbiota in gastric cancer tissues compared with non-cancer tissues. Front Microbiol 2019; 10: 1261.
[http://dx.doi.org/10.3389/fmicb.2019.01261] [PMID: 31231345]

[77] Gantuya B, El Serag HB, Matsumoto T, *et al.* Gastric mucosal microbiota in a Mongolian population with gastric cancer and precursor conditions. Aliment Pharmacol Ther 2020; 51(8): 770-80.
[http://dx.doi.org/10.1111/apt.15675] [PMID: 32133670]

[78] Wang Z, Gao X, Zeng R, *et al.* Changes of the Gastric Mucosal Microbiome Associated With Histological Stages of Gastric Carcinogenesis. Front Microbiol 2020; 11: 997.
[http://dx.doi.org/10.3389/fmicb.2020.00997] [PMID: 32547510]

[79] Liu X, Shao L, Liu X, *et al.* Alterations of gastric mucosal microbiota across different stomach microhabitats in a cohort of 276 patients with gastric cancer. EBioMedicine 2019; 40: 336-48.
[http://dx.doi.org/10.1016/j.ebiom.2018.12.034] [PMID: 30584008]

[80] Ravegnini G, Fosso B, Saverio VD, *et al.* Gastric Adenocarcinomas and Signet-Ring Cell Carcinoma: Unraveling Gastric Cancer Complexity through Microbiome Analysis—Deepening Heterogeneity for a Personalized Therapy. Int J Mol Sci 2020; 21(24): 9735.
[http://dx.doi.org/10.3390/ijms21249735] [PMID: 33419357]

[81] Hsieh YY, Tung SY, Pan HY, *et al.* Increased abundance of *Clostridium* and *Fusobacterium* in gastric microbiota of patients with gastric cancer in Taiwan. Sci Rep 2018; 8(1): 158.
[http://dx.doi.org/10.1038/s41598-017-18596-0] [PMID: 29317709]

[82] Ferreira RM, Pereira-Marques J, Pinto-Ribeiro I, *et al.* Gastric microbial community profiling reveals a dysbiotic cancer-associated microbiota. Gut 2018; 67(2): 226-36.
[http://dx.doi.org/10.1136/gutjnl-2017-314205] [PMID: 29102920]

[83] Bali P, Coker J, Lozano-Pope I, Zengler K, Obonyo M. Microbiome signatures in a fast-and slow-progressing gastric cancer murine model and their contribution to gastric carcinogenesis. Microorganisms 2021; 9(1): 189.
[http://dx.doi.org/10.3390/microorganisms9010189] [PMID: 33477306]

[84] Yang J, Zhou X, Liu X, Ling Z, Ji F. Role of the Gastric Microbiome in Gastric Cancer: From Carcinogenesis to Treatment. Front Microbiol 2021; 12641322
[http://dx.doi.org/10.3389/fmicb.2021.641322] [PMID: 33790881]

[85] Park JY, Seo H, Kang CS, *et al.* Dysbiotic change in gastric microbiome and its functional implication in gastric carcinogenesis. Sci Rep 2022; 12(1): 4285.
[http://dx.doi.org/10.1038/s41598-022-08288-9] [PMID: 35277583]

[86] Coker OO, Dai Z, Nie Y, *et al.* Mucosal microbiome dysbiosis in gastric carcinogenesis. Gut 2018; 67(6): 1024-32.
[http://dx.doi.org/10.1136/gutjnl-2017-314281] [PMID: 28765474]

[87] Ganguly NK, Bhattacharya SK, Sesikeran B, Nair GB, Ramakrishna BS, Sachdev HPS, *et al.* ICMR-DBT guidelines for evaluation of probiotics in food. Indian J Med Res 2011; 134(1): 22-5.
[PMID: 21808130]

[88] Tamtaji OR, Taghizadeh M, Daneshvar Kakhaki R, *et al.* Clinical and metabolic response to probiotic administration in people with Parkinson's disease: A randomized, double-blind, placebo-controlled trial. Clin Nutr 2019; 38(3): 1031-5.
[http://dx.doi.org/10.1016/j.clnu.2018.05.018] [PMID: 29891223]

[89]   Tamtaji OR, Heidari-soureshjani R, Mirhosseini N, *et al*. Probiotic and selenium co-supplementation, and the effects on clinical, metabolic and genetic status in Alzheimer's disease: A randomized, double-blind, controlled trial. Clin Nutr 2019; 38(6): 2569-75.
[http://dx.doi.org/10.1016/j.clnu.2018.11.034] [PMID: 30642737]

[90]   Alipour Nosrani E, Tamtaji OR, Alibolandi Z, *et al*. Neuroprotective effects of probiotics bacteria on animal model of Parkinson's disease induced by 6-hydroxydopamine: A behavioral, biochemical, and histological study. J Immunoassay Immunochem 2021; 42(2): 106-20.
[http://dx.doi.org/10.1080/15321819.2020.1833917] [PMID: 33078659]

[91]   Davoodvandi A, Fallahi F, Tamtaji OR, *et al*. An Update on the Effects of Probiotics on Gastrointestinal Cancers. Front Pharmacol 2021; 12680400
[http://dx.doi.org/10.3389/fphar.2021.680400] [PMID: 34992527]

[92]   Servin AL. Antagonistic activities of lactobacilli and *bifidobacteria* against microbial pathogens. FEMS Microbiol Rev 2004; 28(4): 405-40.
[http://dx.doi.org/10.1016/j.femsre.2004.01.003] [PMID: 15374659]

[93]   Javanmard A, Ashtari S, Sabet B, *et al*. Probiotics and their role in gastrointestinal cancers prevention and treatment; an overview. Gastroenterol Hepatol Bed Bench 2018; 11(4): 284-95.
[PMID: 30425806]

[94]   Cotter PD, Hill C, Ross RP. Bacteriocins: developing innate immunity for food. Nat Rev Microbiol 2005; 3(10): 777-88.
[http://dx.doi.org/10.1038/nrmicro1273] [PMID: 16205711]

[95]   Liong MT. Roles of probiotics and prebiotics in colon cancer prevention: Postulated mechanisms and *in-vivo* evidence. Int J Mol Sci 2008; 9(5): 854-63.
[http://dx.doi.org/10.3390/ijms9050854] [PMID: 19325789]

[96]   Zuccotti GV, Meneghin F, Raimondi C, *et al*. Probiotics in clinical practice: an overview. J Int Med Res 2008; 36(1_suppl) (Suppl. 1): 1A-53A.
[http://dx.doi.org/10.1177/14732300080360S101] [PMID: 18230282]

[97]   Kumar M, Kumar A, Nagpal R, *et al*. Cancer-preventing attributes of probiotics: an update. Int J Food Sci Nutr 2010; 61(5): 473-96.
[http://dx.doi.org/10.3109/09637480903455971] [PMID: 20187714]

[98]   De Preter V, Hamer HM, Windey K, Verbeke K. The impact of pre- and/or probiotics on human colonic metabolism: Does it affect human health? Mol Nutr Food Res 2011; 55(1): 46-57.
[http://dx.doi.org/10.1002/mnfr.201000451] [PMID: 21207512]

[99]   Asemi Z, Jazayeri S, Najafi M, *et al*. Effect of daily consumption of probiotic yogurt on oxidative stress in pregnant women: a randomized controlled clinical trial. Ann Nutr Metab 2012; 60(1): 62-8.
[http://dx.doi.org/10.1159/000335468] [PMID: 22338626]

[100] Asemi Z, Samimi M, Tabasi Z, *et al*. Effect of daily consumption of probiotic yoghurt on lipid profiles in pregnant women: a randomized controlled clinical trial. J Matern Fetal Neonatal Med 2012; 25(9): 1552-6.
[http://dx.doi.org/10.3109/14767058.2011.640372] [PMID: 22098090]

[101] Tajadadi-Ebrahimi M, Bahmani F, Shakeri H, *et al*. Effects of daily consumption of synbiotic bread on insulin metabolism and serum high-sensitivity C-reactive protein among diabetic patients: a double-blind, randomized, controlled clinical trial. Ann Nutr Metab 2014; 65(1): 34-41.
[http://dx.doi.org/10.1159/000365153] [PMID: 25196301]

[102] Bahmani F, Tajadadi-Ebrahimi M, Kolahdooz F, *et al*. The consumption of synbiotic bread containing *Lactobacillus sporogenes* and inulin affects nitric oxide and malondialdehyde in patients with type 2 diabetes mellitus: randomized, double-blind, placebo-controlled trial. J Am Coll Nutr 2016; 35(6): 506-13.
[http://dx.doi.org/10.1080/07315724.2015.1032443] [PMID: 26430929]

[103] Rondanelli M, Faliva MA, Perna S, Giacosa A, Peroni G, Castellazzi AM. Using probiotics in clinical practice: Where are we now? A review of existing meta-analyses. Gut Microbes 2017; 8(6): 521-43.
[http://dx.doi.org/10.1080/19490976.2017.1345414] [PMID: 28640662]

[104] Zitvogel L, Ma Y, Raoult D, Kroemer G, Gajewski TF. The microbiome in cancer immunotherapy: Diagnostic tools and therapeutic strategies. Science 2018; 359(6382): 1366-70.
[http://dx.doi.org/10.1126/science.aar6918] [PMID: 29567708]

[105] Mego M, Holec V, Drgona L, Hainova K, Ciernikova S, Zajac V. Probiotic bacteria in cancer patients undergoing chemotherapy and radiation therapy. Complement Ther Med 2013; 21(6): 712-23.
[http://dx.doi.org/10.1016/j.ctim.2013.08.018] [PMID: 24280481]

[106] Mahkonen A, Putaala H, Mustonen H, Rautonen N, Puolakkainen P. *Lactobacillus acidophilus* 74-2 and butyrate induce cyclooxygenase (COX)-1 expression in gastric cancer cells. Immunopharmacol Immunotoxicol 2008; 30(3): 503-18.
[http://dx.doi.org/10.1080/08923970802135229] [PMID: 18618313]

[107] Linsalata M, Cavallini A, Messa C, Orlando A, Refolo M, Russo F. *Lactobacillus rhamnosus* GG influences polyamine metabolism in HGC-27 gastric cancer cell line: a strategy toward nutritional approach to chemoprevention of gastric cance. Curr Pharm Des 2010; 16(7): 847-53.
[http://dx.doi.org/10.2174/138161210790883598] [PMID: 20388096]

[108] Orlando A, Refolo MG, Messa C, *et al.* Antiproliferative and proapoptotic effects of viable or heat-killed *Lactobacillus paracasei* IMPC2.1 and *Lactobacillus rhamnosus* GG in HGC-27 gastric and DLD-1 colon cell lines. Nutr Cancer 2012; 64(7): 1103-11.
[http://dx.doi.org/10.1080/01635581.2012.717676] [PMID: 23061912]

[109] Cousin FJ, Jouan-Lanhouet S, Dimanche-Boitrel MT, Corcos L, Jan G. Milk fermented by *Propionibacterium freudenreichii* induces apoptosis of HGT-1 human gastric cancer cells. PLoS One 2012; 7(3)e31892
[http://dx.doi.org/10.1371/journal.pone.0031892] [PMID: 22442660]

[110] Nekouian R, Rasouli BS, Ghadimi-Darsajini A, Iragian GR. *In vitro* activity of probiotic *Lactobacillus reuteri* against gastric cancer progression by downregulation of urokinase plasminogen activator/urokinase plasminogen activator receptor gene expression. J Cancer Res Ther 2017; 13(2): 246-51.
[http://dx.doi.org/10.4103/0973-1482.204897] [PMID: 28643742]

[111] Salas-Jara MJ, Sanhueza EA, Retamal-Díaz A, González C, Urrutia H, García A. Probiotic *Lactobacillus fermentum* UCO-979C biofilm formation on AGS and Caco-2 cells and *Helicobacter pylori* inhibition. Biofouling 2016; 32(10): 1245-57.
[http://dx.doi.org/10.1080/08927014.2016.1249367] [PMID: 27834106]

[112] Liang S, Xu L, Zhang D, Wu Z. Effect of probiotics on small intestinal bacterial overgrowth in patients with gastric and colorectal cancer. Turk J Gastroenterol 2016; 27(3): 227-32.
[http://dx.doi.org/10.5152/tjg.2016.15375] [PMID: 27210778]

[113] Gianotti L, Morelli L, Galbiati F, *et al.* A randomized double-blind trial on perioperative administration of probiotics in colorectal cancer patients. World J Gastroenterol 2010; 16(2): 167-75.
[http://dx.doi.org/10.3748/wjg.v16.i2.167] [PMID: 20066735]

[114] Lalla RV, Bowen J, Barasch A, *et al.* MASCC/ISOO clinical practice guidelines for the management of mucositis secondary to cancer therapy. Cancer 2014; 120(10): 1453-61.
[http://dx.doi.org/10.1002/cncr.28592] [PMID: 24615748]

[115] Taremi M, Khoshbaten M, Gachkar L, EhsaniArdakani M, Zali M. Hepatitis E virus infection in hemodialysis patients: A seroepidemiological survey in Iran. BMC Infect Dis 2005; 5(1): 36.
[http://dx.doi.org/10.1186/1471-2334-5-36] [PMID: 15904504]

[116] Sanders ME, Guarner F, Guerrant R, *et al.* An update on the use and investigation of probiotics in health and disease. Gut 2013; 62(5): 787-96.

[http://dx.doi.org/10.1136/gutjnl-2012-302504] [PMID: 23474420]

[117] Russo F, Linsalata M, Orlando A. Probiotics against neoplastic transformation of gastric mucosa: Effects on cell proliferation and polyamine metabolism. World J Gastroenterol 2014; 20(37): 13258-72.
[http://dx.doi.org/10.3748/wjg.v20.i37.13258] [PMID: 25309063]

[118] Khoder G, Al-Menhali AA, Al-Yassir F, Karam SM. Potential role of probiotics in the management of gastric ulcer. Exp Ther Med 2016; 12(1): 3-17.
[http://dx.doi.org/10.3892/etm.2016.3293] [PMID: 27347010]

[119] Biasco G, Paganelli GM, Brandi G, *et al.* Effect of *lactobacillus acidophilus* and *bifidobacterium bifidum* on rectal cell kinetics and fecal pH. Ital J Gastroenterol 1991; 23(3): 142.
[PMID: 1742509]

[120] Bernstein H, Bernstein C, Payne CM, Dvorakova K, Garewal H. Bile acids as carcinogens in human gastrointestinal cancers. Mutat Res Rev Mutat Res 2005; 589(1): 47-65.
[http://dx.doi.org/10.1016/j.mrrev.2004.08.001] [PMID: 15652226]

[121] Jia W, Xie G, Jia W. Bile acid–microbiota crosstalk in gastrointestinal inflammation and carcinogenesis. Nat Rev Gastroenterol Hepatol 2018; 15(2): 111-28.
[http://dx.doi.org/10.1038/nrgastro.2017.119] [PMID: 29018272]

[122] Górska A, Przystupski D, Niemczura MJ, Kulbacka J. Probiotic bacteria: a promising tool in cancer prevention and therapy. Curr Microbiol 2019; 76(8): 939-49.
[http://dx.doi.org/10.1007/s00284-019-01679-8] [PMID: 30949803]

[123] Lidbeck A, Övervik E, Rafter J, Nord CE, Gustafsson JÅ. Effect of *Lactobacillus acidophilus* Supplements on Mutagen Excretion in Faeces and Urine in Humans. Microb Ecol Health Dis 1992; 5(1): 59-67.

[124] Hayatsu H, Hayatsu T. Suppressing effect of *Lactobacillus casei* administration on the urinary mutagenicity arising from ingestion of fried ground beef in the human. Cancer Lett 1993; 73(2-3): 173-9.
[http://dx.doi.org/10.1016/0304-3835(93)90261-7] [PMID: 8221630]

[125] Garrett WS. Cancer and the microbiota. Science 2015; 348(6230): 80-6.
[http://dx.doi.org/10.1126/science.aaa4972] [PMID: 25838377]

[126] Requena T, Martínez-Cuesta MC, Peláez C. Diet and microbiota linked in health and disease. Food Funct 2018; 9(2): 688-704.
[http://dx.doi.org/10.1039/C7FO01820G] [PMID: 29410981]

[127] Canducci F, Armuzzi A, Cremonini F, *et al.* A lyophilized and inactivated culture of *Lactobacillus acidophilus* increases *Helicobacter pylori* eradication rates. Aliment Pharmacol Ther 2000; 14(12): 1625-9.
[http://dx.doi.org/10.1046/j.1365-2036.2000.00885.x] [PMID: 11121911]

[128] Armuzzi A, Cremonini F, Bartolozzi F, *et al.* The effect of oral administration of *Lactobacillus GG* on antibiotic-associated gastrointestinal side-effects during *Helicobacter pylori* eradication therapy. Aliment Pharmacol Ther 2001; 15(2): 163-9.
[http://dx.doi.org/10.1046/j.1365-2036.2001.00923.x] [PMID: 11148433]

[129] Armuzzi A, Cremonini F, Ojetti V, *et al.* Effect of *Lactobacillus* GG supplementation on antibiotic-associated gastrointestinal side effects during *Helicobacter pylori* eradication therapy: a pilot study. Digestion 2001; 63(1): 1-7.
[http://dx.doi.org/10.1159/000051865] [PMID: 11173893]

[130] Sheu BS, Cheng HC, Kao AW, *et al.* Pretreatment with Lactobacillus and *Bifidobacterium*-containing yogurt can improve the efficacy of quadruple therapy in eradicating residual *Helicobacter pylori* infection after failed triple therapy. Am J Clin Nutr 2006; 83(4): 864-9.
[http://dx.doi.org/10.1093/ajcn/83.4.864] [PMID: 16600940]

[131] Cremonini F, Caro S, Covino M, *et al.* Effect of different probiotic preparations on anti-*Helicobacter pylori* therapy-related side effects: a parallel group, triple blind, placebo-controlled study. Am J Gastroenterol 2002; 97(11): 2744-9.
[http://dx.doi.org/10.1111/j.1572-0241.2002.07063.x] [PMID: 12425542]

[132] Tursi A, Brandimarte G, Giorgetti GM, Modeo ME. Effect of *Lactobacillus casei* supplementation on the effectiveness and tolerability of a new second-line 10-day quadruple therapy after failure of a first attempt to cure *Helicobacter pylori* infection. Med Sci Monit 2004; 10(12): CR662-6.
[PMID: 15567983]

[133] Sýkora J, Valecková K, Amlerová J, *et al.* Effects of a specially designed fermented milk product containing probiotic *Lactobacillus casei* DN-114 001 and the eradication of *H. pylori* in children: a prospective randomized double-blind study. J Clin Gastroenterol 2005; 39(8): 692-8.
[http://dx.doi.org/10.1097/01.mcg.0000173855.77191.44] [PMID: 16082279]

[134] Lionetti E, Miniello VL, Castellaneta SP, *et al. Lactobacillus reuteri* therapy to reduce side-effects during anti-*Helicobacter pylori* treatment in children: a randomized placebo controlled trial. Aliment Pharmacol Ther 2006; 24(10): 1461-8.
[http://dx.doi.org/10.1111/j.1365-2036.2006.03145.x] [PMID: 17032283]

[135] Goldman CG, Barrado DA, Balcarce N, *et al.* Effect of a probiotic food as an adjuvant to triple therapy for eradication of *Helicobacter pylori* infection in children. Nutrition 2006; 22(10): 984-8.
[http://dx.doi.org/10.1016/j.nut.2006.06.008] [PMID: 16978844]

[136] Myllyluoma E, Veijola L, Ahlroos T, *et al.* Probiotic supplementation improves tolerance to *Helicobacter pylori* eradication therapy - a placebo-controlled, double-blind randomized pilot study. Aliment Pharmacol Ther 2005; 21(10): 1263-72.
[http://dx.doi.org/10.1111/j.1365-2036.2005.02448.x] [PMID: 15882248]

[137] Ojetti V, Bruno G, Ainora ME, *et al.* Impact of *Lactobacillus reuteri* Supplementation on Anti-*Helicobacter pylori* Levofloxacin-Based Second-Line Therapy. Gastroenterol Res Pract 2012; 2012: 1-6.
[http://dx.doi.org/10.1155/2012/740381] [PMID: 22690211]

CHAPTER 8

Probiotic-based Anticancer Immunity In Hepatocellular Carcinoma (liver Cancer)

Firdosh Shah[1] and **Mitesh Kumar Dwivedi**[1,*]

[1] *C. G. Bhakta Institute of Biotechnology, Faculty of Science, Uka Tarsadia University, Tarsadi, Bardoli, District Surat, Gujarat, India*

Abstract: One of the most dreaded outcomes of chronic liver illness is hepatocellular carcinoma (HCC), and it is the most prevalent primary liver cancer. The gut-liver axis has been shown to play a key role in the emergence of chronic liver disorders, including HCC, in recent experimental and clinical studies. The altered gut microbiota is becoming well recognised as an important factor in the progression of chronic liver disorders, such as HCC. Probiotics administration has been proposed as a new, safe and cost-effective strategy for preventing or treating HCC. Probiotics' ability to bind carcinogens, regulation of gut microbiota, improvement of intestinal barrier integrity, and immunomodulation are the mechanisms by which they exert anticancer benefits. This chapter discusses the alterations in gut microbiota linked to HCC and the implications of probiotics and prebiotics for anticancer mechanisms towards HCC.

Keywords: Carcinogens, Gut microbiota, Hepatocellular cancer, Liver cancer, Probiotics, Prebiotics, Short chain fatty acids (SCFAs).

1. INTRODUCTION

Hepatocellular carcinoma (HCC) is primary liver cancer among the most fatal health conditions which are rapidly expanding across the globe [1, 2]. It has been predicted that by the year 2025, more than 1 million individuals will be annually affected by hepatocellular carcinoma [3]. HCC accounts for approximately 90% of cases and among this, 50% of cases results due to Hepatitis B virus (HBV) infection, which is an important risk factor for HCC [4]. HCC is majorly caused due to chronic liver disease, non-alcoholic fatty liver disease (NAFLD), alcohol abuse, diabetes, *etc* [5 - 7]. HCC can be treated well upon early diagnosis of HCC in patients [8]. But unfortunately, the diagnosis of HCC is often made in later disease stages, which is mostly accompanied by liver failure [9].

---

[*] **Corresponding author Mitesh Kumar Dwivedi:** C. G. Bhakta Institute of Biotechnology, Faculty of Science, Uka Tarsadia University, Bardoli, Surat-Gujarat, India; E-mail: mitesh_dwivedi@yahoo.com

Mitesh Kumar Dwivedi, Alwarappan Sankaranarayanan & Sanjay Tiwari (Eds.)

The human gut consists of 100 trillion microorganisms of diverse taxonomy collectively known as gut microbiota, but the human gut contains more genes than the human genome [10]. Immediately after birth, commensal bacteria colonize within the host and support the overall maintenance of health. Intestinal microbiota helps in degrading bile acids, aids in digestion, produces vitamins, helps in modulating immunity, and also helps in treating diseases such as cancer [11 - 13]. In a healthy individual, *Firmicutes, Bacteroidetes* and *Actinobacteria* account for the majority of the bacterial phyla [12]. Studies have revealed that gut microbiota and gut microbiota-derived products play an indispensable role in the pathogenesis and treatment of HCC. For example, lipoteichoic acid and deoxycholic acid induced the expression of prostaglandin-endoperoxide synthase 2 or cyclooxygenase-2 (COX-2) in senescent hepatic stellate cells (HSCs) *via* Toll-like receptor 2 (TLR-2) to amplify prostaglandin E2 (PGE2)-mediated inhibition of antitumor immunity, resulting in HCC [14]. It has been observed that gut microbiota-derived products can influence non-alcoholic steatohepatitis (NASH) and virus-induced HCC progression *via* modulating hepatic inflammation and immunology [15]. In comparison to non-responders, HCC patients who responded to anti-programmed cell death protein 1 (anti-PD-1) treatment showed a higher taxonomic richness in faeces [16]. Maintaining a balanced microbiota composition is critical. Intestinal dysbiosis occurs when this micro-ecology is disrupted, resulting in an overgrowth of particular harmful bacteria that can cause a number of disorders, including liver pathology. Indeed, the gut microbiota composition is altered in many liver disorders, making gut microbiota remodelling a promising therapeutic target. Probiotics, as a functional food ingredient, may have a positive impact on the gut microbiota and alter the aetiology of chronic liver illnesses [17], and new research suggests that probiotics could be utilised as a treatment for HCC [18] (Table 1). The interaction of gut microbiota with HCC and the potential therapeutic implications of probiotics for HCC are discussed in this chapter.

Table 1. Clinical studies of probiotics and prebiotics in liver cancer (HCC).

Title of the Study	Status	Condition	Interventions	Clinical Trials.gov Identifier
Probiotics enhance the treatment of PD-1 inhibitors in patients with liver cancer	Recruiting	Liver cancer	Experimental: probiotics group The oral probiotic (*Lactobacillus rhamnosus* Probio-M9, one times a day during the whole treatment)	NCT05032014

(Table 1) cont.....

Title of the Study	Status	Condition	Interventions	Clinical Trials.gov Identifier
Integrative nutrition care plan for the patient with liver and colorectal cancer	Enrolling	Liver and colorectal cancer	Powdered supplement 1 (containing β-glucan and gamma-aminobutyric acid) and nutritional products and powdered supplement 2 (contains water-soluble dietary fibre and probiotics)	NCT05030090
Influence of probiotics administration before liver resection in liver disease	Completed	Liver fibrosis, liver cirrhosis and hepatocellular carcinoma	Probiotics- Lactibiane Tolerance Active substance mixture of lactic 10% *Bifidobacterium lactis* LA 303, 10% *Lactobacillus acidophilus* LA 201, LA 40% *Lactobacillus plantarum* 301, 20% *Lactobacillus salivarius* LA 302, LA 20% *Bifidobacterium lactis* 304 Dosage: 10×10^9 probiotic / capsule Composition: One capsule of 560 mg contains Lactibiane tolerance: • 345 mg of corn starch • 114 mg premix lactic • 6 mg of magnesium stearate	NCT02021253
Probiotics in the prevention of hepatocellular carcinoma in cirrhosis	Not yet recruiting	Hepatocellular carcinoma	Each 50 ml bottle contains *Lactobacillus casei* 3.3×10^7 CFU / day, *Lactobacillus plantarum* 3.3×10^7 CFU / day, *Streptococcus faecalis* 3.3×10^7 CFU / day and *Bifidobacterium brevis* 1.0×10^6 CFU / day (BIOFLORA®, BIOSIDUS SA, Argentina)	NCT03853928
Prebiotic effect of eicosapentaenoic acid treatment for colorectal cancer liver metastases	Recruiting	Liver cancer	Drug: Icosapent Ethyl Oral Capsule Soft gelatin capsules containing 1g pure EPA-EE	NCT04682665

2. ROLE OF GUT MICROBIOTA IN LIVER DISEASES

For nutrient absorption and metabolism, the stomach and liver are critical organs. According to new findings, there is a strong link between the liver and the intestines. The hepatic portal vein supplies the liver with roughly 75% of its blood supply. The intestinal blood transports nutrients from the gut to the liver, where they stimulate liver functions and aid in nutrient digestion. By secreting bile into the intestinal lumen, the liver regulates intestinal processes [19]. Once the intestinal barrier is breached, intestinal permeability increases, allowing gut-derived bacterial compounds such as lipopolysaccharides (LPSs) to pass through the portal vein [20] (Fig. **1**).

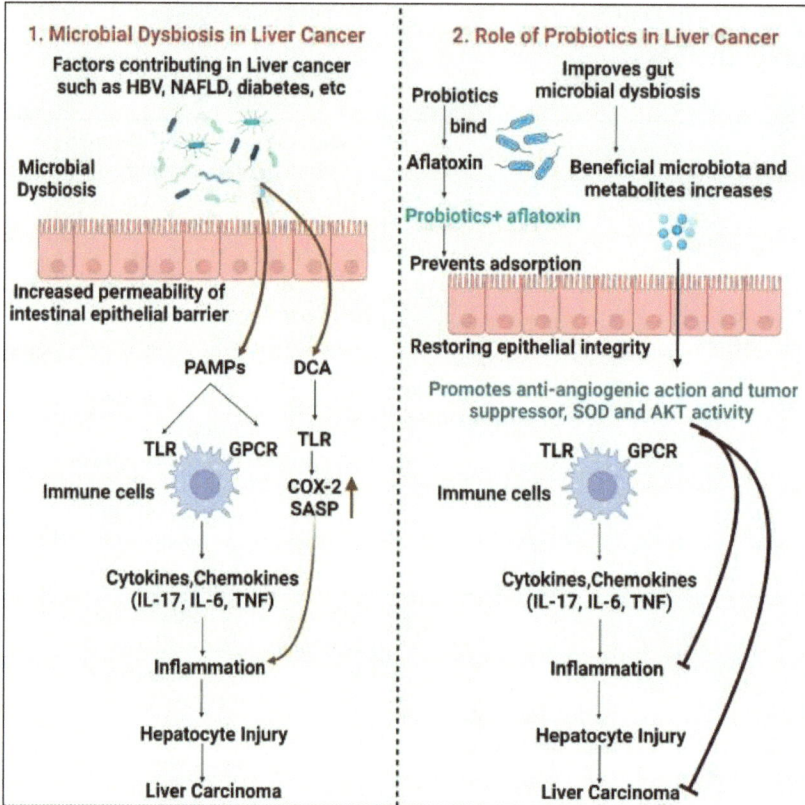

Fig. (**1**). **Role of gut microbiota in pathogenesis of liver cancer and role of probiotics in the treatment of liver cancer. 1. Microbial dysbiosis in liver cancer** Risk factors involved in liver cancer such as NAFLD, HBV virus, obesity, epigenetics, *etc* . create a state of microbial dysbiosis leading to a leaky intestinal epithelial barrier within liver cancer patient. This dysbiosis further results into increase in pro-inflammatory cytokines, pathogen-associated molecular patterns (PAMPs), primary bile acids and secondary bile acids such as deoxycholic acid (DCA). DCA induces the expression of prostaglandin-endoperoxide synthase 2 or cyclooxygenase-2 (COX-2) in senescent hepatic stellate cells (HSCs) *via* Toll-like receptor 2 (TLR-2) to amplify prostaglandin E2 (PGE2)-mediated inhibition of antitumor immunity, resulting in inflammation and leading to liver cancer. **2. Role of probiotics in liver cancer** Probiotics help in increasing beneficial microbiota and their metabolites which prevents adsorption of pathogenic bacteria and restores epithelial integrity. Probiotic bacteria can reduce aflatoxin-induced cytotoxicity while binding to the carcinogens. Probiotics also promote the anti-angiogenic, tumor suppressor, SOD and AKT activity which reduce inflammation, and hepatocyte injury, thereby leading to suppression of liver cancer.

According to mounting data, the gut-liver axis appears to play a key role in the aetiology of liver illnesses such as liver cirrhosis, hepatitis, non-alcoholic steatohepatitis (NASH), and HCC [20 - 24]. Liver illnesses have long been linked to alterations in the gut microbiota's quality and quantity [25]. Almost a decade ago, changes in the gut microbiota were discovered in patients with chronic liver disease. In a substantial percentage of individuals with chronic liver disease (20–75%), the gut flora was disrupted, particularly small intestinal bacterial overgrowth [21]. Endotoxemia seems to be responsible for the onset of liver destruction, most likely *via* interacting with particular recognition receptors such as toll-like receptors (TLRs) [26], while TLR-independent ways by which the gut microbiota causes liver injury have been documented [27] (Fig. **1**). The changes in gut microbiota can increase intestinal permeability to LPSs, which activate kupffer cells and liver macrophages, causing them to release pro-inflammatory cytokines like tumour necrosis factor-α (TNF-α) and reactive oxygen intermediates, resulting in the pathogenesis of a variety of acute and chronic liver diseases [19]. However, it is yet unclear how the changes in the gut microbiota play a role in the aetiology of chronic liver disease and HCC in humans.

3. ROLE OF GUT MICROBIOTA IN HEPATOCELLULAR CARCINO-GENESIS

HCC is becoming more common, and it is frequently associated with a high mortality rate. Cirrhosis caused by HBV or HCV is the most common cause of HCC [28]. Moreover, chronic liver inflammation is assumed to be associated to hepatocarcinogenesis in viral hepatitis; however, the specific mechanism underlying the cause of HCC in NAFLD patients has yet to be understood.

Studies from human research and animal models suggest that the gut microbiota has a role in the development of HCC. Later on, intestinal dysbiosis was discovered in patients with HCC, as well as in mice treated with diethylnitrosamine (DEN). A large suppression of *Lactobacillus* species, *Bifidobacterium* species, and *Enterococcus* species, as well as a significant expansion of *E. coli* and *Atopobium* cluster, indicated an imbalance in gut microbiota composition [29]. When mice were given DEN and the hepatotoxin carbon tetrachloride (CCl_4), a paradigm that matches the milieu of the majority of human HCC, gut sterilisation reduced HCC development. Reduced hepatocarcinogenesis in germ-free (GF) mice compared to particular pathogen-free mice further highlighted the role of the gut microbiota [30]. In addition, Fox *et al.* found a link between *Helicobacter hepaticus* colonization of the intestine and the development of HCC [31]. Huang *et al.* discovered *Helicobacter* sp. 16S rDNA in the livers of HCC patients but not in those of healthy people [32]. Krüttgen *et al.*, on the other hand, failed to discover *Helicobacter hepaticus* in the fecal samples from HCC patients infected with HBV or HCV [33]. As a result, more detailed research into a putative relationship between gut microbiota and HCC in humans is required.

3.1. Gut Microbial Dysbiosis and Bacterial Metabolite Production in Hepatocellular Carcinogenesis

Earlier, chronic DEN therapy resulted in intestinal dysbiosis in rats. This was frequently linked to an increase in harmful bacteria and a decrease in helpful bacteria [29]. Penicillin or dextran sulphate sodium (DSS) administration was demonstrated to disturb gut microbiota balance and damage mucosa, resulting in endotoxemia, systemic inflammation, and tumour formation [29].

Furthermore, intestinal microbial dysbiosis appears to influence the development of HCC through bacterial metabolite production. According to Yoshimoto *et al.*, dietary or hereditary obesity changes the gut microbiota, which raises the levels of deoxycholic acid (DCA), a gut bacterial metabolite that causes DNA damage. After exposure to a chemical carcinogen, DCA rendered the liver to produce a variety of inflammatory and tumor-promoting factors, increasing the development of HCC in mice. Moreover, blocking DCA synthesis or lowering gut microbiota effectively reduced HCC in obese mice in the same scenario [34]. Propionate, a metabolite of the gut microbiota, on the other hand, has been demonstrated to inhibit cancer cell proliferation in the liver [35].

3.2. Immunomodulation in Hepatocellular Carcinogenesis

Immunological state may have a significant impact on HCC progression. Tumor-associated macrophages [36], neutrophils [37], natural killer (NK) cells [38, 39], regulatory T cells (Tregs) [40, 41], and interleukin-6 (IL-6) [42] have all been linked to poor prognosis in HCC patients.

Th17 cell is a new type of T helper cell that produces pro-inflammatory and pro-angiogenic mediators like IL-17A and IL-22. Th17 cells were found in high numbers in the tumours and blood of HCC patients [43.44], and linked to poor survival rate in these patients. Th17 cell by producing IL-17A, promotes tumour angiogenesis by secreting angiogenic mediators and cytokines, and play a pro-tumor role [45]. Th17 cells are not abundant in healthy livers, and the bulk of these cells are created in the gut through interactions with the gut microbiota [46]. As a result, it is thought that IL-17 produced in the intestine may have a role in the development of HCC. The findings reveal that immunological state can vary in distinct tumour microenvironments and have different effects on disease progression, and that gut microbiota can have a significant impact on the development of HCC *via* immunomodulation [47 - 50]. Microbiota shapes the host immune system through modulating both local and systemic immune responses. Microbes activate local immunological responses by interacting with immune cells that express pattern recognition receptors (PRRs) such as TLRs [51]. Local DCs are activated by microbes or microbe-derived components (*e.g.*, constituents, products, metabolites) *via* interactions with PRRs [52]. These interactions allow activated DCs to migrate from the gastrointestinal tract (GIT) to the mesenteric lymph nodes (mLNs), where they present microbe-derived antigens and drive the development of naive T cells into effector T cells, especially Tregs and Th17 cells [53]. A portion of these effector T cells returns to the gastrointestinal system, where they regulate local immune responses. The rest of the population enters the circulatory system and influences systemic immunity. The release of anti-inflammatory cytokines (*e.g.*, IL-10 & TGF-β) or the engagement of DCs by Tregs mediates the conversion of a pro-inflammatory state to an anti-inflammatory state [54]. Th17 cells, on the other hand, orchestrate the immune system's change to a pro-inflammatory state by secreting immunostimulatory cytokines (such as IL-17) or activating and attracting neutrophils [55]. The lamina propria of GF mice lacks these pro-inflammatory Th17 cells, but a particular bacterial subset known as segmented filamentous bacteria can restore their production. This fascinating link clearly shows that microorganisms play a critical role in Th17 cell activation [56]. Because there are few pharmaco-preventive techniques and few chemotherapeutic choices for treating liver cancer, therapeutic regulation of the gut microflora with prebiotics or probiotics could be a novel way to prevent the progression of HCC.

3.3. Toll-like Receptors (TLRs) in Hepatocellular Carcinogenesis

TLR2 activity has been linked to a reduction in the development of HCC in a number of studies [57 - 60]. TLR2 expression was found to be higher in the central zone of HCC compared to the peripheral zone, suggesting that TLR2 signalling may have an indispensable role in preventing hepato-carcinogenesis by restricting the build-up of reactive oxygen species (ROS) and endoplasmic reticulum (ER) stress [58]. TLR2-mediated immune networks may play a role in an integrated defence against HCC and HCC progression by promoting p21- and p16/pRb-dependent senescence and autophagy flux in the liver [60]. Another study found that senescence and the loss of TLR2-mediated immunological activity reduce autophagic flux, which cannot remove sequestome 1 (SQSTM1) aggregates and DNA damage, thereby facilitating the formation and progression of HCC [57]. Moreover, TLR2 decreased the production of the proinflammatory cytokine IL 18 and protected mice from DEN-induced liver carcinogenesis, according to a recent study [59].

TLRs are pattern recognition receptors that identify endotoxins and signals *via* MyD88-dependent and MyD88-independent pathways, thereby activating the innate immunity [61]. Kupffer cells are more responsive to endotoxins than hepatocytes, indicating that the liver is well-equipped to respond to endotoxins [62]. TLR4 has been implicated in hepatocarcinogenesis according to recent research. The TLR4 over expression was observed in the tumour tissues of HCC patients [63, 64]. TLR4 expression levels were found to be strongly linked to microvascular invasion, early recurrence, and poor survival in HCC patients in a recent study by Liu *et al.* [65]. TLR4 signalling triggered by LPS was also found to boost cancer cell survival and proliferation in HCC cells, in another investigation [66].

4. BENEFICIAL ROLE OF PREBIOTICS IN TREATMENT OF HEPATOCELLULAR CARCINOMA

Prebiotics are essential for maintaining a healthy microbial balance in the intestine. They are classified as non-absorbent and indigestible food ingredients, such as lactulose, which has been shown to enhance the growth and activity of gut friendly microbiota [67, 68]. Experts are well-versed for the benefits of prebiotics in cancer prevention [67]. The two primary classes of prebiotics are inulin-type fructans (ITF) and galactooligosaccharides (GOS), based on the chemical structure [69]. Due to its beneficial impacts on health, dietary fibre has always been regarded a vital component of a nutritious meal [70]. It promotes the growth of gut-friendly bacteria like *Prevotella* and *Xylanibacter*, as well as *Bifidobacterium,* the *clostridial* cluster XIVa, and *Faecalibacterium prausnitzii*, while making conditions difficult for harmful bacteria like *Firmicutes* and *Enterobacteriaceae* [71]. A sudden increase in the population of *Bifidobacteria* and *Lactobacilli* is one of the gold standards for gauging gut health and identifying prebiotics. In addition, certain fungal compounds have also been discovered for future usage as prebiotic agents based on recent research. As an energy booster, *Antrodia cinnamomea*, *Hirsutella sinensis*, and *Ganoderma lucidum* have been demonstrated to attenuate LPS-induced endotoxemia, in high-fat diet rats [72].

Several prebiotics discovered and evaluated in laboratories so far, are non-digestible oligosaccharides [73, 74]. For example, lactosucrose, glucooli-gosaccharides, xylooligosaccharides, gentiooligosaccharides, mannan oligosacc-harides, arabinoxylan oligosaccharide, chitooligosaccharide, pectin-derived oligosaccharides, fructooligosaccharides, isomaltooligosaccharides, soybean oligosaccharides, *etc*. The most frequent non-digestible oligosaccharides that have been discovered as functional in nature are xanthan-derived oligosaccharides (XDOs) [74 - 76].

Downregulation of low-grade inflammatory cytokines such as IFN-γ, and IL-1β can be achieved by increasing short chain fatty acids (SCFAs) fabrication in the gut, which can be easily accomplished by incorporating a diet supplemented with 10% (w/v) XOS-supplemented in regular meals to increase *Bifidobacterium* colonies throughout the intestine to an impressive number. Moreover, *in vitro*, the similar rise in the number of *Bifidobacteria* and *Lactobacilli* colonies can be achieved by providing acidic oligosaccharides derived from apple pectin, which also results in an increase in acetic, propionic, and lactic acid concentrations [77].

4.1. Role of Prebiotics Fructans and Butyrate in Hepatocellular Carcinoma

Prebiotics have an indispensable role in maintaining the intestinal flora. They are known as indigestible food ingredients such as lactulose which promotes the growth and activity of various beneficial intestinal bacteria [78]. Several studies reveal that prebiotics have hepatoprotective properties; hence, they may prevent progression of liver damage [79]. Fructans, among other prebiotics, are the most extensively utilised in hepatocellular carcinoma [80]. By stimulating the growth of *Bifidobacteria*, oligofructose and inulin considerably modify the composition of the microbiota, *in vivo* [81]. Inulin-type fructans (ITF) are indigestible carbohydrates that when given orally, reduced the tumour size in hepatic and mammary tumour mice models [82, 83].

Furthermore, the intestinal microbiota altered the metabolome of BaF3 cells, and influences their proliferation. Propionate was found to be higher in the portal vein of rats fed with ITF and mediated a protective effect [83] and entered the liver [84] due to enhanced gut microbiota generated metabolites that particularly target liver tissue. In cancer, altered gut microbiota composition or reduced food intake resulted into lower butyrate and propionate levels [85]. Propionate's antiproliferative impact on BaF3 cells suggests that it is the most powerful mediator of the anticancer effect of the ITF. Hence, the propionate uptake by the liver indicates that ITF may impact BaF3 cell development in the liver. The antitumor effect of prebiotic foods may be due to gut microorganisms-based propionate production [86].

Additionally, butyrate and other SCFAs have been shown to disrupt the cell cycle in human cancer cells, causing cell death, differentiation, and inhibition of proliferation [87 - 89]. Intracellular mechanisms linked to cell proliferation and death have been studied extensively [87, 88]. Free fatty acid receptor 2 (FFAR2) and FFAR3, also known as GPR43 and GPR41, are the two G-protein-coupled receptors that have been identified as SCFA receptors. Propionate is the most effective endogenous agonist for the free fatty acid receptors, and it is found in a variety of cell types including the gut, adipocytes, endocrine cells, and immunological cells [90, 91].

5. PROBIOTICS AS A THERAPEUTIC APPROACH FOR TREATING HEPATOCELLULAR CARCINOMA

The United Nations and WHO describe probiotics as *"live microorganisms which when administered in adequate amounts confer a health benefit for the host"* [92]. However, before an organism can be considered as a probiotic, it must be isolated, purified, described, and proven to be helpful to human health when provided. Probiotic strains must be able to survive passage through the upper gastrointestinal system, reproduce, colonise, and function in the gut in order to be considered as successful probiotic strain [93, 94]. Lactic acid bacteria (LAB) strains, particularly *Lactobacillus* and *Bifidobacterium*, are commonly used as probiotics in fermented dairy products [95].

Probiotics' popularity has skyrocketed in recent years, thanks to their health-promoting properties and ability to prevent or treat a variety of ailments [96, 97]. Because the composition of the gut microbiota is altered in many liver illnesses, redesigning the gut microbiota could be a novel therapeutic target. Probiotics have been shown to be beneficial not only in gastrointestinal but also in liver diseases. Several studies have summarised the benefits of probiotics in the treatment of liver diseases [26, 95, 97 - 103]. Probiotics may exert their therapeutic effects on the gut-liver axis through variety of mechanisms, such as: (I) modulation of gut microbiota composition and antimicrobial factor production; (II) improvement of gut barrier function; and (III) modulation of local and systemic immunity. However, the exact mechanisms of probiotics' beneficial effects on the gut-liver axis are still unknown [95]. Probiotics' positive benefits are often species- or even strain-specific [104]. As a result, the strain or combination of strains used is critical for therapeutic success.

There is limited research on the use of probiotic supplements as a dietary therapy to minimise the risk of HCC caused by aflatoxins in the liver. El-Nezami *et al.* found that dietary supplementation with probiotics such as live *Lactobacillus rhamnosus* LC705 and *Propionibacterium freudenreichii subsp. Shermani* successfully reduced the excretion of aflatoxin-DNA adduct (AFB1-N7-guanine) in urine [105]. In a rat study, administration of VSL#3 (comprised of four *Lactobacilli*, three *Bifidobacteria*, and one *Streptococcus thermophilus subsp salivarius)* repressed the progression of cirrhosis to HCC by restoring gut homeostasis and alleviating intestinal and hepatic inflammation, and thus inhibited DEN-induced hepatocarcinogenesis [29]. In another rat study, which assessed the chemo-preventive effect of probiotic-fermented milk and chlorophyllin on AFB1-induced HCC, the probiotics treatment reduced the tumour incidence, and decreased the c-myc, bcl-2, cyclin D1, and rasp-21 levels, indicating that probiotics can protect against AFB1-induced hepatocarcinogenesis [106].

Probiotics have been shown to slow the course of HCC in mice, according to Li *et al* [18]. The probiotics combo Prohep, (which includes *Lactobacillus rhamnosus* GG, *Escherichia coli Nissle* 1917, and heat-inactivated VSL#3) could change the gut microbiota composition and shrink liver tumours in tumor-injected rats [18]. Moreover, the angiogenic factors were down-regulated by probiotics delivery in addition to reduced tumour size [18]. With respect to molecular pathways, probiotic-treated mice had reduced the levels of Th17 cells in the stomach and less Th17 cells' recruitment to the tumour site [18]. The anticancer activity of probiotics was also linked to the formation of SCFAs, as evidenced by the enrichment of SCFA-related pathways in probiotics-treated mice.

Probiotic effects on aflatoxin toxicity in liver dysfunction and HCC have only been studied in a few trials. El-Nezami *et al.* [107] noticed a decrease in aflatoxin concentration in faeces after administration of *Lactobacillus rhamnosus* LC705. They collected *L. rhamnosus* LC705 together with *Propionibacterium freudenreichii* subspecies, five weeks later. The presence of *L. rhamnosus* LC705 in faeces confirmed that the probiotic capsule had been consumed. The bacterium *L. rhamnosus* LC705 represented the majority of the faecal *Lactobacillus* population in the patients who received the probiotic mixture, but the bacterium was absent in the group who did not get the probiotic mixture. The authors of this study found that taking a probiotic supplement lowered the biological dosage of aflatoxin exposure, suggesting that it could be a useful dietary strategy for reducing the risk of HCC [107].

5.1 Probiotics Helps In Improving Intestinal Dysbiosis

Since the liver is constantly exposed to gut-derived bacterial products, maintaining a functional gut barrier that limits the amounts of bacterial components reaching the liver is critical. The intestinal barrier function is impaired in advanced liver disorders, resulting in an increase in intestinal permeability to gut-derived LPS. The LPS accumulation aids in the progression of HCC by inducing pro-inflammatory responses in the liver [62]. Zhang *et al.* found that probiotics might modify the gut microbiota composition, inhibiting Gram-negative bacteria expansion and improving the intestinal barrier, which reduces endotoxin transmission. As a result, there was less tumorigenic inflammation in the liver [29].

5.2 Probiotics Mediate Modulation of SCFAs Production

The gut microbiota is alone responsible for various key metabolic tasks, including the breakdown of non-digestible carbohydrates in the diet. The end products of carbohydrate fermentation in the human gut include a variety of organic acids, namely acetate, propionate, and butyrate, as well as SCFAs [108]. Colonocytes use butyrate as their principal source of energy. Acetate enters the peripheral circulation and is mostly processed by peripheral tissues, whereas propionate is virtually entirely taken up by the liver from the bloodstream [109]. Certain probiotic strains, such as *Bifidobacteria* and *Lactobacilli*, can change the composition of the gut microbiota, and, consequently the synthesis of SCFAs [110]. This bacterial mediated production of SCFAs may lower the chance of acquiring cancer, particularly HCC. The anti-cancer effect of probiotics was linked to SCFAs synthesis, according to Li *et al.* [18]. Anti-inflammatory fatty acids such as butyrate and propionate can be produced by some bacterial genera, including *Butyricimonas* and *Prevotella*. Probiotics have been demonstrated to boost metabolism associated to SCFAs synthesis, the tricarboxylic acid cycle, carboxylate degradation, and other processes [18], thereby protecting against the development of HCC.

5.3 Probiotics Help in The Regulation of Th17 Response in HCC

Th17 cells, as previously mentioned, have emerged as an important T helper cell subset distinguished by the production of pro-inflammatory and pro-angiogenic mediators, including IL17A and IL22. The Th17 cells' frequency increases within HCC tumours, and has been linked with poor prognosis. HCC accumulates IL17-producing cells, which may aid tumour growth by promoting angiogenesis [29,111]. In mice, Li*et al.* [18] showed that a probiotics mixture that slowed HCC growth decreased the levels of pro-inflammatory cytokines, such as IL-17. Moreover, the probiotics shifted the composition of the gut microbiota toward specific beneficial bacteria, such as *Prevotella* and *Oscillibacter*.

Anti-inflammatory chemicals produced by these bacteria were found to reduce Th17 cells' polarisation and favour the development of anti-inflammatory Treg/Type 1 regulatory T (Tr1) cells in the gut [18]. Interestingly, probiotics controlled the proliferation of segmented filamentous bacteria (SFB), the main Th17-inducing bacteria, in addition to modulating T cell polarisation [18]. The SFB was significantly reduced when probiotics were given. As a result, the production of IL-17 was lowered [18]. As IL-17A generated by Th17 cells promotes angiogenesis [112], lowering Th17 and IL17 levels may aid to slow tumor growth.

5.4. Role of Probiotics in Binding or Adsorption to Carcinogens

There are very few studies that reveal probiotics' ability to bind and immobilise harmful substances in the gut lumen. The harmful effects of dietary toxic chemicals could be decreased, leading to better gut and liver health. Several strains of lactic acid bacteria isolated from dairy products or healthy human individuals have been examined over the last 20 years, and various bacterial strains capable of binding to a variety of mycotoxins have been found [112 - 115]. These bacteria were then shown to bind mycotoxins *ex vivo* in ligated duodenal loops of one-week-old chicks, reducing their absorption into the intestinal tissue by 74% [116].

In the presence of probiotic bacteria, the damage to intestinal epithelia caused by mycotoxins may be reduced. When cytochrome P450 3A4 (CYP3A4) induced Caco-2 monolayers were incubated with aflatoxin B1 (AFB1), the trans-epithelial electrical resistance (TEER) was considerably reduced [117]. This aflatoxin-induced drop in TEER was reduced in the presence of probiotic bacteria, demonstrating that probiotic bacteria could reduce aflatoxin-induced cytotoxicity. Following the above *in vitro* findings, a series of *in vivo* tests were conducted to see if certain strains could bind to AFB1 as a mycotoxin model and if the binding strength was strong enough to reduce AFB1 bioavailability. The probiotic supplementation reduced both AFB1 toxicity and bioavailability, according to the findings from animal model research [118]. Moreover, probiotic bacteria supplementation was demonstrated to successfully lower the urinary excretion of the aflatoxin-DNA adduct (AFB1-N7-guanine), a well-validated biomarker for liver cancer risk, in Chinese participants exposed to AFB1 *via* food [119]. These findings demonstrate that probiotics lower the bioavailability of the carcinogen AFB1 and hence reduce the risk of HCC.

6. FUTURE PERSPECTIVES

Several studies have demonstrated that prebiotics and probiotics play a role in altering gut microbiota and lowering pro-carcinogenic factors in the liver. In view of probiotics' anticancer characteristics, it is possible that modulating gut microbiota using prebiotics could be a unique strategy for preventing the progression of chronic liver disease to HCC (Table **1**). However, more research is needed to validate and clarify the putative pathways involved, and new probiotic and prebiotic-based therapeutic techniques to prevent HCC may be developed in the near future. In addition, with the advancement of high-throughput sequencing technologies, it is now possible to integrate multiple disciplines into molecular pathological epidemiology (MPE), which can provide important etiologic and pathogenic insights into any disease, including HCC, and potentially contribute to precision medicine [120].

CONCLUSION

Overall, the gut-liver axis plays a critical role in the pathophysiology of liver diseases such as HCC. The gut microbiota's significance in the development of HCC is becoming increasingly clear. As a result, tinkering with the gut microbiome could be a unique strategy to treat or prevent HCC. Probiotics, along with prebiotics, could be a novel, safe, and low-cost strategy for preventing or treating HCC. However, more laboratory-based mechanistic studies, as well as extensive human clinical trials evaluating gut microbiota and appropriately selected useful bacterial strains, are needed to gain broader medical acceptance and investigate the possibility of using probiotics as an alternative cancer treatment.

CONSENT FOR PUBLICATION

Not applicable.

CONFLICT OF INTEREST

The authors declare no conflict of interest, financial or otherwise.

ACKNOWLEDGMENT

We are thankful to Uka Tarsadia University, Maliba Campus, Tarsadi, Gujarat, India for providing the facilities needed for the preparation of this chapter.

REFERENCES

[1]   Llovet JM, Zucman-Rossi J, Pikarsky E, *et al.* Hepatocellular carcinoma. Nat Rev Dis Primers 2016; 2(1): 16018.
        [http://dx.doi.org/10.1038/nrdp.2016.18] [PMID: 27158749]

[2]   Villanueva A. Hepatocellular Carcinoma. N Engl J Med 2019; 380(15): 1450-62.
        [http://dx.doi.org/10.1056/NEJMra1713263] [PMID: 30970190]

[3]   International Agency for Research on Cancer. GLOBOCAN 2018. IARC
        https://gco.iarc.fr/today/onlineanalysismap?v=2020&mode=population&mode_population=continents
        &population=900&populations=900&key=asr&sex=0&cancer=11&type=0&statistic=5&prevalence=
        0&population_groupearth&color_palette=default&map_scale=quantile&map_nb_colors=5&continent
        =0&rotate= %255B10%252C0%255D (2020).

[4]   Akinyemiju T, Abera S, Ahmed M, *et al.* The burden of primary liver cancer and underlying etiologies from 1990 to 2015 at the global, regional, and national level. JAMA Oncol 2017; 3(12): 1683-91.
        [http://dx.doi.org/10.1001/jamaoncol.2017.3055] [PMID: 28983565]

[5]   Yu LX, Schwabe RF. The gut microbiome and liver cancer: mechanisms and clinical translation. Nat Rev Gastroenterol Hepatol 2017; 14(9): 527-39.

[http://dx.doi.org/10.1038/nrgastro.2017.72] [PMID: 28676707]

[6]   Sia D, Villanueva A, Friedman SL, Llovet JM. Liver cancer cell of origin, molecular class, and effects on patient prognosis. Gastroenterology 2017; 152(4): 745-61.
[http://dx.doi.org/10.1053/j.gastro.2016.11.048] [PMID: 28043904]

[7]   Zhang C, Yang M, Ericsson AC. Antimicrobial peptides: potential application in liver cancer. Front Microbiol 2019; 10: 1257.
[http://dx.doi.org/10.3389/fmicb.2019.01257] [PMID: 31231341]

[8]   Erstad DJ, Tanabe KK. Hepatocellular carcinoma: early-stage management challenges. J Hepatocell Carcinoma 2017; 4: 81-92.
[http://dx.doi.org/10.2147/JHC.S107370] [PMID: 28721349]

[9]   Balogh J, Victor D III, Asham EH, *et al.* Hepatocellular carcinoma: a review. J Hepatocell Carcinoma 2016; 3: 41-53.
[http://dx.doi.org/10.2147/JHC.S61146] [PMID: 27785449]

[10]   Qin J, Li R, Raes J, *et al.* A human gut microbial gene catalogue established by metagenomic sequencing. Nature 2010; 464(7285): 59-65.
[http://dx.doi.org/10.1038/nature08821] [PMID: 20203603]

[11]   Pennisi E. Biomedicine. Cancer therapies use a little help from microbial friends. Science 2013; 342(6161): 921.
[http://dx.doi.org/10.1126/science.342.6161.921] [PMID: 24264971]

[12]   Tremaroli V, Bäckhed F. Functional interactions between the gut microbiota and host metabolism. Nature 2012; 489(7415): 242-9.
[http://dx.doi.org/10.1038/nature11552] [PMID: 22972297]

[13]   Abt MC, Artis D. The intestinal microbiota in health and disease: the influence of microbial products on immune cell homeostasis. Curr Opin Gastroenterol 2009; 25(6): 496-502.
[http://dx.doi.org/10.1097/MOG.0b013e328331b6b4] [PMID: 19770652]

[14]   Loo TM, Kamachi F, Watanabe Y, *et al.* Gut microbiota promotes obesity-associated liver cancer through PGE (2)-mediated suppression of antitumor immunity. Cancer Discov 2017; 7(5): 522-38.
[http://dx.doi.org/10.1158/2159-8290.CD-16-0932] [PMID: 28202625]

[15]   Schwabe RF, Greten TF. Gut microbiome in HCC – Mechanisms, diagnosis and therapy. J Hepatol 2020; 72(2): 230-8.
[http://dx.doi.org/10.1016/j.jhep.2019.08.016] [PMID: 31954488]

[16]   Zheng Y, Wang T, Tu X, *et al.* Gut microbiome affects the response to anti-PD-1 immunotherapy in patients with hepatocellular carcinoma. J Immunother Cancer 2019; 7(1): 193.
[http://dx.doi.org/10.1186/s40425-019-0650-9] [PMID: 31337439]

[17]   Loguercio C, Simone T, Federico A, *et al.* Gut-liver axis: a new point of attack to treat chronic liver damage? Am J Gastroenterol 2002; 97(8): 2144-6.
[http://dx.doi.org/10.1111/j.1572-0241.2002.05942.x] [PMID: 12190198]

[18]   Li J, Sung CYJ, Lee N, *et al.* Probiotics modulated gut microbiota suppresses hepatocellular carcinoma growth in mice. Proc Natl Acad Sci USA 2016; 113(9): E1306-15.
[http://dx.doi.org/10.1073/pnas.1518189113] [PMID: 26884164]

[19]   Zeuzem S. Gut-liver axis. Int J Colorectal Dis 2000; 15(2): 59-82.
[http://dx.doi.org/10.1007/s003840050236] [PMID: 10855547]

[20]   Seki E, Schnabl B. Role of innate immunity and the microbiota in liver fibrosis: crosstalk between the liver and gut. J Physiol 2012; 590(3): 447-58.
[http://dx.doi.org/10.1113/jphysiol.2011.219691] [PMID: 22124143]

[21]   Compare D, Coccoli P, Rocco A, *et al.* Gut–liver axis: The impact of gut microbiota on non alcoholic fatty liver disease. Nutr Metab Cardiovasc Dis 2012; 22(6): 471-6.

[http://dx.doi.org/10.1016/j.numecd.2012.02.007] [PMID: 22546554]

[22] Chassaing B, Etienne-Mesmin L, Gewirtz AT. Microbiota-liver axis in hepatic disease. Hepatology 2014; 59(1): 328-39.
[http://dx.doi.org/10.1002/hep.26494] [PMID: 23703735]

[23] Szabo G. Gut-liver axis in alcoholic liver disease. Gastroenterology 2015; 148(1): 30-6.
[http://dx.doi.org/10.1053/j.gastro.2014.10.042] [PMID: 25447847]

[24] Szabo G, Bala S. Alcoholic liver disease and the gut-liver axis. World J Gastroenterol 2010; 16(11): 1321-9.
[http://dx.doi.org/10.3748/wjg.v16.i11.1321] [PMID: 20238398]

[25] Schnabl B, Brenner DA. Interactions between the intestinal microbiome and liver diseases. Gastroenterology 2014; 146(6): 1513-24.
[http://dx.doi.org/10.1053/j.gastro.2014.01.020] [PMID: 24440671]

[26] Cesaro C, Tiso A, Del Prete A, *et al.* Gut microbiota and probiotics in chronic liver diseases. Dig Liver Dis 2011; 43(6): 431-8.
[http://dx.doi.org/10.1016/j.dld.2010.10.015] [PMID: 21163715]

[27] Bilzer M, Roggel F, Gerbes AL. Role of Kupffer cells in host defense and liver disease. Liver Int 2006; 26(10): 1175-86.
[http://dx.doi.org/10.1111/j.1478-3231.2006.01342.x] [PMID: 17105582]

[28] Mittal S, El-Serag HB. Epidemiology of HCC: Consider the population. J Clin Gastroenterol 2013; 47: S2-6.
[http://dx.doi.org/10.1097/MCG.0b013e3182872f29] [PMID: 23632345]

[29] Zhang HL, Yu LX, Yang W, *et al.* Profound impact of gut homeostasis on chemically-induced pro-tumorigenic inflammation and hepatocarcinogenesis in rats. J Hepatol 2012; 57(4): 803-12.
[http://dx.doi.org/10.1016/j.jhep.2012.06.011] [PMID: 22727732]

[30] Dapito DH, Mencin A, Gwak GY, *et al.* Promotion of hepatocellular carcinoma by the intestinal microbiota and TLR4. Cancer Cell 2012; 21(4): 504-16.
[http://dx.doi.org/10.1016/j.ccr.2012.02.007] [PMID: 22516259]

[31] Fox JG, Feng Y, Theve EJ, *et al.* Gut microbes define liver cancer risk in mice exposed to chemical and viral transgenic hepatocarcinogens. Gut 2010; 59(1): 88-97.
[http://dx.doi.org/10.1136/gut.2009.183749] [PMID: 19850960]

[32] Huang Y, Fan XG, Wang ZM, Zhou JH, Tian XF, Li N. Identification of *helicobacter* species in human liver samples from patients with primary hepatocellular carcinoma. J Clin Pathol 2004; 57(12): 1273-7.
[http://dx.doi.org/10.1136/jcp.2004.018556] [PMID: 15563667]

[33] Krüttgen A, Horz HP, Weber-Heynemann J, *et al.* Study on the association of *helicobacter* species with viral hepatitis-induced hepatocellular carcinoma. Gut Microbes 2012; 3(3): 228-33.
[http://dx.doi.org/10.4161/gmic.19922] [PMID: 22572832]

[34] Yoshimoto S, Loo TM, Atarashi K, *et al.* Obesity-induced gut microbial metabolite promotes liver cancer through senescence secretome. Nature 2013; 499(7456): 97-101.
[http://dx.doi.org/10.1038/nature12347] [PMID: 23803760]

[35] Bindels LB, Porporato P, Dewulf EM, *et al.* Gut microbiota-derived propionate reduces cancer cell proliferation in the liver. Br J Cancer 2012; 107(8): 1337-44.
[http://dx.doi.org/10.1038/bjc.2012.409] [PMID: 22976799]

[36] Zhu XD, Zhang JB, Zhuang PY, *et al.* High expression of macrophage colony-stimulating factor in peritumoral liver tissue is associated with poor survival after curative resection of hepatocellular carcinoma. J Clin Oncol 2008; 26(16): 2707-16.
[http://dx.doi.org/10.1200/JCO.2007.15.6521] [PMID: 18509183]

[37]   Li YW, Qiu SJ, Fan J, *et al.* Intratumoral neutrophils: A poor prognostic factor for hepatocellular carcinoma following resection. J Hepatol 2011; 54(3): 497-505.
[http://dx.doi.org/10.1016/j.jhep.2010.07.044] [PMID: 21112656]

[38]   Chew V, Chen J, Lee D, *et al.* Chemokine-driven lymphocyte infiltration: an early intratumoural event determining long-term survival in resectable hepatocellular carcinoma. Gut 2012; 61(3): 427-38.
[http://dx.doi.org/10.1136/gutjnl-2011-300509] [PMID: 21930732]

[39]   Taketomi A, Shimada M, Shirabe K, Kajiyama K, Gion T, Sugimachi K. Natural killer cell activity in patients with hepatocellular carcinoma. Cancer 1998; 83(1): 58-63.
[http://dx.doi.org/10.1002/(SICI)1097-0142(19980701)83:1<58::AID-CNCR8>3.0.CO;2-A] [PMID: 9655293]

[40]   Gao Q, Qiu SJ, Fan J, *et al.* Intratumoral balance of regulatory and cytotoxic T cells is associated with prognosis of hepatocellular carcinoma after resection. J Clin Oncol 2007; 25(18): 2586-93.
[http://dx.doi.org/10.1200/JCO.2006.09.4565] [PMID: 17577038]

[41]   Fu J, Xu D, Liu Z, *et al.* Increased regulatory T cells correlate with CD8 T-cell impairment and poor survival in hepatocellular carcinoma patients. Gastroenterology 2007; 132(7): 2328-39.
[http://dx.doi.org/10.1053/j.gastro.2007.03.102] [PMID: 17570208]

[42]   Pang XH, Zhang JP, Zhang YJ, *et al.* Preoperative levels of serum interleukin-6 in patients with hepatocellular carcinoma. Hepatogastroenterology 2011; 58(110-111): 1687-93.
[http://dx.doi.org/10.5754/hge10799] [PMID: 21940335]

[43]   Zhang JP, Yan J, Xu J, *et al.* Increased intratumoral IL-17-producing cells correlate with poor survival in hepatocellular carcinoma patients. J Hepatol 2009; 50(5): 980-9.
[http://dx.doi.org/10.1016/j.jhep.2008.12.033] [PMID: 19329213]

[44]   Liao R, Sun J, Wu H, *et al.* High expression of IL-17 and IL-17RE associate with poor prognosis of hepatocellular carcinoma. J Exp Clin Cancer Res 2013; 32(1): 3.
[http://dx.doi.org/10.1186/1756-9966-32-3] [PMID: 23305119]

[45]   Ye J, Livergood RS, Peng G. The role and regulation of human Th17 cells in tumor immunity. Am J Pathol 2013; 182(1): 10-20.
[http://dx.doi.org/10.1016/j.ajpath.2012.08.041] [PMID: 23159950]

[46]   Ivanov II, Atarashi K, Manel N, *et al.* Induction of intestinal Th17 cells by segmented filamentous bacteria. Cell 2009; 139(3): 485-98.
[http://dx.doi.org/10.1016/j.cell.2009.09.033] [PMID: 19836068]

[47]   Rastelli M, Cani PD, Knauf C. The gut microbiome influences host endocrine functions. Endocr Rev 2019; 40(5): 1271-84.
[http://dx.doi.org/10.1210/er.2018-00280] [PMID: 31081896]

[48]   Tang WHW, Li DY, Hazen SL. Dietary metabolism, the gut microbiome, and heart failure. Nat Rev Cardiol 2019; 16(3): 137-54.
[http://dx.doi.org/10.1038/s41569-018-0108-7] [PMID: 30410105]

[49]   Mazmanian SK, Liu CH, Tzianabos AO, Kasper DL. An immunomodulatory molecule of symbiotic bacteria directs maturation of the host immune system. Cell 2005; 122(1): 107-18.
[http://dx.doi.org/10.1016/j.cell.2005.05.007] [PMID: 16009137]

[50]   Hooper LV, Littman DR, Macpherson AJ. Interactions between the microbiota and the immune system. Science 2012; 336(6086): 1268-73.
[http://dx.doi.org/10.1126/science.1223490] [PMID: 22674334]

[51]   Takeda K, Kaisho T, Akira S. Toll-Like Receptors. Annu Rev Immunol 2003; 21(1): 335-76.
[http://dx.doi.org/10.1146/annurev.immunol.21.120601.141126] [PMID: 12524386]

[52]   Iwasaki A, Medzhitov R. Control of adaptive immunity by the innate immune system. Nat Immunol 2015; 16(4): 343-53.

[http://dx.doi.org/10.1038/ni.3123] [PMID: 25789684]

[53]   Lathrop SK, Bloom SM, Rao SM, *et al.* Peripheral education of the immune system by colonic commensal microbiota. Nature 2011; 478(7368): 250-4.
[http://dx.doi.org/10.1038/nature10434] [PMID: 21937990]

[54]   Lindau D, Gielen P, Kroesen M, Wesseling P, Adema GJ. The immunosuppressive tumour network: myeloid-derived suppressor cells, regulatory T cells and natural killer T cells. Immunology 2013; 138(2): 105-15.
[http://dx.doi.org/10.1111/imm.12036] [PMID: 23216602]

[55]   Weaver CT, Elson CO, Fouser LA, Kolls JK. The Th17 pathway and inflammatory diseases of the intestines, lungs, and skin. Annu Rev Pathol 2013; 8(1): 477-512.
[http://dx.doi.org/10.1146/annurev-pathol-011110-130318] [PMID: 23157335]

[56]   Ivanov II, Atarashi K, Manel N, *et al.* Induction of intestinal Th17 cells by segmented filamentous bacteria. Cell 2009; 139(3): 485-98.
[http://dx.doi.org/10.1016/j.cell.2009.09.033] [PMID: 19836068]

[57]   Lin H, Hua F, Hu ZW. Autophagic flux, supported by toll-like receptor 2 activity, defends against the carcinogenesis of hepatocellular carcinoma. Autophagy 2012; 8(12): 1859-61.
[http://dx.doi.org/10.4161/auto.22094] [PMID: 22996042]

[58]   Lin H, Liu X, Yu J, Hua F, Hu Z. Antioxidant N-acetylcysteine attenuates hepatocarcinogenesis by inhibiting ROS/ER stress in TLR2 deficient mouse. PLoS One 2013; 8(10)e74130
[http://dx.doi.org/10.1371/journal.pone.0074130] [PMID: 24098333]

[59]   Lin H, Yan J, Wang Z, *et al.* Loss of immunity-supported senescence enhances susceptibility to hepatocellular carcinogenesis and progression in Toll-like receptor 2-deficient mice. Hepatology 2013; 57(1): 171-82.
[http://dx.doi.org/10.1002/hep.25991] [PMID: 22859216]

[60]   Li S, Sun R, Chen Y, Wei H, Tian Z. TLR2 limits development of hepatocellular carcinoma by reducing IL18-mediated immunosuppression. Cancer Res 2015; 75(6): 986-95.
[http://dx.doi.org/10.1158/0008-5472.CAN-14-2371] [PMID: 25600646]

[61]   Akira S, Takeda K. Toll-like receptor signalling. Nat Rev Immunol 2004; 4(7): 499-511.
[http://dx.doi.org/10.1038/nri1391] [PMID: 15229469]

[62]   Yu LX, Yan HX, Liu Q, *et al.* Endotoxin accumulation prevents carcinogen-induced apoptosis and promotes liver tumorigenesis in rodents. Hepatology 2010; 52(4): 1322-33.
[http://dx.doi.org/10.1002/hep.23845] [PMID: 20803560]

[63]   Yang J, Zhang JX, Wang H, Wang GL, Hu QG, Zheng QC. Hepatocellular carcinoma and macrophage interaction induced tumor immunosuppression *via* Treg requires TLR4 signaling. World J Gastroenterol 2012; 18(23): 2938-47.
[http://dx.doi.org/10.3748/wjg.v18.i23.2938] [PMID: 22736917]

[64]   Eiró N, Altadill A, Juárez LM, *et al.* Toll-like receptors 3, 4 and 9 in hepatocellular carcinoma: Relationship with clinicopathological characteristics and prognosis. Hepatol Res 2014; 44(7): 769-78.
[http://dx.doi.org/10.1111/hepr.12180] [PMID: 23742263]

[65]   Liu WT, Jing YY, Yu G, *et al.* Toll like receptor 4 facilitates invasion and migration as a cancer stem cell marker in hepatocellular carcinoma. Cancer Lett 2015; 358(2): 136-43.
[http://dx.doi.org/10.1016/j.canlet.2014.12.019] [PMID: 25511737]

[66]   Wang L, Zhu R, Huang Z, Li H, Zhu H. Lipopolysaccharide-induced toll-like receptor 4 signaling in cancer cells promotes cell survival and proliferation in hepatocellular carcinoma. Dig Dis Sci 2013; 58(8): 2223-36.
[http://dx.doi.org/10.1007/s10620-013-2745-3] [PMID: 23828139]

[67]   Fotiadis CI, Stoidis CN, Spyropoulos BG, Zografos ED. Role of probiotics, prebiotics and synbiotics in chemoprevention for colorectal cancer. World J Gastroenterol 2008; 14(42): 6453-7.

[http://dx.doi.org/10.3748/wjg.14.6453] [PMID: 19030195]

[68]   Davis CD, Milner JA. Gastrointestinal microflora, food components and colon cancer prevention. J Nutr Biochem 2009; 20(10): 743-52.
[http://dx.doi.org/10.1016/j.jnutbio.2009.06.001] [PMID: 19716282]

[69]   Martinez FD. The human microbiome. Early life determinant of health outcomes. Ann Am Thorac Soc 2014; 11(Suppl 1) (Suppl. 1): S7-S12.
[http://dx.doi.org/10.1513/AnnalsATS.201306-186MG] [PMID: 24437411]

[70]   Kaczmarczyk MM, Miller MJ, Freund GG. The health benefits of dietary fiber: Beyond the usual suspects of type 2 diabetes mellitus, cardiovascular disease and colon cancer. Metabolism 2012; 61(8): 1058-66.
[http://dx.doi.org/10.1016/j.metabol.2012.01.017] [PMID: 22401879]

[71]   Shen Q, Zhao L, Tuohy KM. High-level dietary fibre up-regulates colonic fermentation and relative abundance of saccharolytic bacteria within the human faecal microbiota *in vitro*. Eur J Nutr 2012; 51(6): 693-705.
[http://dx.doi.org/10.1007/s00394-011-0248-6] [PMID: 21952691]

[72]   Weijers CAGM, Franssen MCR, Visser GM. Glycosyltransferase-catalyzed synthesis of bioactive oligosaccharides. Biotechnol Adv 2008; 26(5): 436-56.
[http://dx.doi.org/10.1016/j.biotechadv.2008.05.001] [PMID: 18565714]

[73]   Saad N, Delattre C, Urdaci M, Schmitter JM, Bressollier P. An overview of the last advances in probiotic and prebiotic field. Lebensm Wiss Technol 2013; 50(1): 1-16.
[http://dx.doi.org/10.1016/j.lwt.2012.05.014]

[74]   Wang Y. Prebiotics: Present and future in food science and technology. Food Res Int 2009; 42(1): 8-12.
[http://dx.doi.org/10.1016/j.foodres.2008.09.001]

[75]   He X, Li R, Huang G, Hwang H, Jiang X. Influence of marine oligosaccharides on the response of various biological systems to UV irradiation. J Funct Foods 2013; 5(2): 858-68.
[http://dx.doi.org/10.1016/j.jff.2013.01.035]

[76]   Patel S, Goyal A. Functional oligosaccharides: production, properties and applications. World J Microbiol Biotechnol 2011; 27(5): 1119-28.
[http://dx.doi.org/10.1007/s11274-010-0558-5]

[77]   Chen J, Liang R, Liu W, *et al.* Pectic-oligosaccharides prepared by dynamic high-pressure microfluidization and their *in vitro* fermentation properties. Carbohydr Polym 2013; 91(1): 175-82.
[http://dx.doi.org/10.1016/j.carbpol.2012.08.021] [PMID: 23044120]

[78]   Fotiadis CI, Stoidis CN, Spyropoulos BG, Zografos ED. Role of probiotics, prebiotics and synbiotics in chemoprevention for colorectal cancer. World J Gastroenterol 2008; 14(42): 6453-7.
[http://dx.doi.org/10.3748/wjg.14.6453] [PMID: 19030195]

[79]   Davis CD, Milner JA. Gastrointestinal microflora, food components and colon cancer prevention. J Nutr Biochem 2009; 20(10): 743-52.
[http://dx.doi.org/10.1016/j.jnutbio.2009.06.001] [PMID: 19716282]

[80]   Roberfroid MB. Prebiotics and probiotics: are they functional foods? Am J Clin Nutr 2000; 71(6) (Suppl.): 1682S-7S.
[http://dx.doi.org/10.1093/ajcn/71.6.1682S] [PMID: 10837317]

[81]   Gibson GR, Roberfroid MB. Dietary modulation of the human colonic microbiota: introducing the concept of prebiotics. J Nutr 1995; 125(6): 1401-12.
[http://dx.doi.org/10.1093/jn/125.6.1401] [PMID: 7782892]

[82]   Kondegowda NG, Meaney MP, Baker C, Ju YH. Effects of non-digestible carbohydrates on the growth of estrogen-dependent human breast cancer (MCF-7) tumors implanted in ovariectomized athymic mice. Nutr Cancer 2011; 63(1): 55-64.

[PMID: 21170812]

[83] Taper HS, Delzenne NM, Roberfroid MB. Growth inhibition of transplantable mouse tumors by non-digestible carbohydrates. Int J Cancer 1997; 71(6): 1109-12.
[http://dx.doi.org/10.1002/(SICI)1097-0215(19970611)71:6<1109::AID-IJC30>3.0.CO;2-5] [PMID: 9185718]

[84] Daubioul C, Rousseau N, Taper H, *et al.* Dietary fructans, but not cellulose, decrease triglyceride accumulation in the liver of obese Zucker fa/fa rats. J Nutr 2002; 132(5): 967-73.
[http://dx.doi.org/10.1093/jn/132.5.967] [PMID: 11983823]

[85] Guarner F, Malagelada JR. Gut flora in health and disease. Lancet 2003; 361(9356): 512-9.
[http://dx.doi.org/10.1016/S0140-6736(03)12489-0] [PMID: 12583961]

[86] Bindels LB, Porporato P, Dewulf EM, *et al.* Gut microbiota-derived propionate reduces cancer cell proliferation in the liver. Br J Cancer 2012; 107(8): 1337-44.
[http://dx.doi.org/10.1038/bjc.2012.409] [PMID: 22976799]

[87] Aoyama M, Kotani J, Usami M. Butyrate and propionate induced activated or non-activated neutrophil apoptosis *via* HDAC inhibitor activity but without activating GPR-41/GPR-43 pathways. Nutrition 2010; 26(6): 653-61.
[http://dx.doi.org/10.1016/j.nut.2009.07.006] [PMID: 20004081]

[88] Tang Y, Chen Y, Jiang H, Nie D. Short-chain fatty acids induced autophagy serves as an adaptive strategy for retarding mitochondria-mediated apoptotic cell death. Cell Death Differ 2011; 18(4): 602-18.
[http://dx.doi.org/10.1038/cdd.2010.117] [PMID: 20930850]

[89] Siavoshian S, Segain JP, Kornprobst M, *et al.* Butyrate and trichostatin A effects on the proliferation/differentiation of human intestinal epithelial cells: induction of cyclin D3 and p21 expression. Gut 2000; 46(4): 507-14.
[http://dx.doi.org/10.1136/gut.46.4.507] [PMID: 10716680]

[90] Brown AJ, Goldsworthy SM, Barnes AA, *et al.* The Orphan G protein-coupled receptors GPR41 and GPR43 are activated by propionate and other short chain carboxylic acids. J Biol Chem 2003; 278(13): 11312-9.
[http://dx.doi.org/10.1074/jbc.M211609200] [PMID: 12496283]

[91] Le Poul E, Loison C, Struyf S, *et al.* Functional characterization of human receptors for short chain fatty acids and their role in polymorphonuclear cell activation. J Biol Chem 2003; 278(28): 25481-9.
[http://dx.doi.org/10.1074/jbc.M301403200] [PMID: 12711604]

[92] Guidelines for the Evaluation of Probiotics in Food. Available online: http://www.who.int/foodsafety/fs_management/en/probiotic_guidelines.pdf

[93] Saarela M, Mogensen G, Fondén R, Mättö J, Mattila-Sandholm T. Probiotic bacteria: safety, functional and technological properties. J Biotechnol 2000; 84(3): 197-215.
[http://dx.doi.org/10.1016/S0168-1656(00)00375-8] [PMID: 11164262]

[94] Reuter G. The *Lactobacillus* and *Bifidobacterium* microflora of the human intestine: composition and succession. Curr Issues Intest Microbiol 2001; 2(2): 43-53.
[PMID: 11721280]

[95] Kirpich IA, McClain CJ. Probiotics in the treatment of the liver diseases. J Am Coll Nutr 2012; 31(1): 14-23.
[http://dx.doi.org/10.1080/07315724.2012.10720004] [PMID: 22661622]

[96] Sanders ME, Guarner F, Guerrant R, *et al.* An update on the use and investigation of probiotics in health and disease. Gut 2013; 62(5): 787-96.
[http://dx.doi.org/10.1136/gutjnl-2012-302504] [PMID: 23474420]

[97] De Moreno MA. The administration of probiotics and fermented products containing lactic acid bacteria exert beneficial effects against intestinal and non-intestinal cancers. J Food Nutr Disor 2014;

S1-005.

[98]   Nitin J, Mithun S, Pn R, Reddy DN. Liver diseases: The role of gut microbiota and probiotics. J Probiotics Health 2016; 4(3): 2.
[http://dx.doi.org/10.4172/2329-8901.1000154]

[99]   Elzouki AN. Probiotics and liver disease: Where are we now and where are we going? J Clin Gastroenterol 2016; 50 (Suppl. 2): S188-90.
[http://dx.doi.org/10.1097/MCG.0000000000000712] [PMID: 27741172]

[100]   Gratz SW, Mykkanen H, El-Nezami HS. Probiotics and gut health: A special focus on liver diseases. World J Gastroenterol 2010; 16(4): 403-10.
[http://dx.doi.org/10.3748/wjg.v16.i4.403] [PMID: 20101763]

[101]   Imani Fooladi AA, Hosseini HM, Nourani MR, Khani S, Alavian SM. Probiotic as a novel treatment strategy against liver disease. Hepat Mon 2013; 13(2)e7521
[http://dx.doi.org/10.5812/hepatmon.7521] [PMID: 23610585]

[102]   Sheth AA, Garcia-Tsao G. Probiotics and liver disease. J Clin Gastroenterol 2008; 42 (Suppl. 2): S80-4.
[http://dx.doi.org/10.1097/MCG.0b013e318169c44e] [PMID: 18542037]

[103]   Sharma V, Garg S, Aggarwal S. Probiotics and liver disease. Perm J 2013; 17(4): 62-7.
[http://dx.doi.org/10.7812/TPP/12-144] [PMID: 24361022]

[104]   Hill C, Guarner F, Reid G, *et al.* The International Scientific Association for Probiotics and Prebiotics consensus statement on the scope and appropriate use of the term probiotic. Nat Rev Gastroenterol Hepatol 2014; 11(8): 506-14.
[http://dx.doi.org/10.1038/nrgastro.2014.66] [PMID: 24912386]

[105]   De LeBlanc AM, Matar C, Perdigón G. The application of probiotics in cancer. Br J Nutr 2007; 98(S1) (Suppl. 1): S105-10.
[http://dx.doi.org/10.1017/S0007114507839602] [PMID: 17922945]

[106]   Kumar M, Verma V, Nagpal R, *et al.* Effect of probiotic fermented milk and chlorophyllin on gene expressions and genotoxicity during AFB1-induced hepatocellular carcinoma. Gene 2011; 490(1-2): 54-9.
[http://dx.doi.org/10.1016/j.gene.2011.09.003] [PMID: 21963996]

[107]   El-Nezami HS, Polychronaki NN, Ma J, *et al.* Probiotic supplementation reduces a biomarker for increased risk of liver cancer in young men from Southern China. Am J Clin Nutr 2006; 83(5): 1199-203.
[http://dx.doi.org/10.1093/ajcn/83.5.1199] [PMID: 16685066]

[108]   Neish AS. Microbes in gastrointestinal health and disease. Gastroenterology 2009; 136(1): 65-80.
[http://dx.doi.org/10.1053/j.gastro.2008.10.080] [PMID: 19026645]

[109]   Wong JMW, de Souza R, Kendall CWC, Emam A, Jenkins DJA. Colonic health: fermentation and short chain fatty acids. J Clin Gastroenterol 2006; 40(3): 235-43.
[http://dx.doi.org/10.1097/00004836-200603000-00015] [PMID: 16633129]

[110]   LeBlanc JG, Chain F, Martín R, Bermúdez-Humarán LG, Courau S, Langella P. Beneficial effects on host energy metabolism of short-chain fatty acids and vitamins produced by commensal and probiotic bacteria. Microb Cell Fact 2017; 16(1): 79.
[http://dx.doi.org/10.1186/s12934-017-0691-z] [PMID: 28482838]

[111]   Numasaki M, Fukushi J, Ono M, *et al.* Interleukin-17 promotes angiogenesis and tumor growth. Blood 2003; 101(7): 2620-7.
[http://dx.doi.org/10.1182/blood-2002-05-1461] [PMID: 12411307]

[112]   Murugaiyan G, Saha B. Protumor vs antitumor functions of IL-17. J Immunol 2009; 183(7): 4169-75.
[http://dx.doi.org/10.4049/jimmunol.0901017] [PMID: 19767566]

[113] El-Nezami H, Kankaanpää P, Salminen S, Ahokas J. Physicochemical alterations enhance the ability of dairy strains of lactic acid bacteria to remove aflatoxin from contaminated media. J Food Prot 1998; 61(4): 466-8.
[http://dx.doi.org/10.4315/0362-028X-61.4.466] [PMID: 9709211]

[114] El-Nezami H, Kankaanpaa P, Salminen S, Ahokas J. Ability of dairy strains of lactic acid bacteria to bind a common food carcinogen, aflatoxin B1. Food Chem Toxicol 1998; 36(4): 321-6.
[http://dx.doi.org/10.1016/S0278-6915(97)00160-9] [PMID: 9651049]

[115] El-Nezami H, Polychronaki N, Salminen S, Mykkänen H. Binding rather than metabolism may explain the interaction of two food-Grade *Lactobacillus* strains with zearalenone and its derivative (')alpha-earalenol. Appl Environ Microbiol 2002; 68(7): 3545-9.
[http://dx.doi.org/10.1128/AEM.68.7.3545-3549.2002] [PMID: 12089040]

[116] El-Nezami HS, Chrevatidis A, Auriola S, Salminen S, Mykkänen H. Removal of common Fusarium toxins *in vitro* by strains of *Lactobacillus* and *Propionibacterium*. Food Addit Contam 2002; 19(7): 680-6.
[http://dx.doi.org/10.1080/02652030210134236] [PMID: 12113664]

[117] El-Nezami H, Mykkänen H, Kankaanpää P, Salminen S, Ahokas J. Ability of *Lactobacillus* and *Propionibacterium* strains to remove aflatoxin B, from the chicken duodenum. J Food Prot 2000; 63(4): 549-52.
[http://dx.doi.org/10.4315/0362-028X-63.4.549] [PMID: 10772225]

[118] Gratz S, Wu QK, El-Nezami H, Juvonen RO, Mykkänen H, Turner PC. *Lactobacillus* rhamnosus strain GG reduces aflatoxin B1 transport, metabolism, and toxicity in Caco-2 Cells. Appl Environ Microbiol 2007; 73(12): 3958-64.
[http://dx.doi.org/10.1128/AEM.02944-06] [PMID: 17449679]

[119] Gratz S, Täubel M, Juvonen RO, *et al. Lactobacillus rhamnosus* strain GG modulates intestinal absorption, fecal excretion, and toxicity of aflatoxin B(1) in rats. Appl Environ Microbiol 2006; 72(11): 7398-400.
[http://dx.doi.org/10.1128/AEM.01348-06] [PMID: 16980432]

[120] Ogino S, Nishihara R, VanderWeele TJ, *et al.* The role of molecular pathological epidemiology in the study of neoplastic and non-neoplastic diseases in the era of precision medicine. Epidemiology 2016; 27(4): 602-11.
[http://dx.doi.org/10.1097/EDE.0000000000000471] [PMID: 26928707]

CHAPTER 9

Probiotics-based Anticancer Immunity In Cervical Cancer

Mehran Mahooti[1,2]**, Elahe Abdolalipour**[1]**, Seyed Mohammad Miri**[1] **and Amir Ghaemi**[1,*]

[1] *Department of Influenza and other respiratory viruses, Pasteur Institute of Iran, Tehran, Iran*

[2] *Department of Biotechnology, Iranian Research Organization for Science and Technology, Tehran, Iran*

Abstract: In the recent past, many investigations have been directed toward finding the possible relationship between probiotic preventive-therapeutic effects and different cancers. Among different cancers, human papillomavirus (HPV)-induced cancer is the third most frequent cancer among women, resulting in being the second cause of death worldwide. Current treatments, such as chemotherapy and radiotherapy, have been shown to have some limitations, and the available effective cervical vaccines are costly, particularly in developing countries. Therefore, the researchers seek alternatives, such as natural components, as a new approach to treating and cure HPV-induced cancer. Among several natural components, probiotics have increasingly gained more attention due to the probiotic-associated immunomodulation and therapeutic efficacy shown in several studies, as well as their lower risk for human health. In this chapter, we have reviewed the association between probiotics and cervical cancer and discussed how probiotics could exert their effects to suppress or even inhibit the growth of cervical tumors, preclinically or clinically. The different aspects of probiotic application have been precisely studied to assess the potential of probiotics in improving or treating HPV-induced cancer. In addition, the effects of probiotics on immune responses have been described.

Keywords: Anti-cancer effect, Cervical cancer, Human papillomavirus, Immunomodulatory effect, Immune response, Probiotics.

1. INTRODUCTION

A survey in 2018 demonstrated that about 311,000 women out of 570,000 women diagnosed with cervical cancer died from this disease [1, 2]. Notably, the incidence and mortality of cervical cancer are believed to be positively related to

---

* **Corresponding author Amir Ghaemi:** Department of Influenza and other respiratory viruses, Pasteur Institute of Iran, Tehran, Iran; E-mails: ghaem_amir@yahoo.com and A_ghaemi@pasteur.ac.ir

Mitesh Kumar Dwivedi, Alwarappan Sankaranarayanan & Sanjay Tiwari (Eds.)

human papillomavirus (HPV) and human immunodeficiency virus (HIV) infection, whereas being negatively associated with cervical cancer screening coverage [3]. During the 1990s, HPV was recognized as a key cause of cervical cancer, and this association is equally important as the discovery of the relation between cigarette smoking and lung cancer, or between chronic infections with hepatitis B virus (HBV) [4]. According to reports, genital HPV infection is responsible for approximately 500,000 cervical cancer cases and 275,000 associated deaths each year globally [5, 6]. Moreover, HPV has been attributed to playing a role, in varying degrees, in different diseases ranging from benign papillomas or warts to distinct cancers, including cancer of the anus, vulva, vagina, penis, and head and neck [7 - 10].

Papillomavirus, which is a member of the *Papovaviridae* family, is a relatively small, non-enveloped virus with a double-stranded DNA approximately 8 kilobases in length, and its genome is enclosed by a spherical capsid with icosahedral harmony and a diameter of about 55 nm. The genomic particle of this virus is hitched to cellular histones and contained in a protein capsid composed of 72 pentameric capsomers [11]. Three segments, including early, late and genomic regions, compose the genome of papillomavirus. E1, E2 and E4-E8, which are considered early regions, constitute half of the HPV genome. The E1 and E2 are involved in the regulation of DNA replication, E2 in transcription, and E5, E6 and E7 in cell transformation. The late region (L), including L1 and L2 capsid proteins, comprises 40% of the genome, while the genomic regulatory region, involving the structural proteins of the virion, forms the rest of the genome [12, 13].

Although there are more than 100 types of HPV, at least 14 types are known to cause cancer (also known as the high-risk type). In comparison to low-risk HPV 6 and 11, which cause genital warts and respiratory papillomatosis, long time infections with high-risk HPV types, including 16, 18, 31, 33, 34, 35, 39, 45, 51, 52, 56, 58, 59, 66, 68, and 70, particularly 16 and 18, which together contribute to more than 70% of cervical cancers worldwide, result in cervical cancer [11, 14]. HPV primarily transmits through skin-to-skin contact, and studies have revealed that sexual activity influences the risk of being infected with HPV infection and cervical cancer [15]. There are four stages of cervical cancer occurrence; first, HPV infection of the transformation zone (TZ); second, HPV infection persistence; third, clonal expansion of HPV-infected cells to high-grade cervical intraepithelial neoplasia (CIN 3) or adenocarcinoma *in situ* (AIS); and forth, their progression to invasive cancer [16].

2. PATHOGENESIS OF HPV AND CERVICAL CANCER

When the virus particle anchors to the epithelial basal layer through its receptor, heparan sulfate proteoglycans (HSPGs), and enters the dividing basal cells, infection with papillomaviruses begins [1]. Following the entry of the virus, the viral genome is maintained and amplified in the nuclei of infected basal epithelial cells. In order to have a persistent infection of basal cells, viral genomes approximately replicate once per cell cycle during the S phase, making HPV genomes persist in basal epithelial cells for years to decades [1, 17]. Although the basal cells become infected, these cells keep dividing and generating daughter cells, one of which remains in the basal layer to continue replication, which is required for the replication of the virus. The other daughter cell goes upward toward the suprabasal layer and differentiates there till it is finally shed from the epithelial surface [18, 19]. E5, E6, and E7 actions, which lead to induction and propagation of cell growth, result in constant cervical cells' growth and division, to stimulate the late viral genes expressed in the suprabasal layer, needed for capsid structure formation. HPV life cycle continues over time, and carcinogenic progression is not often the normal HPV life cycle, so the vast majority of infections are benign and transitory, which ultimately become undetectable in 12-24 months [20, 21]. Compared to genital HPV infections caused by low-risk (LR) non-oncogenic HPVs, which show higher rates of viral clearance (clearance of 90% of infections within 2 years) and disease regression, the high-risk (HR) types like HPV 16 and 18, belonging to the α genus, are associated with cancers of the cervix [22]. In other words, infection with HR HPV leads to lesions in the cervix, inclining to progress toward invasive cervical cancer over time [23]. Among oncogenic HPV types, HPV types 16 and 18 have been shown to be in high-grade cervical dysplastic lesions and the majority of invasive cervical cancers. Additionally, HR HPVs have some strategies to overcome the dependency on host cellular DNA synthesis machinery as compared to LR HPV with a normal life cycle. One strategy is to integrate their genome into a host chromosome, which normally occurs near common fragile sites of the human genome [24]. In this process, *E6* and *E7* genes tend to constantly express while other portions of the viral DNA are deleted or their expression is disturbed [25]. While E2 and E1, the two proteins playing an important role in the transcription and replication control, lose their activities, the deregulation of E6 and E7 oncoproteins begins [26]. Studies have demonstrated that the expression of high-risk HPV *E6* and *E7* genes in primary human keratinocytes facilitates their immortalization [27]. In addition, the E6 and E7 proteins are pivotal for the inhibition of tumor suppressor genes such as *p53* and *pRb* (retinoblastoma protein) [28]. E6-mediated inhibition of p53 allows several cellular changes to turn a cell oncogenic. One of the changes is to elicit uncontrolled cell proliferation by evading the cellular checkpoints. The degradation of p53 occurs when HPV E6, with the help of E6AP, binds to a motif, the LxxLL consensus sequence, in the conserved domain of E6AP, forming a heterotrimeric complex of E6/E6AP/p53 leading the cells to undergo uncontrolled cell division; thereby, evading the preventive checkpoints [29]. On the other hand, E7-mediated suppression of pRb is another pivotal step for achieving unrestrained cell proliferation. Of note, pRb–E2F interaction is a mandatory checkpoint for the cells to travel through a G1-S phase transition, and this pRb-E2F complex remains unchanged when the cells are not prepared to enter the S-phase. However, during infection with HPV, E7 targets pRb for ubiquitination, resulting in the release of E2F transcription factors, which in turn transcribe cyclin A, cyclin E, and $p16^{INK4A}$ together to make the cells undergo to premature S-phase entry [30]. Importantly, in addition to the induction of expression of $p16^{INK4A}$ through pRb disintegration, E7 does the same thing by epigenetic derepression through KDM6B (H3K27-specific demethylase 6B) [31]. Moreover, two studies confirmed that E6 and E7 are crucial for the persistence of HPV-mediated cancer, since the absence of E6 and E7 activity results in cancer cells' senescence or apoptosis [32, 33]. Following several findings which showed that E6 and E7 are the key players in the process of HPV-mediated cervical tumorgenesis, many vaccine approaches have tried to target these proteins [34]. In the context of prophylactic HPV vaccines, Cervarix and Gardasil are two well-known vaccines for cervical cancer prevention. While Cervarix proved to be an efficient vaccine against HPV16, 18, 31, 33, and 45, for which screen methods are not adequate, Gardasil is effective against HPV 16, 18, and 31. Both vaccines contain a protein of the L1 protein capsid in the form of a virus-like particle (VLP), and are used particularly against two HR HPV types causing cervical cancer. Moreover, both vaccines induce memory B cells, and for those individuals who got vaccinated with each vaccine four years before, specific memory T lymphocytes against type 16 VLPs were elicited in them [35, 36]. However, prophylactic-based vaccines are not only costly but also do not protect infected individuals, and they do not cover all types of HPV infections [37]. Therefore, due to the pivotal role of E6 and E7 in cervical cancer and limitations of prophylactic vaccines, therapeutic vaccines as another strategy to overcome cervical cancer challenges have been developed. This type of vaccine ranges from live vector, protein, or peptide to cell-based vaccines. One advantage of therapeutic vaccine over prophylactic vaccines is that infected patients can also utilize this type of vaccine due to the effect of therapeutic vaccines against pre-existing HPV infections and HPV-associated lesions [38]. The important role of all these types of vaccine is to bring E6 or E7 antigens in various forms and deliver them to antigen-presenting cells (APCs), where antigens stimulate antigen presentation through major histocompatibility complex class I and class II, resulting in the generation of $CD8^+$ cytotoxic T cell or $CD4^+$ helper T cell responses [39, 40]. However, to date, there are no approved therapeutic vaccines exist [41]. Therefore, alternatives besides prophylactic and therapeutic vaccines are required. These alternatives are approaches like chemotherapy, radiotherapy, and surgery that have been utilized as primary treatment methods for cervical cancer. However, the application of these treatments often is challenged by limited efficacy, increased toxicity, and side effects [42]. Hence, there is great attention towards employing agents that activate immune responses and overcome the associated limitations of conventional therapies against cervical cancer [43]. Among different approaches against distinct cancers, the use of natural components or immune-stimulatory agents to reinforce the immune system to recognize, attack, and destroy cancer cells with low side effects has recently been developed [44, 45]. For instance, several studies have shown that curcumin has the ability to induce and modulate immune responses while it seems to be safe for use [46, 47], or cinnamon, as a safe natural component has been shown to act as an immunomodulatory agent with the ability to be even used against different cancers [48, 49].

3. PROBIOTICS

Probiotics are the other immunomodulatory natural components, which can be considered as a treatment option for different cancers. The word probiotic comes from Latin, meaning "for life" and multiple fermented products such as cheese, wine, beer, kefir, and Doogh (Yogurt Drink) included in the human diet are rich in probiotics [50]. World Health Organization (WHO) and the Food and Agriculture Organization (FAO) define Probiotics as "live microorganisms which, when administered in proper amounts, confer a health benefit on the host" [51]. The two most studied probiotics are *Lactobacillus* and *Bifidobacterium* spp [52 - 54] and earlier investigations focused mainly on the role of probiotics as a dietary supplement or food nutrition [55]. However, recently, the application of probiotics has changed toward utilizing them in medical fields as either prophylactic or therapeutic agents against a wide range of diseases such as influenza [56] and cancers like colon cancer [57]. With more studies demonstrating the ability of probiotics to induce and modulate immune responses, more investigations have been conducted to elucidate the exact role of probiotics against distinct diseases, including cancers. Since then, different studies have demonstrated an association between increased consumption of probiotics and reduced cancer progression [58, 59]. This chapter further discusses the function of probiotics against cervical cancer.

4. PROBIOTIC AND CERVICAL CANCER (WITH A FOCUS ON POSSIBLE ANTI-CERVICAL CANCER MECHANISM OF PROBIOTICS)

It has been well understood that probiotics exert some immune responses mainly through different pathways that subsequently result in the secretion of many cytokines and modulation of immune cells such as dendritic cells (DCs), T cells, and B cells in the gut-associated lymphoid tissue (GALT) [60]. Additionally, the immune-modulatory properties of probiotics, including regulatory impact on innate and adaptive immune responses, is partly due to the interaction of probiotics and their associated fragments with pattern recognition receptors (PRRs) such as different toll-like reporters (TLRs) [61]. For instance, TLR2, 4, 5, and TLR9 have been proven to be activated by different probiotics or their fragments like flagellin (TLR5 agonist) or LPS (TLR4 agonist), including *Lactobacilli* and *Bifidobacteria* which further result in induction of immune responses [62 - 66]. These patterns exist on intestinal epithelial cells and link innate and adaptive immunity by recognizing pathogen-associated molecular patterns (PAMPs) and therefore conveying pathogen-related molecular signals into cells through transmembrane (TM) protein that ultimately results in many changes in signaling pathways as well as in the production of pro-inflammatory or anti-inflammatory cytokines [67].

It may be possible that these probiotic-induced immune cells migrate from the gut to other organs, such as the cervix of the vagina, through a less studied axis, named the gut-vagina axis, and exert probiotic's beneficial effects in that organ [68, 69]. Based on the interaction of PRRs with probiotics and their fragments, different types of immune cells reach the infected site, such as the cervix, and start functioning against cancer. However, most studies have been devoted to surveying the possible effects of probiotics on cervical cancer cells or cervical cancer treatment-associated complications. For instance, some investigations on the impact of the probiotic on cervical cancer cell lines proved that different probiotics can elicit a range of functions such as apoptosis, proliferation inhibition, inflammation reduction, as well as metastasis suppression [70]. In addition, Rahbar Saadat *et al.* [71] showed that vaginal-isolated *Lactococcus lactis* can elicit apoptosis against cancer through an alternation of microRNAs. This apoptosis was due to the down-regulation of induction of TLR4, miR-21, and miR-200b expression levels [71]. Reduction in miR-21 expression could be important for the treatment of cervical cancer with probiotics, because it has been reported that miR-21 expression increases in invasive cancer tissues [72]. However, further research is needed to explore the relationship between the effect of probiotics on microRNAs and probiotic-associated anti-cancer effects. Although more studies are required based on the probable existence of the gut-vaginal axis and the role of TLRs in immune cells' trafficking, the probiotics can be considered as an option for treatment of the cancer, alone or along with other anti-cervical cancer agents.

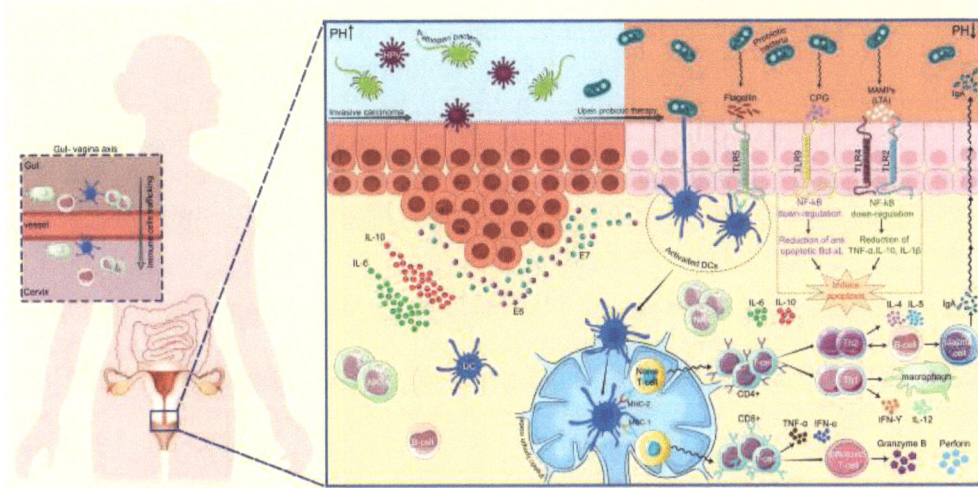

Fig. (1). The different possible mechanisms of probiotics in the prevention of cervical cancer. Probiotics and their fragments confer immunomodulation through direct and indirect interaction with epithelial cells. One possible indirect effect of probiotics on cervical cancer could attribute to immune cell trafficking *via* the gut-vagina axis through which probiotic-induced immune cells migrate to the site of infection. Moreover, probiotics and their fragments as MAMPs may directly interact with different pattern recognition receptors (PRRs) like TLRs to induce different immune cells. Additionally, probiotics have been shown to treat bacterial vaginosis and to keep the pH of the vagina balanced.

It has been demonstrated that nuclear factor kappa-B (NF-kB) plays roles in the proliferation, metastasis, angiogenesis and cell immortality of cervical cancer [73]. Some probiotics have been proven to suppress the NF-kB pathway or/and hamper the activation of NF-kB [74, 75]. In this context, anti-inflammatory *Lactobacillus plantarum* NK3 and *Bifidobacterium longum* NK49 could induce a decline in vaginal and uterus TNF-α levels and NF-kB activation, suggesting these probiotics as potential candidates in alleviating cervical cancer outcomes [76]. Additionally, the inhibition of NF-κB signaling pathways was observed by *Lactobacillus rhamnosus* GG components such as CpG in mouse macrophage RAW264.7 cells. The authors demonstrated that pre-incubation of the cell line with CPG of probiotics suppressed the activation of the MAPK and NF-κB signaling pathways, and then down-regulated TNF-α and IL-6 cytokines' production [77]. Moreover, other probiotic fragments can also suppress NF-κB signaling. For example, lipoteichoic acid (LTA) of *Lactobacillus plantarum* has been shown to inhibit poly I:C-induced IL-8 production through attenuation of NF-κB activation [78]. This LTA down-regulation effect on NF-κB activation was also shown in another study in which six out of eight *Bifidobacteria* suppressed the NF-κB activation by lipopolysaccharide [79]. Signal transducer and activator of transcription 3 (STAT3) is another signaling pathway, which is activated in cervical cancer, especially in HPV⁺ type. This pathway mediates the up-regulation of anti-apoptotic genes such as *Bcl-xL* and *survivin* at the tumor site, resulting in the development of cervical cancer [80]. A number of studies have reported the inhibitory effect of some probiotics, such as VSL#3 (a mixture of 8 probiotics), and *Lactobacillus plantarum* NCU116 exopolysaccharides (EPSs) on STAT3 signaling pathway, introducing these probiotics as therapeutic options for future anti-cervical cancer studies [81, 82]. The distinct possible probiotic mechanisms involved in the prevention of cervical cancer are shown in Fig. (**1**).

Moreover, in order to acquire more knowledge about the impact of probiotics on cervical cancer, the following sections deal with the probiotics' effects on cervical cancer in three distinct parts, including *in vitro*, preclinical, and clinical categories.

5. PROBIOTIC AND CERVICAL CANCER (*IN VITRO* STUDIES)

Most primary studies have assessed the potential anti-cervical cancer impact of probiotics on different cell lines prior to the preclinical and clinical studies. For example, there has been an association between the vaginal and cervical ecosystem with *Lactobacillus* spp, and some evidence confirmed that the presence of these bacteria in healthy women is critical in preventing and inhibiting the growth of pathogens and bacterial vaginosis (BV) [83, 84]. Few studies utilized the common vaginal *lactobacillus* as probiotics to evaluate the pathogen-inhibitory effect of probiotics. Motevaseli *et al.* [85] evaluated the cytotoxic effect of live *Lactobacilli*, their components, and supernatants on HeLa (cervical tumor), and then compared their result with the results derived from human normal fibroblast-like cervical (HNCF). They demonstrated that *Lactobacilli* supernatants exert cytotoxic effects on cervical tumor cells through the reduction of caspase-3 activity, and the apoptosis was inhibited by supernatants of bacteria, and this was confirmed through the increased levels of human chorionic gonadotropin b (hCGb), which is known to inhibit apoptosis [85]. In 2014, some researchers sought to reveal the mechanisms through which *Lactobacillus crispatus* and *Lactobacillus rhamnosus* culture supernatants exert their anti-proliferative effects on HeLa cervical cancer cells. They observed that upon treatment with both strains' supernatants, mRNA levels of *CASP3* and two autophagy genes, *TG14* and *BECN1*, were down-regulated. Moreover, both the supernatants led to the down-regulation of HPV *E6* oncogenes. They concluded that due to the dual role of autophagy in either suppression or pro-survival of tumor cells, the cytotoxicity effect of studied *Lactobacilli* supernatants on HeLa cells can be partially in response to the down-regulation of HPV oncogenes [86]. Moreover, an investigation on SiHa cervical cancer cell, known to express HPV type 16, revealed that the probiotic, *Bifidobacterium adolescentis* SPM1005-A can repress *E6* and *E7* oncogenes, and consequently be a potential antiviral agent against HPV-associated cancer [87]. Similarly, *L. crispatus*, *L. jensenii*, and *L. gasseri* have been shown to suppress cervical cancer cells proliferation accompanied by a reduction in expression of HPV *E6* and *E7* oncogenes, *CDK2*, and *cyclin A*, as well as an increase in *p21*. In addition, these supernatants exerted their effects through the significant elevation of cell number in the S phase and a high reduction in cell number in the G2/M phase in Caski Cells [88]. Another study by Nouri *et al*. demonstrated that the supernatants of two *Lactobacilli*, *Lactobacillus rhamnosus* and *Lactobacillus crispatus,* exerted cytotoxic effect on HeLa cell line through the reduction of *CASP3* gene expression, as well as down-regulation of matrix metalloproteinases' expression (MMP-2 & MMP-9) and up-regulation of two tissue inhibitors of MMP-9 and MMP-2 genes (*i.e.*, *TIMP-1* & *TIMP-2*) [89]. In addition, *Enterococcus lactis* IW5 obtained from the human gut, and its metabolites secretions have been evaluated on HeLa cancer cells. The researchers observed that *E. lactis* IW5 inhibited HeLa cancer cell line but did not inhibit the normal cell line. This inhibition was not only due to the amount of annexinV+/PI+ (late apoptotic cells) in HeLa cell after the treatment with *E. lactis* IW5, but also was due to down-regulation of the expression of anti-apoptotic genes (*ERBB2* & *ERBB3*), intrinsic apoptosis blocker genes (*BCL2* & *BCL-XL*), and *CASP8* gene [90]. Investigation on the possible anti-cervical cancer effects of the probiotic isolated from vaginal fluid, *i.e.*, *Lactobacillus brevis*, on HeLa cells showed an increase in the level of casp3 and casp8 expression, suggesting that it could be a safe and cost-effective strategy against cancer [91]. To discover whether the byproducts of the strain isolated from the human vagina exert an anticancer effect, Sungur *et al*. [92] assessed the potential effect of EPSs of *L. gasseri* on HeLa cervical cancer and reported that the cell proliferation of HeLa cells was inhibited by EPS and live *L. gasseri* through up-regulation of Bax and Caspase 3 [92]. Furthermore, a study assessing the anticancer effect of the probiotics isolated from human breast milk revealed that three cell-free culture supernatant of isolated strains, including *Lactobacillus casei* SR1, *Lactobacillus casei* SR2, and *Lactobacillus paracasei* SR4 not only up-regulated the expression of apoptotic genes (*BAX, BAD, caspase3, caspase8,* & *caspase9*) but also down-regulated the *BCl2* gene expression in HeLa cell line, thereby proving the anti-cervical cancer effect of probiotics [93]. To indicate whether the anti-cancer effects of probiotics are associated with the change in the level of cancer-testis antigens (CTAs; highly expressed in human malignancies), supernatants of *Lactobacillus rhamnosus* GG and *Lactobacillus crispatus* SJ-3C-US were shown to down-regulate the expression of four CTAs, including Testis specific 10 (*TSGA10*), Aurora kinase C (*AURKC*), Opa interacting protein 5 (*OIP5*) and A-Kinase anchoring protein 4 (*AKAP4*) in HeLa cell line, and inhibited HeLa cell growth, thus confirming the anti-cervical cancer effect of these probiotics [94]. Additionally, Lee *et al.* observed that supernatants of probiotic *Bacillus polyfermenticus* KU3 isolated from kimchi, suppressed the proliferation of HeLa (92.93%), while no inhibition effect was detected on normal MRC-5 cells proliferation [95]. As for the anti-cervical cancer effect of cell-free extracts of probiotics, Kim *et al.* [96] showed that *L. casei* extract did not affect the growth of cervical cancer cell lines, including CaSki and HeLa, though when *L. casei* extract combined with anticancer drugs elicited the S-phase cell cycle arrest in HeLa and CaSki cell lines, which could be associated with its anticancer effects, as the cell cycle is correlated with growth rate in cancers. Further, to assess the mechanisms through which probiotics exert anti-tumor activity against HeLa and U14 cells, *L. debrueckii* probiotic was shown to prevent the migration of cervical cancer cells *in vitro*. This migration to the extracellular matrix (ECM) was claimed to be associated with one pivotal step in tumor metastasis [97]. Additionally, this live *Lactobacilli* up-regulated the E-cadherin, and its levels were conversely related to various human malignancies, as a low level of this glycoprotein has been observed in distinct human malignancies [98, 99]. Moreover, Nami *et al.* [100] demonstrated that *L. acidophilus* secretions exert an anti-proliferative effect on HeLa carcinoma cells, mainly through the induction of apoptosis [100]. Studies reporting the effects of probiotic bacteria on cervical cancer cell lines are shown in Table. **1**.

Table. (1). *In vitro* **studies associated with probiotics effects on cervical cancer.**

Probiotic Strain	Cell Line	Main Findings	Reference
Live *Lactobacilli* (supernatants)	HeLa	Reduction of caspase-3 activity; Inhibition of apoptosis; Increase level of human chorionic gonadotropin b (hCGb)	[70]
Lactobacillus crispatus and *Lactobacillus rhamnosus* (supernatants)	HeLa	Reduction of proliferation of HeLa cell; Down-regulation of mRNA level of CASP3 and two autophagy genes, TG14 and BECN1; Down-regulation of HPV E6 oncogenes	[71]
Bifidobacterium adolescentis SPM1005-A	SiHa	Suppression of *E6* and *E7* oncogene expression	[72]
L. crispatus, L. jensenii, and L. gasseri (supernatants)	Caski	Reduction of the proliferation of Caski cell; Reduction in expression of HPV *E6* and *E7* oncogenes; Reduction in expression of *CDK2* and *cyclin A;* Increase in expression of *p21*	[73]

(Table 1) cont.....

Probiotic Strain	Cell Line	Main Findings	Reference
Lactobacillus rhamnosus and Lactobacillus crispatus (supernatants)	HeLa	Reduction of *CASP3* gene expression; Down-regulation of matrix metalloproteinases expression (MMP-2 & MMP-9); Up-regulation of two tissue inhibitors of MMP-9 and MMP-2 genes (TIMP-1 & TIMP-2)	[74]
Enterococcus lactis IW5	HeLa	Inhibition of HeLa cell proliferation; Down-regulation of the expression of anti-apoptotic genes (*ERBB2* & *ERBB3*); Down-regulation of intrinsic apoptosis blocker genes (*BCL2* & *BCL-XL*); Down-regulation of *CASP8* gene	[75]
Lactobacillus brevis	HeLa	Increase the expression of casp3 and casp8	[76]
Live *L.gasseri* & its EPS	HeLa	Inhibition of HeLa cell proliferation; Up-regulation of Bax and Caspase 3; Induction of apoptosis	[77]
Lactobacillus rhamnosus GG and *Lactobacillus crispatus SJ-3C-US* (supernatants)	HeLa	Down-regulatation of expression of Testis specific 10 (*TSGA10*), Aurora kinase C (*AURKC*), Opa interacting protein 5 (*OIP5*) & A-Kinase anchoring protein 4 (*AKAP4*); Inhibition of HeLa cell growth	[79]
Bacillus polyfermenticus KU3 (supernatants)	HeLa	Suppuration of HeLa proliferation	[80]
L. casei extract (cell free extract)	CaSki & HeLa	Elicit S-phase cell cycle arrest in HeLa and CaSki cell lines when used along with anticancer drugs	[81]
L.debrueckii	HeLa & U14	Prevention of migration of cervical cancer cells; Up-regulation of E-cadherin	[84]
L. acidophilus (secretion)	HeLa	Inhibition of HeLa cell proliferation	[85]

6. ANTI-CERVICAL CANCER EFFECT OF PROBIOTICS IN THE CONTEXT OF PRECLINICAL STUDIES

Most preclinical studies on this subject are devoted to using Lactic acid bacteria as a good delivery vehicle for mucosal immunization. Studies suggested that oncoproteins or capsid proteins of HPV like E6 or E7 are expressed on lactic acid bacteria to induce sufficient specific cellular immunity [101 - 104]. On the other hand, utilizing probiotics as natural components against cervical cancer has been investigated in a few studies. One study, which demonstrated the effect of probiotics on HeLa cell growth inhibition, examined *Lactobacilli* impact on E-cadherin expression in U14 cervical carcinoma to find the possible relation between probiotic anti-cervical effects and the expression of E-cadherin, and then utilized U14 tumor-burdened mice to further investigate this relationship, *in vivo*. They observed that upon *Lactobacilli* treatment, the expression of E-cadherin was increased, and the tumor weight and volume declined in cervical carcinoma-bearing mice [99]. Moreover, Jacouton *et al.* [105] evaluated the anti-tumoral effect and associated mechanism of probiotic *L. casei* BL23 against cervical cancer, *in vivo*. The TC-1 tumor-bearing mice were intranasally (i.n.) administrated with the probiotic, and the results revealed that these bacteria inhibited the tumor growth in mice through distinct mechanisms ranging from systemic expression of NK cells and expression of immune T cells subpopulations like CD4$^+$, CD3$^+$, and CD8$^+$ T cells to an elevation in local FOXP3 levels in tumor-bearing mice, as well as an increase in IL-2, which together led to tumor size reduction and inhibition of cervical cancer, *in vivo* [105]. Additionally, one study has evaluated the possible anti-cervical cancer effect of the probiotic *Bifidobacterium bifidum* in TC-1 tumor-bearing mice, and it was observed that 5 times administration of this probiotic either orally or intravenously (i.v.) leads to the prevention and inhibition of cervical cancer growth, respectively.

The potent efficacy of i.v. injection of the probiotic seems to be associated with an increased level of tumor-specific IL-12 and IFN-γ, lymphocyte proliferation and CD8$^+$ cytolytic responses. Of note, in this study oral administration of the same probiotic increased the level of IL-12 and IFN-γ, as well as induction of CD8$^+$ CTLs. More importantly, induction of IL-10 and IL-6 in the TME and systematic level of IL-4 significantly elevated both orally and i.v. Administrated mice [106]. This study also assessed the impact of oral administration of probiotic *Lactobacillus casei TD-2* on mice challenged with TC-1 induced-cervical cancer and observed that this probiotic alone or in combination with GM-CSF can increase the levels of IFN-γ, IL-4, and IL-12 in the spleen of mice, as well as the level of TRAIL in the TME, while decreasing the level of IL-10 in the TME of mice. The results of this study confirmed the protective effect of probiotics against cervical cancer [107]. Studies associated with probiotics-induced immune response in *in vivo* preclinical studies are summarized in Table **2**.

Table. (2). Probiotics-mediated immune response in *in vivo* preclinical studies.

Probiotic Strain	Study Design	Main Findings	Reference
Live *Lactobacilli*	Upon U14 cell challenge, BALB/c mice, were intraperitoneally administrated with probiotics for a continuous 20 days	Increased expression of E-cadherin; Decline in the tumor weight and tumor volume	[99]

(Table 2) cont.....

Probiotic Strain	Study Design	Main Findings	Reference
L. casei BL23	C57 BL/6 mice were intranasally administered with the probiotic prior to the subcutaneous TC-1 challenge	Inhibition of tumor growth expression of NK cells and immune T cells subpopulation (CD4$^+$, CD3$^+$, and CD8$^+$); Elevation of local Foxp3 levels and IL-2; Reduction of tumor size	[105]
Bifidobacterium bifidum	C57 BL/6 mice, 5 times administration of this probiotic either orally or intravenously before and after TC-1 challenge	Inhibition of cervical cancer growth; Elevation of systemic IL-4; Increase in systemic IFN-γ and IL-12 and CD8$^-$CTL	[106]
Lactobacillus casei TD-2	C57 BL/6 mice, were administered with probiotics orally alone or combined with GM-CSF before and after TC-1 Challenge for 21 days	Inhibition of cervical cancer growth; Increased level of TRAIL in the TME; Elevation of systemic IL-4; Increase in systemic IFN-γ and IL-12; Decreased level of IL-10 in the TME	[107]

7. PROBIOTICS AGAINST CERVICAL CANCER AND SIDE EFFECTS ASSOCIATED WITH CLINICAL CERVICAL CANCER THERAPIES

Most of the clinical studies on probiotics and cervical cancer are allocated to the role of probiotics in the reduction of the incidence of radiation-induced diarrhoea and the evaluation of probiotic influence on HPV clearance and cervical smear quality.

One strategy for cervical cancer treatment is to carry out radiation alone or along with different anticancer agents. This method of therapy is a standard and easy-to-deliver option for advanced cervical cancer cases and those with contraindications to surgery [108, 109]. However, diarrhoea always occurs in patients undergoing radiotherapy. Hence, several studies have used probiotics to reduce the incidence of the rate of diarrhoea in radiated patients. For instance, Chitapanarux *et al.* [110] observed that individuals with pelvic radiotherapy along with weekly cisplatin when administered with live *Lactobacillus acidophilus* and *Bifidobacterium bifidum* before and during the radiotherapy, showed improved diarrhoea incidence rate and significantly improved the stool consistency compared to a placebo group. In a randomized double-blind placebo-controlled study, live *Lactobacillus acidophilus* LA-5 and *Bifidobacterium animalis* subsp. *lactis* BB-12 significantly reduced the prevalence of radiotherapy-associated diarrhoea [111]. The same results with distinct probiotics were observed, thereby proving the efficacy of probiotics as a cost-effective and facile approach to overcome this kind of diarrhoea in cervical cancer patients [112 - 114]. In a clinical study, 62 out of 123 women with genital HR-HPV infection were subjected to probiotics and results showed that in comparison to the control group, there was a significant reduction in mildly abnormal cervical smear and unsatisfactory smear rates in the probiotic group, although the genital HR-HPV clearance was not affected in the study group [115]. In a case report, a man with HIV, confirmed anal condylomatosis, as well as positive HPV18, was treated with multi-strain probiotics and it was observed that HPV-related anal condylomas were diminished. This anal condylomatosis in HIV-infected patients was correlated with a lower level

of HPV clearance in response to the immune deficiency as well as gut intraepithelial lymphocytes [116]. Additionally, Verhoeven *et al.* [117] reported that 54 women with an HPV$^+$ low-grade squamous intraepithelial lesion who consumed probiotics, showed a high clearance of cytological abnormalities along with HPV clearance in 29% of the study group. A phase-I trial study involving recombinant *L. lactis* and expressing E7 of HPV16 in the form of an oral vaccine was conducted to evaluate the safety, tolerability, and immunogenicity of the probiotic. The results indicated no adverse effects in the volunteers, while CTL responses in cervical lymphocytes and PBMCs were increased in the probiotic group. Moreover, the oral vaccine based on this *L. lactis* was shown to elicit a faster increase in serum IgG, vaginal IgA, and vaginal IFN-γ concentrations in healthy volunteer women [118]. Table **3** shows studies related to probiotic effects on cervical cancer-associated treatments and complications in clinical studies.

Table. (3). Probiotic effects on cervical cancer-associated treatment and complications in clinical studies.

Probiotic Strain	Subject/ Study Design	Main Findings	Reference
Live Lactobacillus acidophilus plus *Bifidobacterium bifidum*	Patients diagnosed with locally advanced cervical cancer/ before and during radiotherapy probiotic were given to radiotherapy -undergone patients	Reduction of diarrhoea-associated radiotherapy Improved stool consistency	[95]
Live Lactobacillus acidophilus LA-5 plus *Bifidobacterium animalis subsp. lactis BB-12*	Cervical cancer patients/ at the beginning until the end of radiotherapy probiotic were given to radiotherapy - undergone patients	Reduction of the prevalence of the Radiotherapy-associated diarrhoea	[96]

(Table 3) cont.....

Probiotic Strain	Subject/ Study Design	Main Findings	Reference
Lactic acid bacteria (VSL#3)	Cervical cancer patients/ probiotic were given from the start until the end of radiotherapy	Reduction of daily bowel movement; Reduction of diarrhoea -associated radiotherapy	[97]
Lactobacillus rhamnosus GR-1 plus *Lactobacillus reuteri RC-14*	Women with genital HR-HPV infection/ probiotic were administrated orally (daily) until the negative HR-HPV testing	Reduction in mildly abnormal cervical smear and unsatisfactory smear rates	[100]
Lactobacillus plantarum **DSM 24730**, *Streptococcus thermophilus* **DSM 24731**, *Bifidobacterium breve* **DSM 24732**, *Lactobacillus paracasei* **DSM 24733**, *Lactobacillus delbrueckii* **subsp,** *bulgaricus* **DSM 24734**, *Lactobacillus acidophilus* **DSM 24735**, *Bifidobacterium longum* DSM 24736, and*Bifidobacterium infantis* **DSM 24737;**	A man with positive HPV-18/ 4 months administration of multi-strain probiotic	Diminishing of HPV-related anal condylomas	[101]
Lactobacillus casei Shirota	Women with HPV+ low-grade squamous intraepithelial lesion/ studied group were received probiotics during the study period	High clearance of cytological abnormalities along with HPV clearance in 29% of the study group	[102]

CONCLUSION

According to a wide range of *in vitro* studies, preclinical and clinical trials, probiotics have been proven to at least inhibit cervical cancer proliferation partly due to their effect on reduction in expression of HPV *E6* and *E7* oncogenes and up-regulation of apoptotic genes like caspases or even decline in the expression of some apoptosis blocker genes. Moreover, increases in lymphocyte proliferation, CD8+ cytolytic responses, and some cytokines such as IL-12 and IFN-γ have been shown to be associated with the use of probiotics. Although more clinical trials on the direct use of probiotics on the distinct models of HPV are required for a better understanding of the efficacy of probiotics on HPV, several studies suggested that the use of probiotics as an alternative strategy or in combination with different anti-cancer methods can be cost-effective and beneficial against cervical cancer.

Fig. (**2**) shows an overview of the role of probiotics in cervical cancer.

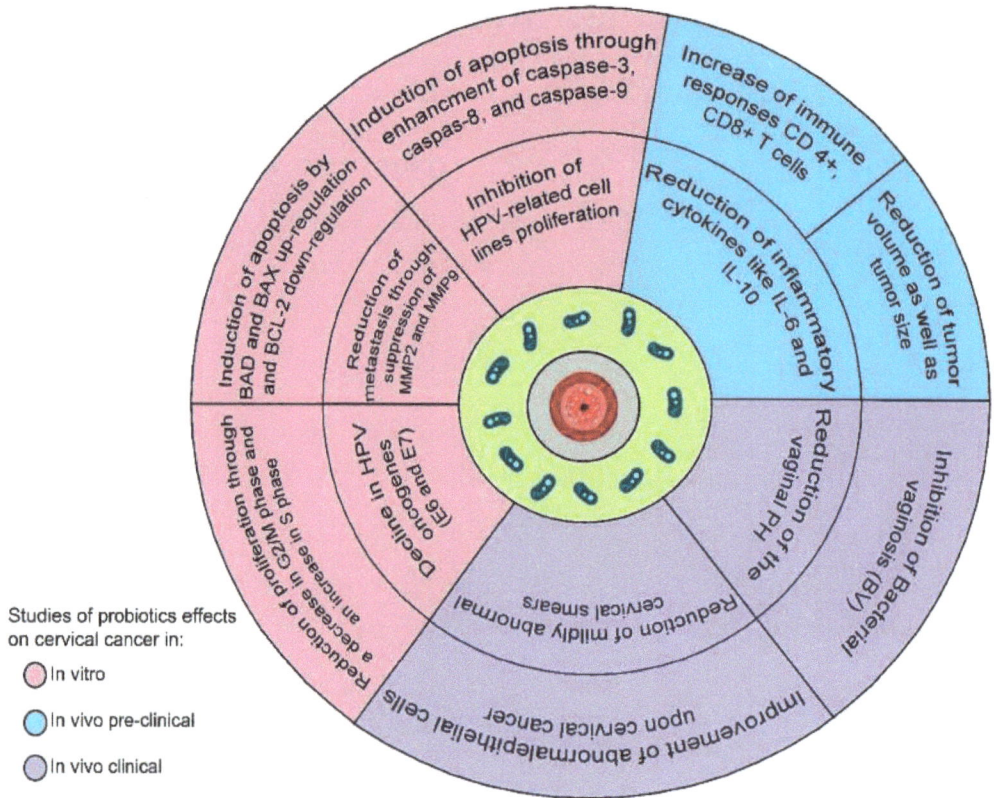

Fig. (2). Role of probiotics in prevention and treatment of cervical cancer.

CONSENT FOR PUBLICATION

Not applicable.

CONFLICT OF INTEREST

The authors declare no conflict of interest, financial or otherwise.

ACKNOWLEDGEMENT

Declared none.

REFERENCES

[1]   Harden ME, Munger K. Human papillomavirus molecular biology. Mutat Res Rev Mutat Res 2017; 772: 3-12.
[http://dx.doi.org/10.1016/j.mrrev.2016.07.002] [PMID: 28528688]

[2]   Arbyn M, Weiderpass E, Bruni L, *et al.* Estimates of incidence and mortality of cervical cancer in
       2018: a worldwide analysis. Lancet Glob Health 2020; 8(2): e191-203.
       [http://dx.doi.org/10.1016/S2214-109X(19)30482-6] [PMID: 31812369]

[3]   He WQ, Li C. Recent global burden of cervical cancer incidence and mortality, predictors, and
       temporal trends. Gynecol Oncol 2021; 163(3): 583-92.
       [http://dx.doi.org/10.1016/j.ygyno.2021.10.075] [PMID: 34688503]

[4]   Bosch FX, Lorincz A, Muñoz N, Meijer CJLM, Shah KV. The causal relation between human
       papillomavirus and cervical cancer. J Clin Pathol 2002; 55(4): 244-65.
       [http://dx.doi.org/10.1136/jcp.55.4.244] [PMID: 11919208]

[5]   Parkin DM, Bray F, Ferlay J, Pisani P. Global cancer statistics, 2002. CA Cancer J Clin 2005; 55(2):
       74-108.
       [http://dx.doi.org/10.3322/canjclin.55.2.74] [PMID: 15761078]

[6]   Walboomers JM, Jacobs MV, Manos MM, *et al.* Human papillomavirus is a necessary cause of
       invasive cervical cancer worldwide. J Pathol 1999; 189(1): 12-9.
       [http://dx.doi.org/10.1002/(SICI)1096-9896(199909)189:1<12::AID-PATH431>3.0.CO;2-F] [PMID:
       10451482]

[7]   Handisurya A, Schellenbacher C, Kirnbauer R. Diseases caused by human papillomaviruses (HPV). J
       Dtsch Dermatol Ges 2009; 7(5): 453-66.
       [PMID: 19302229]

[8]   Gillison ML, Koch WM, Capone RB, *et al.* Evidence for a causal association between human
       papillomavirus and a subset of head and neck cancers. J Natl Cancer Inst 2000; 92(9): 709-20.
       [http://dx.doi.org/10.1093/jnci/92.9.709] [PMID: 10793107]

[9]   Carter JJ, Madeleine MM, Shera K, *et al.* Human papillomavirus 16 and 18 L1 serology compared
       across anogenital cancer sites. Cancer Res 2001; 61(5): 1934-40.
       [PMID: 11280749]

[10]   De Martel C, Plummer M, Vignat J, Franceschi S. Worldwide burden of cancer attributable to HPV by
       site, country and HPV type. Int J Cancer 2017; 141(4): 664-70.
       [http://dx.doi.org/10.1002/ijc.30716] [PMID: 28369882]

[11]   Burd EM. Human papillomavirus and cervical cancer. Clin Microbiol Rev 2003; 16(1): 1-17.
       [http://dx.doi.org/10.1128/CMR.16.1.1-17.2003] [PMID: 12525422]

[12]   Hafkamp HC, Manni JJ, Speel EJM. Role of human papillomavirus in the development of head and
       neck squamous cell carcinomas. Acta Otolaryngol 2004; 124(4): 520-6.
       [http://dx.doi.org/10.1080/00016480310016893] [PMID: 15224887]

[13]   Devaraj K, Gillison ML, Wu TC. Development of HPV vaccines for HPV-associated head and neck
       squamous cell carcinoma. Crit Rev Oral Biol Med 2003; 14(5): 345-62.
       [http://dx.doi.org/10.1177/154411130301400505] [PMID: 14530303]

[14]   Clifford GM, Smith JS, Aguado T, Franceschi S. Comparison of HPV type distribution in high-grade
       cervical lesions and cervical cancer: a meta-analysis. Br J Cancer 2003; 89(1): 101-5.
       [http://dx.doi.org/10.1038/sj.bjc.6601024] [PMID: 12838308]

[15]   Faridi R, Zahra A, Khan K, Idrees M. Oncogenic potential of Human Papillomavirus (HPV) and its
       relation with cervical cancer. Virol J 2011; 8(1): 269.
       [http://dx.doi.org/10.1186/1743-422X-8-269] [PMID: 21635792]

[16]   Braaten KP, Laufer MR. Human Papillomavirus (HPV), HPV-Related Disease, and the HPV Vaccine.
       Rev Obstet Gynecol 2008; 1(1): 2-10.
       [PMID: 18701931]

[17]   Maglennon GA, McIntosh P, Doorbar J. Persistence of viral DNA in the epithelial basal layer suggests
       a model for papillomavirus latency following immune regression. Virology 2011; 414(2): 153-63.

[http://dx.doi.org/10.1016/j.virol.2011.03.019] [PMID: 21492895]

[18]   Letian T, Tianyu Z. Cellular receptor binding and entry of human papillomavirus. Virol J 2010; 7(1): 2.
[http://dx.doi.org/10.1186/1743-422X-7-2] [PMID: 20051141]

[19]   Giroglou T, Florin L, Schäfer F, Streeck RE, Sapp M. Human papillomavirus infection requires cell surface heparan sulfate. J Virol 2001; 75(3): 1565-70.
[http://dx.doi.org/10.1128/JVI.75.3.1565-1570.2001] [PMID: 11152531]

[20]   Brianti P, De Flammineis E, Mercuri SR. Review of HPV-related diseases and cancers. New Microbiol 2017; 40(2): 80-5.
[PMID: 28368072]

[21]   Insinga RP, Dasbach EJ, Elbasha EH. Epidemiologic natural history and clinical management of Human Papillomavirus (HPV) Disease: a critical and systematic review of the literature in the development of an HPV dynamic transmission model. BMC Infect Dis 2009; 9(1): 119.
[http://dx.doi.org/10.1186/1471-2334-9-119] [PMID: 19640281]

[22]   Forcier M, Musacchio N. An overview of human papillomavirus infection for the dermatologist: disease, diagnosis, management, and prevention. Dermatol Ther 2010; 23(5): 458-76.
[http://dx.doi.org/10.1111/j.1529-8019.2010.01350.x] [PMID: 20868401]

[23]   Ibeanu OA. Molecular pathogenesis of cervical cancer. Cancer Biol Ther 2011; 11(3): 295-306.
[http://dx.doi.org/10.4161/cbt.11.3.14686] [PMID: 21239888]

[24]   Thorland EC, Myers SL, Gostout BS, Smith DI. Common fragile sites are preferential targets for HPV16 integrations in cervical tumors. Oncogene 2003; 22(8): 1225-37.
[http://dx.doi.org/10.1038/sj.onc.1206170] [PMID: 12606949]

[25]   Baker CC, Phelps WC, Lindgren V, Braun MJ, Gonda MA, Howley PM. Structural and transcriptional analysis of human papillomavirus type 16 sequences in cervical carcinoma cell lines. J Virol 1987; 61(4): 962-71.
[http://dx.doi.org/10.1128/jvi.61.4.962-971.1987] [PMID: 3029430]

[26]   Zerfass K, Schulze A, Spitkovsky D, Friedman V, Henglein B, Jansen-Dürr P. Sequential activation of cyclin E and cyclin A gene expression by human papillomavirus type 16 E7 through sequences necessary for transformation. J Virol 1995; 69(10): 6389-99.
[http://dx.doi.org/10.1128/jvi.69.10.6389-6399.1995] [PMID: 7666540]

[27]   Hawley-Nelson P, Vousden KH, Hubbert NL, Lowy DR, Schiller JT. HPV16 E6 and E7 proteins cooperate to immortalize human foreskin keratinocytes. EMBO J 1989; 8(12): 3905-10.
[http://dx.doi.org/10.1002/j.1460-2075.1989.tb08570.x] [PMID: 2555178]

[28]   Tsai TC, Chen SL. The biochemical and biological functions of human papillomavirus type 16 E5 protein. Arch Virol 2003; 148(8): 1445-53.
[http://dx.doi.org/10.1007/s00705-003-0111-z] [PMID: 12898324]

[29]   Scheffner M, Werness BA, Huibregtse JM, Levine AJ, Howley PM. The E6 oncoprotein encoded by human papillomavirus types 16 and 18 promotes the degradation of p53. Cell 1990; 63(6): 1129-36.
[http://dx.doi.org/10.1016/0092-8674(90)90409-8] [PMID: 2175676]

[30]   Boyer SN, Wazer DE, Band V. E7 protein of human papilloma virus-16 induces degradation of retinoblastoma protein through the ubiquitin-proteasome pathway. Cancer Res 1996; 56(20): 4620-4.
[PMID: 8840974]

[31]   McLaughlin-Drubin ME, Park D, Munger K. Tumor suppressor p16INK4A is necessary for survival of cervical carcinoma cell lines. Proc Natl Acad Sci USA 2013; 110(40): 16175-80.
[http://dx.doi.org/10.1073/pnas.1310432110] [PMID: 24046371]

[32]   Yamato K, Yamada T, Kizaki M, *et al.* New highly potent and specific E6 and E7 siRNAs for treatment of HPV16 positive cervical cancer. Cancer Gene Ther 2008; 15(3): 140-53.
[http://dx.doi.org/10.1038/sj.cgt.7701118] [PMID: 18157144]

[33]   Jabbar SF, Abrams L, Glick A, Lambert PF. Persistence of high-grade cervical dysplasia and cervical cancer requires the continuous expression of the human papillomavirus type 16 E7 oncogene. Cancer Res 2009; 69(10): 4407-14.
[http://dx.doi.org/10.1158/0008-5472.CAN-09-0023] [PMID: 19435895]

[34]   De Andrea M, Gheit T, Kiyono T, Kundu R. Human Papillomavirus E6 and E7: The Cervical Cancer Hallmarks and Targets for Therapy.

[35]   Nicol AF, Nuovo GJ, Dillner J. A summary of the 25th International Papillomavirus Conference 2009: Vaccines, screening, epidemiology and therapeutics. J Clin Virol 2010; 47(3): 208-15.
[http://dx.doi.org/10.1016/j.jcv.2009.12.005] [PMID: 20080439]

[36]   Olsson SE, Villa LL, Costa RLR, *et al.* Induction of immune memory following administration of a prophylactic quadrivalent human papillomavirus (HPV) types 6/11/16/18 L1 virus-like particle (VLP) vaccine. Vaccine 2007; 25(26): 4931-9.
[http://dx.doi.org/10.1016/j.vaccine.2007.03.049] [PMID: 17499406]

[37]   Madrid-Marina V, Torres-Poveda K, López-Toledo G, García-Carrancá A. Advantages and disadvantages of current prophylactic vaccines against HPV. Arch Med Res 2009; 40(6): 471-7.
[http://dx.doi.org/10.1016/j.arcmed.2009.08.005] [PMID: 19853187]

[38]   Hung CF, Ma B, Monie A, Tsen SW, Wu T-C. Therapeutic human papillomavirus vaccines: current clinical trials and future directions. Expert Opin Biol Ther 2008; 8(4): 421-39.
[http://dx.doi.org/10.1517/14712598.8.4.421] [PMID: 18352847]

[39]   Yao Y, Huang W, Yang X, *et al.* HPV-16 E6 and E7 protein T cell epitopes prediction analysis based on distributions of HLA-A loci across populations: An *in silico* approach. Vaccine 2013; 31(18): 2289-94.
[http://dx.doi.org/10.1016/j.vaccine.2013.02.065] [PMID: 23499609]

[40]   Yang A, Jeang J, Cheng K, *et al.* Current state in the development of candidate therapeutic HPV vaccines. Expert Rev Vaccines 2016; 15(8): 989-1007.
[http://dx.doi.org/10.1586/14760584.2016.1157477] [PMID: 26901118]

[41]   Smalley Rumfield C, Roller N, Pellom ST, Schlom J, Jochems C. Therapeutic Vaccines for HPV-Associated Malignancies. ImmunoTargets Ther 2020; 9: 167-200.
[http://dx.doi.org/10.2147/ITT.S273327] [PMID: 33117742]

[42]   Tsuda N, Watari H, Ushijima K. Chemotherapy and molecular targeting therapy for recurrent cervical cancer. Chin J Cancer Res 2016; 28(2): 241-53.
[http://dx.doi.org/10.21147/j.issn.1000-9604.2016.02.14] [PMID: 27199523]

[43]   Lee SJ, Yang A, Wu TC, Hung CF. Immunotherapy for human papillomavirus-associated disease and cervical cancer: review of clinical and translational research. J Gynecol Oncol 2016; 27(5)e51
[http://dx.doi.org/10.3802/jgo.2016.27.e51] [PMID: 27329199]

[44]   Cheung AS, Mooney DJ. Engineered materials for cancer immunotherapy. Nano Today 2015; 10(4): 511-31.
[http://dx.doi.org/10.1016/j.nantod.2015.06.007] [PMID: 26640511]

[45]   Ajaya Kumar R, Sridevi K, Vijaya Kumar N, Nanduri S, Rajagopal S. Anticancer and immunostimulatory compounds from Andrographis paniculata. J Ethnopharmacol 2004; 92(2-3): 291-5.
[http://dx.doi.org/10.1016/j.jep.2004.03.004] [PMID: 15138014]

[46]   Yadav VS, Mishra KP, Singh DP, Mehrotra S, Singh VK. Immunomodulatory effects of curcumin. Immunopharmacol Immunotoxicol 2005; 27(3): 485-97.
[http://dx.doi.org/10.1080/08923970500242244] [PMID: 16237958]

[47]   Catanzaro M, Corsini E, Rosini M, Racchi M, Lanni C. Immunomodulators Inspired by Nature: A Review on Curcumin and Echinacea. Molecules 2018; 23(11): 2778.
[http://dx.doi.org/10.3390/molecules23112778] [PMID: 30373170]

[48]   Sadeghi S, Davoodvandi A, Pourhanifeh MH, *et al.* Anti-cancer effects of cinnamon: Insights into its apoptosis effects. Eur J Med Chem 2019; 178: 131-40.
[http://dx.doi.org/10.1016/j.ejmech.2019.05.067] [PMID: 31195168]

[49]   Hamidpour R, Hamidpour M, Hamidpour S, Shahlari M. Cinnamon from the selection of traditional applications to its novel effects on the inhibition of angiogenesis in cancer cells and prevention of Alzheimer's disease, and a series of functions such as antioxidant, anticholesterol, antidiabetes, antibacterial, antifungal, nematicidal, acaracidal, and repellent activities. J Tradit Complement Med 2015; 5(2): 66-70.
[http://dx.doi.org/10.1016/j.jtcme.2014.11.008] [PMID: 26151013]

[50]   Ozen M, Dinleyici EC. The history of probiotics: the untold story. Benef Microbes 2015; 6(2): 159-65.
[http://dx.doi.org/10.3920/BM2014.0103] [PMID: 25576593]

[51]   Mahooti M, Miri SM, Abdolalipour E, Ghaemi A. The immunomodulatory effects of probiotics on respiratory viral infections: A hint for COVID-19 treatment? Microb Pathog 2020; 148104452
[http://dx.doi.org/10.1016/j.micpath.2020.104452] [PMID: 32818576]

[52]   Śliżewska K, Markowiak-Kopeć P, Śliżewska W. The Role of Probiotics in Cancer Prevention. Cancers (Basel) 2020; 13(1): 20.
[http://dx.doi.org/10.3390/cancers13010020] [PMID: 33374549]

[53]   Lee J-E, Lee J, Kim JH, *et al.* Characterization of the Anti-Cancer Activity of the Probiotic Bacterium *Lactobacillus fermentum* Using 2D vs. 3D Culture in Colorectal Cancer Cells. Biomolecules 2019; 9(10): 557.
[http://dx.doi.org/10.3390/biom9100557] [PMID: 31581581]

[54]   Bahmani S, Azarpira N, Moazamian E. Anti-colon cancer activity of *Bifidobacterium* metabolites on colon cancer cell line SW742. Turk J Gastroenterol 2019; 30(9): 835-42.
[http://dx.doi.org/10.5152/tjg.2019.18451] [PMID: 31530527]

[55]   Khalesi S, Bellissimo N, Vandelanotte C, Williams S, Stanley D, Irwin C. A review of probiotic supplementation in healthy adults: helpful or hype? Eur J Clin Nutr 2019; 73(1): 24-37.
[http://dx.doi.org/10.1038/s41430-018-0135-9] [PMID: 29581563]

[56]   Mahooti M, Abdolalipour E, Salehzadeh A, Mohebbi SR, Gorji A, Ghaemi A. Immunomodulatory and prophylactic effects of *Bifidobacterium bifidum* probiotic strain on influenza infection in mice. World J Microbiol Biotechnol 2019; 35(6): 91.
[http://dx.doi.org/10.1007/s11274-019-2667-0] [PMID: 31161259]

[57]   Drago L. Probiotics and colon cancer. Microorganisms 2019; 7(3): 66.
[http://dx.doi.org/10.3390/microorganisms7030066] [PMID: 30823471]

[58]   Amara AA, Shibl A. Role of Probiotics in health improvement, infection control and disease treatment and management. Saudi Pharm J 2015; 23(2): 107-14.
[http://dx.doi.org/10.1016/j.jsps.2013.07.001] [PMID: 25972729]

[59]   Kumar M, Kumar A, Nagpal R, *et al.* Cancer-preventing attributes of probiotics: an update. Int J Food Sci Nutr 2010; 61(5): 473-96.
[http://dx.doi.org/10.3109/09637480903455971] [PMID: 20187714]

[60]   Shida K, Nanno M. Probiotics and immunology: separating the wheat from the chaff. Trends Immunol 2008; 29(11): 565-73.
[http://dx.doi.org/10.1016/j.it.2008.07.011] [PMID: 18835747]

[61]   Wan LYM, Chen ZJ, Shah NP, El-Nezami H. Modulation of intestinal epithelial defense responses by probiotic bacteria. Crit Rev Food Sci Nutr 2016; 56(16): 2628-41.
[http://dx.doi.org/10.1080/10408398.2014.905450] [PMID: 25629818]

[62]   Grabig A, Paclik D, Guzy C, *et al. Escherichia coli* strain Nissle 1917 ameliorates experimental colitis *via* toll-like receptor 2- and toll-like receptor 4-dependent pathways. Infect Immun 2006; 74(7): 4075-82.

[http://dx.doi.org/10.1128/IAI.01449-05] [PMID: 16790781]

[63]   Vijay-Kumar M, Aitken JD, Gewirtz AT. Toll like receptor-5: protecting the gut from enteric microbes. Semin Immunopathol 2008; 30(1): 11-21.
[http://dx.doi.org/10.1007/s00281-007-0100-5] [PMID: 18066550]

[64]   Adam E, Delbrassinne L, Bouillot C, *et al.* Probiotic *Escherichia coli* Nissle 1917 activates DC and prevents house dust mite allergy through a TLR4-dependent pathway. Eur J Immunol 2010; 40(7): 1995-2005.
[http://dx.doi.org/10.1002/eji.200939913] [PMID: 20432233]

[65]   Neville BA, Forde BM, Claesson MJ, *et al.* Characterization of pro-inflammatory flagellin proteins produced by *Lactobacillus ruminis* and related motile *Lactobacilli*. PLoS One 2012; 7(7)e40592
[http://dx.doi.org/10.1371/journal.pone.0040592] [PMID: 22808200]

[66]   Miyake K. Innate recognition of lipopolysaccharide by Toll-like receptor 4–MD-2. Trends Microbiol 2004; 12(4): 186-92.
[http://dx.doi.org/10.1016/j.tim.2004.02.009] [PMID: 15051069]

[67]   de Kivit S, Tobin MC, Forsyth CB, Keshavarzian A, Landay AL. Regulation of Intestinal Immune Responses through TLR Activation: Implications for Pro- and Prebiotics. Front Immunol 2014; 5: 60.
[http://dx.doi.org/10.3389/fimmu.2014.00060] [PMID: 24600450]

[68]   Russo E, Nannini G, Dinu M, Pagliai G, Sofi F, Amedei A. Exploring the food-gut axis in immunotherapy response of cancer patients. World J Gastroenterol 2020; 26(33): 4919-32.
[http://dx.doi.org/10.3748/wjg.v26.i33.4919] [PMID: 32952339]

[69]   Taghinezhad-S S, Keyvani H, Bermúdez-Humarán LG, Donders GGG, Fu X, Mohseni AH. Twenty years of research on HPV vaccines based on genetically modified lactic acid bacteria: an overview on the gut-vagina axis. Cell Mol Life Sci 2021; 78(4): 1191-206.
[http://dx.doi.org/10.1007/s00018-020-03652-2] [PMID: 32979054]

[70]   Jahanshahi M, Maleki Dana P, Badehnoosh B, *et al.* Anti-tumor activities of probiotics in cervical cancer. J Ovarian Res 2020; 13(1): 68.
[http://dx.doi.org/10.1186/s13048-020-00668-x] [PMID: 32527332]

[71]   Rahbar Saadat Y, Pourseif MM, Zununi Vahed S, Barzegari A, Omidi Y, Barar J. Modulatory Role of Vaginal-Isolated *Lactococcus lactis* on the Expression of miR-21, miR-200b, and TLR-4 in CAOV-4 Cells and *In Silico* Revalidation. Probiotics Antimicrob Proteins 2020; 12(3): 1083-96.
[http://dx.doi.org/10.1007/s12602-019-09596-9] [PMID: 31797280]

[72]   Pardini B, De Maria D, Francavilla A, Di Gaetano C, Ronco G, Naccarati A. MicroRNAs as markers of progression in cervical cancer: a systematic review. BMC Cancer 2018; 18(1): 696.
[http://dx.doi.org/10.1186/s12885-018-4590-4] [PMID: 29945565]

[73]   Tilborghs S, Corthouts J, Verhoeven Y, *et al.* The role of Nuclear Factor-kappa B signaling in human cervical cancer. Crit Rev Oncol Hematol 2017; 120: 141-50.
[http://dx.doi.org/10.1016/j.critrevonc.2017.11.001] [PMID: 29198328]

[74]   Lee HJ, Lim SM, Kim DH. *Lactobacillus johnsonii* CJLJ103 attenuates scopolamine-Induced memory impairment in mice by increasing BDNF expression and inhibiting NF-κB activation. J Microbiol Biotechnol 2018; 28(9): 1443-6.
[http://dx.doi.org/10.4014/jmb.1805.05025] [PMID: 30111074]

[75]   Kim WG, Kim HI, Kwon EK, Han MJ, Kim DH. *Lactobacillus plantarum* LC27 and *Bifidobacterium longum* LC67 mitigate alcoholic steatosis in mice by inhibiting LPS-mediated NF-κB activation through restoration of the disturbed gut microbiota. Food Funct 2018; 9(8): 4255-65.
[http://dx.doi.org/10.1039/C8FO00252E] [PMID: 30010169]

[76]   Kim DE, Kim JK, Han SK, Jang SE, Han MJ, Kim DH. *Lactobacillus plantarum* NK3 and *Bifidobacterium longum* NK49 Alleviate Bacterial Vaginosis and Osteoporosis in Mice by Suppressing NF-κB-Linked TNF-α Expression. J Med Food 2019; 22(10): 1022-31.

[http://dx.doi.org/10.1089/jmf.2019.4419] [PMID: 31381476]

[77]   Qi SR, Cui YJ, Liu JX, Luo X, Wang HF. *Lactobacillus rhamnosus* GG components, SLP, gDNA and CpG, exert protective effects on mouse macrophages upon lipopolysaccharide challenge. Lett Appl Microbiol 2020; 70(2): 118-27.
       [http://dx.doi.org/10.1111/lam.13255] [PMID: 31782817]

[78]   Kim KW, Kang SS, Woo SJ, *et al.* Lipoteichoic Acid of Probiotic *Lactobacillus plantarum* Attenuates Poly I:C-Induced IL-8 Production in Porcine Intestinal Epithelial Cells. Front Microbiol 2017; 8: 1827.
       [http://dx.doi.org/10.3389/fmicb.2017.01827] [PMID: 28983294]

[79]   Riedel CU, Foata F, Philippe D, Adolfsson O, Eikmanns B-J, Blum S. Anti-inflammatory effects of *bifidobacteria* by inhibition of LPS-induced NF-κB activation. World J Gastroenterol 2006; 12(23): 3729-35.
       [http://dx.doi.org/10.3748/wjg.v12.i23.3729] [PMID: 16773690]

[80]   Chen C-L, Hsieh F-C, Lieblein JC, *et al.* Stat3 activation in human endometrial and cervical cancers. Br J Cancer 2007; 96(4): 591-9.
       [http://dx.doi.org/10.1038/sj.bjc.6603597] [PMID: 17311011]

[81]   Do E, Hwang SW, Kim SY, *et al.* Suppression of colitis-associated carcinogenesis through modulation of IL-6/STAT3 pathway by balsalazide and VSL#3. J Gastroenterol Hepatol 2016; 31(8): 1453-61.
       [http://dx.doi.org/10.1111/jgh.13280] [PMID: 26711554]

[82]   Zhou X, Qi W, Hong T, *et al.* Exopolysaccharides from *Lactobacillus plantarum* NCU116 regulate intestinal barrier function *via* STAT3 signaling pathway. J Agric Food Chem 2018; 66(37): 9719-27.
       [http://dx.doi.org/10.1021/acs.jafc.8b03340] [PMID: 30134660]

[83]   Anders H, Jarstrand C, Påhlson C. Treatment of bacterial vaginosis with lactobacilli. Sex Transm Dis 1992; 19(3): 146-8.
       [http://dx.doi.org/10.1097/00007435-199205000-00007] [PMID: 1523530]

[84]   Ravel J, Gajer P, Abdo Z, *et al.* Vaginal microbiome of reproductive-age women. Proc Natl Acad Sci USA 2011; 108(Suppl 1) (Suppl. 1): 4680-7.
       [http://dx.doi.org/10.1073/pnas.1002611107] [PMID: 20534435]

[85]   Motevaseli E, Shirzad M, Akrami SM, Mousavi AS, Mirsalehian A, Modarressi MH. Normal and tumour cervical cells respond differently to vaginal lactobacilli, independent of pH and lactate. J Med Microbiol 2013; 62(7): 1065-72.
       [http://dx.doi.org/10.1099/jmm.0.057521-0] [PMID: 23618799]

[86]   Motevaseli E, Azam R, Akrami SM, *et al.* The effect of *Lactobacillus crispatus* and *Lactobacillus rhamnosus* culture supernatants on expression of autophagy genes and HPV E6 and E7 oncogenes in the HeLa cell line. Cell J 2016; 17(4): 601-7.
       [PMID: 26862519]

[87]   Cha MK, Lee DK, An HM, *et al.* Antiviral activity of *Bifidobacterium adolescentis* SPM1005-A on human papillomavirus type 16. BMC Med 2012; 10(1): 72.
       [http://dx.doi.org/10.1186/1741-7015-10-72] [PMID: 22788922]

[88]   Wang KD, Xu DJ, Wang BY, Yan DH, Lv Z, Su JR. Inhibitory effect of vaginal *Lactobacillus* supernatants on cervical cancer cells. Probiotics Antimicrob Proteins 2018; 10(2): 236-42.
       [http://dx.doi.org/10.1007/s12602-017-9339-x] [PMID: 29071554]

[89]   Nouri Z, Karami F, Neyazi N, *et al.* Dual anti-metastatic and anti-proliferative activity assessment of two probiotics on HeLa and HT-29 cell lines. Cell J 2016; 18(2): 127-34.
       [PMID: 27551673]

[90]   Nami Y, Haghshenas B, Haghshenas M, Abdullah N, Yari Khosroushahi A. The prophylactic effect of probiotic *Enterococcus lactis* IW5 against different human cancer cells. Front Microbiol 2015; 6: 1317.

[http://dx.doi.org/10.3389/fmicb.2015.01317] [PMID: 26635778]

[91]   Chobdar N, Ahmadizadeh C. The effect of *Lactobacillus brevis* on Apoptosis and casp (casp8, casp3) gene Expression in HeLa Cancer Cells. Iran J Med Microbiol 2020; 14(1): 84-100.
[http://dx.doi.org/10.30699/ijmm.14.1.84]

[92]   Sungur T, Aslim B, Karaaslan C, Aktas B. Impact of Exopolysaccharides (EPSs) of *Lactobacillus gasseri* strains isolated from human vagina on cervical tumor cells (HeLa). Anaerobe 2017; 47: 137-44.
[http://dx.doi.org/10.1016/j.anaerobe.2017.05.013] [PMID: 28554813]

[93]   Riaz Rajoka MS, Zhao H, Lu Y, *et al.* Anticancer potential against cervix cancer (HeLa) cell line of probiotic *Lactobacillus casei* and *Lactobacillus paracasei* strains isolated from human breast milk. Food Funct 2018; 9(5): 2705-15.
[http://dx.doi.org/10.1039/C8FO00547H] [PMID: 29762617]

[94]   Nouri Z, Neyazi N, Modarressi MH, *et al.* Down-regulation of TSGA10, AURKC, OIP5 and AKAP4 genes by *Lactobacillus rhamnosus* GG and *Lactobacillus crispatus* SJ-3C-US supernatants in HeLa cell line. Klin Onkol 2018; 31(6): 429-33.
[http://dx.doi.org/10.14735/amko2018429] [PMID: 30545223]

[95]   Lee NK, Son SH, Jeon EB, Jung GH, Lee JY, Paik HD. The prophylactic effect of probiotic *acillus polyfermenticus* KU3 against cancer cells. J Funct Foods 2015; 14: 513-8.
[http://dx.doi.org/10.1016/j.jff.2015.02.019]

[96]   Kim SN, Lee WM, Park KS, Kim JB, Han DJ, Bae J. The effect of *Lactobacillus casei* extract on cervical cancer cell lines. Contemp Oncol (Pozn) 2015; 4(4): 306-12.
[http://dx.doi.org/10.5114/wo.2014.45292] [PMID: 26557779]

[97]   Kalluri R, Weinberg RA. The basics of epithelial-mesenchymal transition. J Clin Invest 2009; 119(6): 1420-8.
[http://dx.doi.org/10.1172/JCI39104] [PMID: 19487818]

[98]   Dohadwala M, Yang SC, Luo J, *et al.* Cyclooxygenase-2-dependent regulation of E-cadherin: prostaglandin E(2) induces transcriptional repressors ZEB1 and snail in non-small cell lung cancer. Cancer Res 2006; 66(10): 5338-45.
[http://dx.doi.org/10.1158/0008-5472.CAN-05-3635] [PMID: 16707460]

[99]   Li X, Wang H, Du X, *et al.* Lactobacilli inhibit cervical cancer cell migration *in vitro* and reduce tumor burden *in vivo* through upregulation of E-cadherin. Oncol Rep 2017; 38(3): 1561-8.
[http://dx.doi.org/10.3892/or.2017.5791] [PMID: 28713905]

[100]   Nami Y, Abdullah N, Haghshenas B, Radiah D, Rosli R, Khosroushahi AY. Probiotic potential and biotherapeutic effects of newly isolated vaginal *Lactobacillus acidophilus* 36YL strain on cancer cells. Anaerobe 2014; 28: 29-36.
[http://dx.doi.org/10.1016/j.anaerobe.2014.04.012] [PMID: 24818631]

[101]   Lee TY, Kim YH, Lee KS, *et al.* Human papillomavirus type 16 E6-specific antitumor immunity is induced by oral administration of HPV16 E6-expressing *Lactobacillus casei* in C57BL/6 mice. Cancer Immunol Immunother 2010; 59(11): 1727-37.
[http://dx.doi.org/10.1007/s00262-010-0903-4] [PMID: 20706715]

[102]   Yoon SW, Lee TY, Kim SJ, *et al.* Oral administration of HPV-16 L2 displayed on *Lactobacillus casei* induces systematic and mucosal cross-neutralizing effects in Balb/c mice. Vaccine 2012; 30(22): 3286-94.
[http://dx.doi.org/10.1016/j.vaccine.2012.03.009] [PMID: 22426329]

[103]   Mohseni AH, Taghinezhad-S S, Keyvani H, Razavilar V. Extracellular overproduction of E7 oncoprotein of Iranian human papillomavirus type 16 by genetically engineered *Lactococcus lactis*. BMC Biotechnol 2019; 19(1): 8.
[http://dx.doi.org/10.1186/s12896-019-0499-5] [PMID: 30678667]

[104] Ribelles P, Benbouziane B, Langella P, Suárez JE, Bermúdez-Humarán LG, Riazi A. Protection against human papillomavirus type 16-induced tumors in mice using non-genetically modified lactic acid bacteria displaying E7 antigen at its surface. Appl Microbiol Biotechnol 2013; 97(3): 1231-9.
[http://dx.doi.org/10.1007/s00253-012-4575-1] [PMID: 23212671]

[105] Jacouton E, Michel ML, Torres-Maravilla E, Chain F, Langella P, Bermúdez-Humarán LG. Elucidating the immune-related mechanisms by which probiotic strain *Lactobacillus casei* BL23 displays anti-tumoral properties. Front Microbiol 2019; 9: 3281.
[http://dx.doi.org/10.3389/fmicb.2018.03281] [PMID: 30687269]

[106] Abdolalipour E, Mahooti M, Salehzadeh A, *et al.* Evaluation of the antitumor immune responses of probiotic *Bifidobacterium bifidum* in human papillomavirus-induced tumor model. Microb Pathog 2020; 145104207
[http://dx.doi.org/10.1016/j.micpath.2020.104207] [PMID: 32325236]

[107] Abdolalipour E, Mahooti M, Gorji A, Ghaemi A. Synergistic Therapeutic Effects of Probiotic *Lactobacillus casei* TD-2 Consumption on GM-CSF-Induced Immune Responses in a Murine Model of Cervical Cancer. Nutr Cancer 2020; 1-11.
[PMID: 33356596]

[108] Li Y, Yu T, Yan H, *et al.* Vaginal microbiota and HPV infection: Novel mechanistic insights and therapeutic strategies. Infect Drug Resist 2020; 13: 1213-20.
[http://dx.doi.org/10.2147/IDR.S210615] [PMID: 32431522]

[109] Landoni F, Maneo A, Colombo A, *et al.* Randomised study of radical surgery *versus* radiotherapy for stage Ib-IIa cervical cancer. Lancet 1997; 350(9077): 535-40.
[http://dx.doi.org/10.1016/S0140-6736(97)02250-2] [PMID: 9284774]

[110] Chitapanarux I, Chitapanarux T, Traisathit P, Kudumpee S, Tharavichitkul E, Lorvidhaya V. Randomized controlled trial of live *lactobacillus acidophilus* plus *bifidobacterium bifidum* in prophylaxis of diarrhea during radiotherapy in cervical cancer patients. Radiat Oncol 2010; 5(1): 31.
[http://dx.doi.org/10.1186/1748-717X-5-31] [PMID: 20444243]

[111] Linn YH, Thu KK, Win NHH. Effect of probiotics for the prevention of acute radiation-induced diarrhoea among cervical cancer patients: a randomized double-blind placebo-controlled study. Probiotics Antimicrob Proteins 2019; 11(2): 638-47.
[http://dx.doi.org/10.1007/s12602-018-9408-9] [PMID: 29550911]

[112] Delia P, Sansotta G, Donato V, *et al.* Use of probiotics for prevention of radiation-induced diarrhea. World J Gastroenterol 2007; 13(6): 912-5.
[http://dx.doi.org/10.3748/wjg.v13.i6.912] [PMID: 17352022]

[113] Liu MM, Li ST, Shu Y, Zhan HQ. Probiotics for prevention of radiation-induced diarrhea: A meta-analysis of randomized controlled trials. PLoS One 2017; 12(6)e0178870
[http://dx.doi.org/10.1371/journal.pone.0178870] [PMID: 28575095]

[114] Qiu G, Yu Y, Wang Y, Wang X. The significance of probiotics in preventing radiotherapy-induced diarrhea in patients with cervical cancer: A systematic review and meta-analysis. Int J Surg 2019; 65: 61-9.
[http://dx.doi.org/10.1016/j.ijsu.2019.03.015] [PMID: 30928672]

[115] Ou YC, Fu HC, Tseng CW, Wu CH, Tsai CC, Lin H. The influence of probiotics on genital high-risk human papilloma virus clearance and quality of cervical smear: a randomized placebo-controlled trial. BMC Womens Health 2019; 19(1): 103.
[http://dx.doi.org/10.1186/s12905-019-0798-y] [PMID: 31340789]

[116] Ceccarelli G, Cavallari EN, Savinelli S, *et al.* Clearance of human papillomavirus related anal condylomas after oral and endorectal multistrain probiotic supplementation in an HIV positive male. Medicine (Baltimore) 2018; 97(16)e0329
[http://dx.doi.org/10.1097/MD.0000000000010329] [PMID: 29668581]

[117] Verhoeven V, Renard N, Makar A, *et al.* Probiotics enhance the clearance of human papillomavirus-related cervical lesions. Eur J Cancer Prev 2013; 22(1): 46-51.
[http://dx.doi.org/10.1097/CEJ.0b013e328355ed23] [PMID: 22706167]

[118] Mohseni AH, Taghinezhad-S S, Keyvani H. The first clinical use of a recombinant *Lactococcus lactis* expressing human papillomavirus type 16 E7 oncogene oral vaccine: A phase I safety and immunogenicity trial in healthy women volunteers. Mol Cancer Ther 2020; 19(2): 717-27.
[http://dx.doi.org/10.1158/1535-7163.MCT-19-0375] [PMID: 31645442]

CHAPTER 10

Probiotics-based Anticancer Immunity In Lung Cancer

Rabinarayan Parhi[1,*], Suryakanta Swain[2], Suvendu Kumar Sahoo[3], Sandip Prasad Tiwari[4] and Rajni Yadav[4]

[1] *Department of Pharmaceutical Sciences, Susruta School of Medical and Paramedical Sciences, Assam University (A Central University), Silchar, Assam, India*

[2] *Department of Pharmaceutical Science, School of Health Sciences, Kaziranga University, Jorhat, Assam, India*

[3] *GITAM Institute of Pharmacy, GITAM Deemed to be University, Gandhi Nagar Campus, Visakhapatnam, Andhra Pradesh, India*

[4] *Faculty of Pharmacy, Kalinga University, Naya Raipur, Chhattisgarh, India*

Abstract: Among various death-causing diseases, the morbidity and mortality related to cancer are the highest, with millions of new malignancies added to the tally every year and predicted to increase at a higher rate by 2030. Lung cancer is continued to be the leading cause of cancer death worldwide, with a share of 11.6% of all cancers. Since the start of the millennium, there has been a continuous effort to provide the benefits of probiotics in the management and treatment of cancer, particularly lung cancer. Probiotics are defined as "live microorganisms which, when administered in adequate amounts, confer health benefits on the host". These include specific strains of bacteria and fungi. Bacterial strains belonging to *Lactobacillus* and *Bifidobacterium* have demonstrated promising results in the prevention, attenuation, and treatment of the progression of lung cancer. The present chapter focuses on the types and aetiology of lung cancer and the role and mechanism of action of probiotics in providing immunity against lung cancer.

Keywords: Chemotherapy, Dysbiosis, Dendritic cells, Immunity, Immuno-modulation, Immune checkpoint inhibitor ICI), Interleukins, Lung cancer, Microbiome, Mutagens, Natural killer T (NKT) cell, Probiotics.

1. INTRODUCTION

Lung cancer is categorized as the most common cancer (a share of 11.6% of all cancers), with the highest rate of mortality (1.7 million) out of over 2.09 million

* **Corresponding author Rabinarayan Parhi:** Department of Pharmaceutical Sciences, Susruta School of Medical and Paramedical Sciences, Assam University (A Central University), Silchar, Assam, India; E-mail: bhu_rabi@rediffmail.com

Mitesh Kumar Dwivedi, Alwarappan Sankaranarayanan & Sanjay Tiwari (Eds.)

diagnoses in 2018 [1, 2]. The overall survival rate of five years in lung cancer is very low (≈ 20%) because of reasons such as delayed diagnosis and low response rate to the prescribed treatment [3]. The major factors contributing to lung cancer include genetic factors, smoking, drinking of alcohol, chronic respiratory diseases (such as asthma and chronic obstructive pulmonary disease, COPD), environmental factors (*e.g.*, microbial population in humans, microbiota, *etc.*), heavy metal consumption, exposure to silica dust, radon gas and asbestos [4, 5]. Apart from host microbiota, non-native pathogens also play an important role in the mediation of oncogenesis, including human papillomavirus (HPV), Kaposi's sarcoma virus (KSV), and Epstein-Barr virus (EBV) [6]. In addition, chronic antibiotic therapy can increase the risk of oncogenesis in the lung by killing the helpful microbes involved in the maintenance of homeostasis, providing resistance against disease-causing pathogens, and regulating the normal functioning of the system. Among all the factors, smoking is the major contributor accounting for 80-90% of all lung cancer cases [7].

Treatment options available for lung cancer are surgery, chemotherapy, radiotherapy, targeted therapy, and immunotherapy. But the treatment of lung cancer is based on the stage of cancer and unique health condition [8]. For instance, early-stage lung cancer needs surgery for remedy, whereas, for the advanced stage, the best treatment options have been chemotherapy, radiotherapy, immunotherapy, or a combination thereof [8, 9]. The current management of lung cancer involves systemic chemotherapy, which arbitrarily kills cancer cells and damages healthy cells, and may lead to drug resistance. Furthermore, it also gives birth to life-threatening side effects by compromising immunity and strength and impairing the treatment option, which mostly leads to suffering worse than the malignancy of cancer itself [10]. Despite the modern toll for diagnosis and various methods for treatments, the mortality related to lung cancer is still high. Therefore, to reduce mortality and minimize the suffering due to side effects caused by advanced treatment, scientists are more focused on alternative therapies, including physical activity, lifestyle modification, and nutrition supplements. The outcome of that effort is probiotics, which are currently used extensively in the management of various diseases, including cancers that originate in different body parts [11].

According to the United States-World Health Organization (US-WHO), probiotics are defined as live microorganisms which, when administered adequately, confer health benefits on the host [12, 13]. Probiotics are generally recognized as safe (GRAS) as they are frequently derived from safe microbes, such as *Lactobacillus* (naturally present in the small intestine) and *Bifidobacterium* (natural inhabitant of the large intestine) [14]. They are used to prevent and treat various cancers, including lung cancer, and act by enhancing innate immunity and antagonizing the pathogenic organisms in airways. Thus, probiotics are believed to act as immunomodulatory agents, and host defense activators, and decrease the disease severity [15]. The first probiotics introduced into research were *Lactobacillus acidophilus* by Hull *et al.* in 1984 and then *Bifidobacterium bifidum* in 1991 by Holcombh *et al.* [16]. The present chapter discusses lung cancer, drivers for lung cancer, ideal characteristics, and mechanism of action of probiotics as immunotherapy in preventing and treating lung cancer.

2. LUNG CANCER

Cancer is an uncontrolled cell division caused by unrepairable damage of deoxyribonucleic acid (DNA), and originates from the mutation of the tumor suppressor genes or proto-oncogenes [17]. Cancer is the second leading cause of death globally, with 18.1 million new cancer cases in 2018, and expected to reach 29.4 million by 2040 [18]. As per the World Health Organization (WHO) latest report, 70% of total death due to cancer happen in low and middle-income countries [19]. Cancer is considered a multifactorial disease with genetic defects, including lack of DNA repair or mutation at the time of DNA replication, which contributes to approximately 5-10% of the cases, and external factors such as environmental exposure to UV radiation, toxic substances, and infectious agents contributing the majority (90-95%) of the cases of cancers [20, 21]. Cancer types such as stomach, colorectal, lung, liver, breast, and prostate have a major share in mortality. Cancer cells demonstrate various altered physiological activities, such as apoptosis resistance, insensitivity to growth, growth-inhibiting signals, metastasis, and unlimited proliferation with sustained angiogenesis [21]. Out of various options available for cancer treatment, chemotherapy with drugs having cytotoxic and immunotoxicity seems to be the best option in the present scenario.

Lung cancer is the deadliest and most frequently occurring malignancy with the leading cause of mortality worldwide. Like other cancers, lung cancer involves proliferation, metastasis and invasion [22]. If lung cancer is detected at an early stage, surgery is the best possible solution. However, in most cases, it is detected at the advanced stage. In this scenario, the majority of the patients necessitate systemic chemotherapy. However, systemic chemotherapy frequently leads to side effects such as diarrhoea, nausea, and vomiting. The former may be the result of the changes in the intestinal flora, intestinal barrier dysfunction, and epithelial cell apoptosis of the intestine [23]. Hence, there is a need for additional treatment options, such as maintaining the microbiome population in the lungs and balancing it with the gut microbiome [24].

There are two broad classes of lung cancers such as small-cell lung cancer (SCLC) and non-small cell lung cancer (NSCLC). Out of these two types,

NSCLC spreads slowly but contributes to about 78% of lung cancers. However, SCLC accounts for about 25%, and shows faster growth and metastasis. The NSCLC is of three types: squamous cell carcinoma, adenocarcinoma, with the highest occurrence, and large cell carcinoma, with the least occurrence [25]. The different types of lung cancers are depicted in Fig. (**1**).

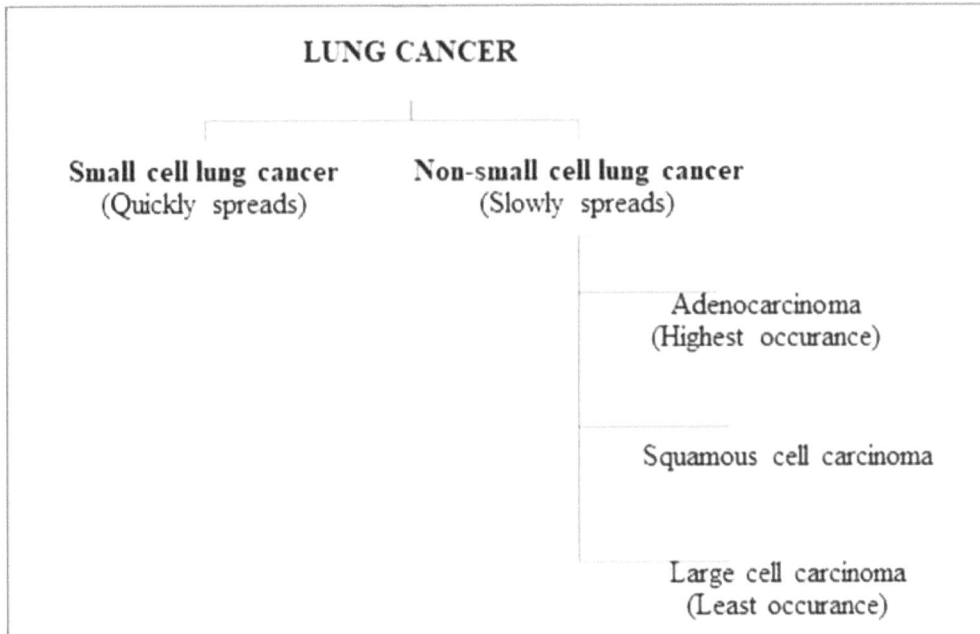

Fig. (1). Types of lung cancer.

3. DRIVERS OF LUNG CANCERS

There are three causes or drivers of lung cancer such as host factors, environmental factors, and microbial factors [26]. The host factors involve aging, susceptibility of the population, weak immune system, and individual gene susceptibility.

3.1. Genetic and Mutation Drivers

The genes responsible for cancer are tumor suppressor genes or proto-oncogenes. When a mutation occurs in these genes, it results in uncontrolled cell division and cancer [17]. Exposure to UV light, smoking, and airborne particles are environmental factors that may contribute to lung cancer by inducing microbiota imbalance (dysbiosis) and gene mutation. However, there is a triple interaction among the three drivers that are in conjunction responsible for lung cancer, as depicted in Fig. (**2**).

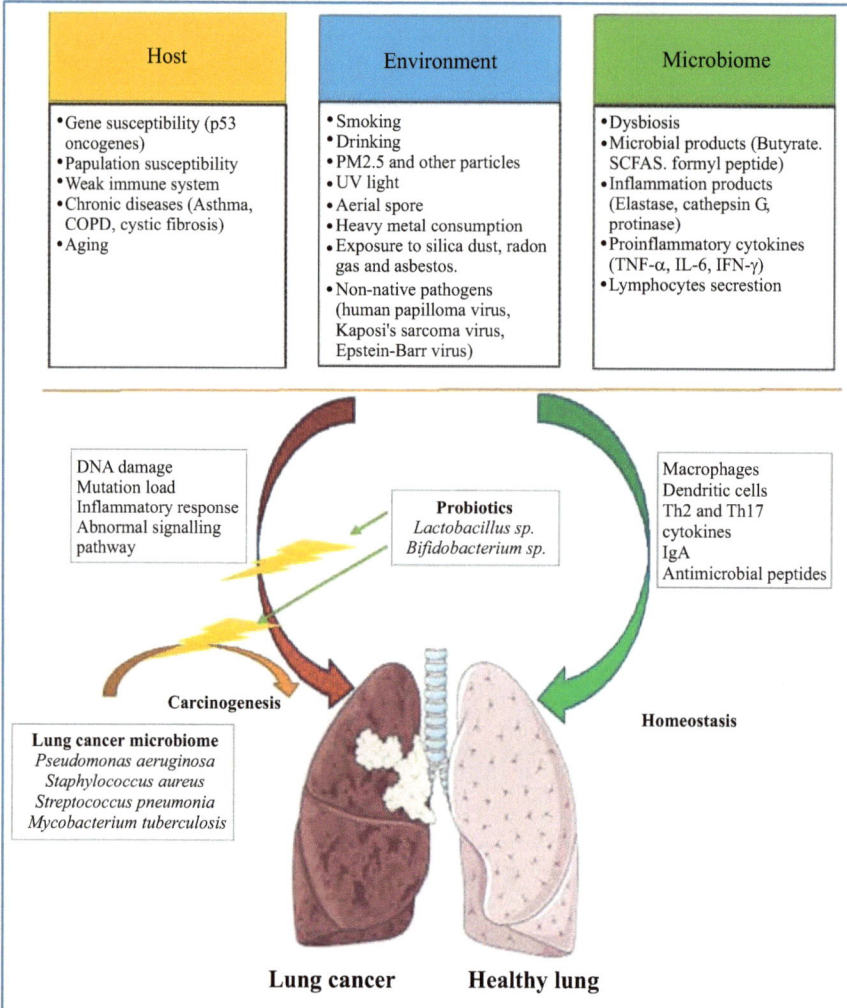

Fig. (2). Triple contributors of lung cancer: Host factors, environment factors and lung microbiome. Host factors such as aging, gene susceptibility or chronic diseases are associated with tumorigenesis. Environmental factors such as UV light, smoking and air-born particles have the potential to cause gene mutation and alter the community of microbiota. Microbiota, by either releasing short-chain fatty acids (SCFAs) or producing inflammatory products, can lead to DNA damage in the host cells or trigger downstream immune signalling pathways, which results into the promotion of malignant behaviour. The probiotics exert their anticancer activity by either modulating the immunomodulatory characteristics of cancer cells *via* NK cells, macrophages, and T cells or by enhancing the formation of cytokines, anti-angiogenic and antioxidant factors, resulting in the reduction of pro-carcinogenic enzymes and cancer-specific proteins. Probiotics also help to reduce the colonization of lung cancer microbiome.

3.2. Microbial Drivers

3.2.1. Lung microbiome and its relation with gut microbiome

The microbiome is the entire gamut of microorganisms such as bacteria, protozoa, fungi, and viruses, and their related gene, genome, as well as their derived metabolites [27]. The human gut microbiome is comprised of majorly (90%) bacteria with species such as *Bacteroides*, *Bifidobacterium*, *Ruminococcus*, *Eubacteria*, and *Clostridium*. In addition, other species, including *Peptococcus*, *Ruminococcus*, and *Peptostreptococcus* are also prevalent in the gut [28]. Bacteria of these species play a crucial role in maintaining human health, such as improvement of digestion, nerve function, as well as angiogenesis [29]. Due to any reason (mainly due to antibiotic intake), if there is an alteration or change in the gut microbiome, it may lead to various chronic diseases, including gastroenteric cancers (*e.g.*, cancer caused by *H. pylori*) [5].

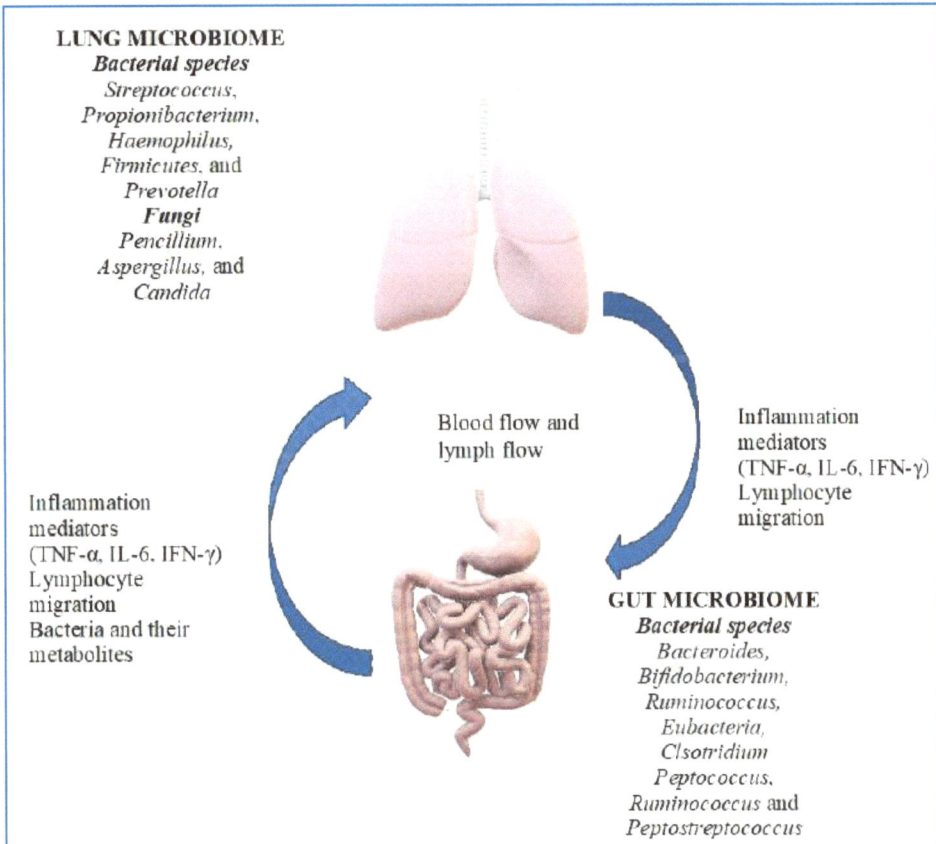

Fig. (3). Relationship between lung microbiome and gut microbiome.

Similar to the gut microbiome, the lung microbiome is composed of bacteria, viruses, and fungi that come inside through air exchanges with the surrounding environment or the inhalation of mucosal secretions. Among the bacterial species, *Streptococcus*, *Propionibacterium*, *Haemophilus,* and *Prevotella* are the major ones. These bacterial species coexist with fungi, including *Penicillium*, *Aspergillus,* and *Candida*, without causing any infections in human lungs [30]. This is because the above bacterial genera resist the colonization of pathogens in the lungs. Recently, it has been hypothesized that there is possible microbial communication between the lung and gut microbiome directly through mucosal, digestive, and respiratory activities or indirectly through metabolites and cytokines in the systemic circulation Fig. (**3**) [26]. Factors such as microbial growth rates, migration, and elimination lead to the alteration of local lung microbiome communities under the situation of health and disease [31]. Microbial disturbance in the gut as well as in the lung, mainly occurs due to frequent antibacterial therapy, resulting in lung cancer as well as COPD, asthma, and cystic fibrosis [26]. Recent studies have shown an association of increased levels of *Enterococcus sp.* and decreased levels of *Actinobacteria sp.* and *Bifidobacterium sp.* with lung cancer. In addition, disturbance of the normal function of the gut microbiome also induces the progression of lung cancer [32].

3.2.2. Immunity of Lung

The lungs maintain their immune system by differentiating beneficial commensal microbiota and self-components from dangerous materials, and responding against foreign harmful invaders in the critical regions such as the upper and lower respiratory tracts. In this lung homeostasis maintenance, there are two layers of defences: (i) Epithelium-macrophage axis, and (ii) tissue-resident lymphoid cells. In the primary line of defence, the pulmonary epithelium plays a crucial role by acting as a barrier against invading pathogenic microorganisms. In addition, mucociliary action on the epithelial cell layer strengthens the protective feature of the pulmonary epithelium with proper regulation [33, 34]. Macrophage is one of the most critical determinants of the lung's immunological tone in association with dendritic cells (DCs). Its major function is to prevent the colonization of microbes, which is the starting point of disease appearance such as cancer. The tissue-resident lymphoid cells include: (a) gamma-delta T cell (γδ T cells), (b) Natural Killer T cell (NKT cell), (c) Innate lymphoid cells (ICLs), (d) Resident memory B and T cells, and (e) Regulatory T cells (Tregs). The latter two types are specialized sub-cells of T cells. Above tissue-resident cells are activated in drainage lymph nodes and participate in the elimination of antigen, in the respiratory tract. Among all, γδ T cells constitute a major population, and its role is believed to be pathogen dependent. Recruitment of γδ T cells is believed to be increased with the inhalation of innocuous bacteria that do not cause bacterial infection or dysbiosis and play an important role in protection against allergy [35, 36]. The ICLs play a critical role in the maintenance of homeostasis in addition to tissue repair and regulation of immunity. Resident memory T (TRM) cells of the lung are involved in the expression of CD4, CD8, CD69, and various T cell receptor repertoire and avail rapid immune response in healthy lungs [37, 38]. DCs regulate the induction of Treg cells through programmed death-ligand 1 (PD-L1) tolerogenic pathways. In addition, invariant natural killer (iNK) T cells are also expressed on DCs. Treg cells play a very crucial role in the development and maintenance of immune tolerance against airborne particles. DCs also induce the production of T helper cells (Th1 & Th17 cells) [39]. The crucial effector and regulator cells of innate immune responses in the host are $\gamma\delta$ T cells [40], whereas activation and regulation of adaptive immune responses are provided by a well-formed network of DCs [41].

3.2.3. Microbial Contribution To Lung Cancer

The factors such as chronic infections (*e.g.*, COPD), overuse of antibiotics or changes in diet, and environmental factors capable of disrupting healthy partnerships between host immunity and microbiota potentially increase the chance of lung cancer [42]. This imbalance between host immunity and microbiota is believed to be the starting point of inflammation caused by hyperresponsive immunity or could be related to a defect in immune surveillance mechanisms [39]. The inflammation-based carcinogenesis in the lung involves multifactorial etiopathogenesis, as mentioned above. This inflammation results in the loss of epithelial integrity and thereby leaking serum protein into the airways. Subsequently, bacterial products such as butyrate, short-chain fatty acids (SCFAs), or formyl peptides are formed, and these act as powerful chemo-attractants for alveolar migrant's neutrophils and monocytes. This induces chronic inflammation, parenchymal lung damage, and loss of alveolar attachments [43, 44]. It was also reported that the inflammation produces elastase, cathepsin G, and proteinase 3, which lead to disruption of the epithelial layer and, thereby, mucous secretion increases and it stimulates the production of chemo-attractant chemokines such as IL8, IL6, and IL-8. These chemo-attractants directly act on epithelium cells and activate the nuclear factor Kappa light chain enhancer of the activated B-cell (NF-κB-1) pathway and induce proliferation, migration, and invasion of cancer cells [45].

4. PROBIOTICS

Probiotics are live non-pathogenic microbes, which play a key role in providing health benefits to the host when administered in desired quantities. However, dead probiotics and their metabolic secretions were found to show the same or higher biological responses [46, 47]. Probiotics are found abundantly in fermented dairy products, including cheese, cultured buttermilk, yogurt, *etc.* They are also rich in fermented products such as rice, barley, soy, maize, wheat, *etc* [48]. In addition, probiotics are found in abundance in breast milk, GIT of humans, and animal. Probiotics are majorly available in the market as functional foods and dietary supplements for the prevention and treatment of various diseases [49]. Probiotics are termed live microbiological ingredients when used as dietary supplements and live biotherapeutic agents when used as drugs [50]. Commercial products, including tablets, capsules, envelopes, vials, *etc.*, are available for probiotics containing varying doses of such microbes [51]. Previous studies reported that probiotics are used as an adjunct therapy in the management of various diseases pertaining to GIT, including irritable bowel syndrome (IBS), ulcerative colitis (UC), encephalopathy, diarrhoea, *etc.* The use of probiotics in gastroenterology has specific documented guidelines and consensus [52]. Probiotics are broadly classified as bacterial and yeast-based probiotics. Furthermore, the bacteria-based probiotics have the following categories: lactic acid and non-lactic acid-forming bacterial strains. The common bacterial probiotics are *Lactobacillus, Lactococcus, Enterococcus, Bifidobacterium, Clsotridiales, Escherichia coli, Bacillus, Weissella,* and *Enterococci* spp [50, 53]. Among the yeast, *Saccharomyces cerevisiae, Pichia, Debaryomyces, Kluyyeromyces, Candida, Hanseniaspora,* and *Metschnikowia* are used as probiotics [54, 55].

4.1. Ideal Properties of Probiotics

The ideal properties of probiotics are: (i) It should have a human origin; (ii) It should be non-pathogenic and show antagonistic activity against pathogens; (iii) It should exhibit resistance to gut pH, particularly to acid resistance in the stomach; (iv) It should show bile tolerance and should have the potential for bile salt hydrolase activity; (v) It should be capable of adhering to mucosal or epithelial cells all along with GIT; (vi) It should provide stability during processing; (vii) It should not have mutagenic and carcinogenic activities; (viii) It should cause immune stimulation; (ix) It should be capable of modulating microbiota, immunity, and metabolism, and (x) It should be able to colonize in the gut and produce host-useful bioactive materials Fig. (**4**) [16, 56, 57].

4.2. Mechanisms of Action of Probiotics

There are many proposed mechanisms of action of probiotics in the prevention (anti-mutagenic activity) and treatment of cancers. These proposed mechanisms of action are listed below and schematically represented in Fig. (**4**) [14, 58, 59].

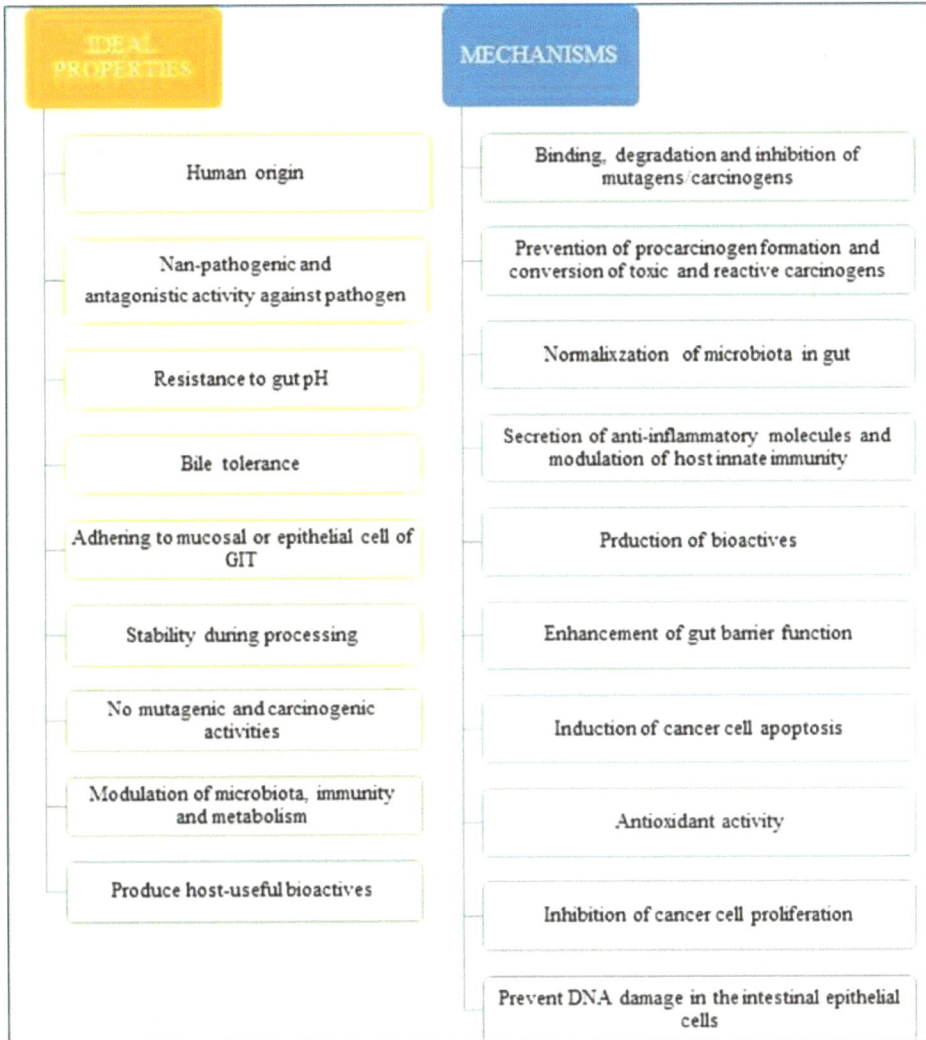

Fig. (4). Schematic diagram for ideal properties of probiotics and their possible mechanisms of action.

i. Binding, degradation, and inhibition of mutagens/carcinogens.

ii. Prevention of procarcinogen formation and conversion of toxic, harmful, and highly reactive carcinogens.

iii. Normalization of disturbed microbiota in the gut.

iv. Modulation of host innate immune and inflammatory system by enhancing the secretion of anti-inflammatory molecules.

v. Production of bioactives (*e.g.*, lactic acid bacteria produce lactic acid, vitamins, bacteriocin, fatty acid, enzymes, peptides, & exopolysaccharides).

vi. Enhancement of gut barrier function.

vii. Lowering of gut pH due to formation of bacteriocins and SCFAs.
viii. Interaction with the gut-brain axis.
 ix. Antioxidant activity.
  x. Inhibition of cancer cell proliferation.
 xi. Induction of cancer cell apoptosis, and
xii. Prevention of DNA damage in the intestinal epithelial cells.

4.3. Probiotics in Lung Cancer

In recent times, probiotic bacteria have attracted many researchers owning to their preventive as well as treatment properties against lung cancer. The major mechanisms of anticancer properties of probiotics include: (i) inhibition of pathogenic bacteria involved in the synthesis of carcinogens and mutagens, (ii) prevention of oxidative damage to the DNA, (iii) altering the metabolism of carcinogens, (iv) immunomodulation through macrophages, NK cells, lymphocytes, cytokines and IFN-γ, (v) promotion of apoptosis by changing the expression of various genes involved, (vi) inhibition of proliferation and metastasis, (vii) controlling cell cycle, and (viii) controlling signalling pathways involved in malignancies [5]. Probiotics are used in the prevention and treatment of lung cancers either by their direct mode of action or by their indirect mode of action, as described below with the case studies.

4.3.1. Direct Action of Probiotics in the Treatment of Lung Cancer

There are certain strains of probiotics with the genus *Lactobacillus*, *Bifidobacterium*, and *Escherichia*, which were successfully investigated for their anticancer potential against lung cancer. In 1985, the first evidence of the probiotic effect on lung cancer was reported. In this study, *L. casei* was used to treat Lewis lung cancer cells and cell line-10 hepatoma in animal models such as mice and guinea pigs. The study revealed that *L. casei* suppressed regional and pulmonary lymph node metastasis [60]. This was followed by the use of seven strains of probiotics, including *L. casei*, *L. plantarum*, *L. acidophilus*, *L. bulgaricus*, *Leuconostoc mesenterides*, *Streptococuss thermophilus* and *B. bifdum* against sarcoma 180 cells and Lewis lung cancer in the mouse. Among all the strains, *L. casei* demonstrated promising antitumor effects in terms of increased body weight and mean survival time when administered intraperitoneally [61].

In another study, *L. lactis KC24* was studied against lung carcinoma cell lines (SK-MES-1) and inhibition of proliferation to a large extent (86.53%), with the use of 3-(4,5-dimethylthiazole-2-yl)-2,5-diphenyltetrazolium bromide (MMT) assay was observed [62]. In a separate study, Han *et al.* [63] reported that *L. lactis*

NK34 (106 CFU/well) exhibited a strong inhibition of proliferation when SK-MES-1 cell lines were used. Sharma *et al.* [64] reported strong cytotoxic activity of two strains of *Lactobacillus* such as *L. lactis NK 34* and *L. lactis KC24,* on SK-MES-1 cell line. Another *Lactobacillus* strain, *L. acidophilus* was also tried for its anticancer potential against Lewis lung cancer in mice models. In this study, the anticancer activity was found to be enhanced in mice treated with *L. acidophilus* (the mice were co-administered with cisplatin) through the upregulation of *Ifng, Prfe* and *Gzmb* mRNA expression [65]. In a different study, administration of milk fermented by *L. casei CRL 431* to tumor-induced BALB/c mice demonstrated a reduction in tumor growth and lung metastasis. The result was attributed to increased $CD4^+$ and $CD8^+$ T cells and decreased the infiltration of macrophages [66]. Zamberi *et al.* [67] employed a probiotic-incorporated milk product (Kefir) and reported that it significantly improved the formation of cytotoxic T cells and T helper cells with the reduction in the metastasis to the lung.

Furthermore, co-administration of various strains of *Bifidobacterium,* including *B. breve, B. lactis, B. bifidum* and *B. longum* through oral route was able to restrain tumor progression in a similar line to PD-L1 specific antibody therapy (*i.e.,* checkpoint inhibitor) [68]. In a very interesting study, a possible synergistic effect of combined administration of probiotics (*Bacillus subtilis*) along with anticancer vaccine was investigated in an animal model *viz.* metastatic Lewis lung carcinoma and solid sarcoma. The results showed an improved inhibition of metastasis by 2 to 2.5 times in combination therapy compared to the mice treated with only vaccines [69].

The probiotic strains of *Enterococcus hirae* and *Barnesiella intestinihominis* were found to exhibit improved efficacy of an anticancer drug, cyclophosphamide, along with Th1-based cell immune reactions, leading to longer progression-free survival in advanced lung cancer cured with chemotherapy. Thus, these two probiotic strains were termed as "oncomicrobiotics" [70]. Diarrhoea is one of the major side effects caused by chemotherapy due to apoptosis of intestinal epithelial cells or alternation in the gut microflora or formation of pro-inflammatory cytokines. To minimize the above-mentioned side effect, the probiotic *Clostridium butyricum* was administered to lung cancer patients. The results demonstrated that the probiotic treatment reduced the chemotherapy-induced diarrhoea and also helped in the maintenance of homeostasis [23]. Co-administration of *Bacillus subtilis* with cancer therapy in a patient suffering from lung cancer was found to refine the intestinal microflora and eliminate the imbalance of gut microflora, thereby resulting in decreased gastrointestinal complications [71]. Similarly, Mlu *et al.* [72] employed combination therapy of probiotics (*Lactobacillus, Bifidobacterium, & Bacteroides*) with anticancer drugs in a lung cancer patient. The therapy improved gut microbiota, and led to a reduction in gut-related complications due to cancer therapy in lung cancer patients. Another study focused on the oral administration of a probiotic cocktail of *Bifidobacterium* genus with strains *B. longum, B. lactis,* and *B. breve* in the mouse induced with cancer. The cocktail probiotic therapy improved the anti-tumor immunity and anti-protein 1 or its ligand 1, thereby reducing the tumor growth considerably. In addition, the enhanced function of DCs, the chemokine-based transmission of immune cells to tumor site, improved T cell activation and CD8+ T cells' stimulation were also observed [73].

4.3.2. Indirect Action of Probiotics in Lung Cancer Therapy

4.3.2.1. Anti-mutagenic Action and Heavy Metal Neutralization

Mutagens-induced lung cancer is linked to a mutation in the *p53* tumor suppressor gene. In the majority of cases of lung cancer, benzopyrene, a polycyclic aromatic hydrocarbon found in cigarette smoke, is the potential mutagen. In particular, benzopyrene diol epoxide, a metabolite of benzopyrene is responsible for inducing the mutation by binding with DNA. This binding is found to be more frequent in lung cancer ($\approx$35%) than that of other cancer (<10%), thus indicating the main link between lung cancer and benzopyrene. Sodium azide is another inorganic mutagenic agent responsible for lung cancer. Both *Bifidobacterium* and *Lactobacillus* strains were studied extensively for their beneficial effects against benzopyrene-induced lung cancer. These strains act by binding to benzopyrone which results in its inactivation.

In one study, various species of *Bifidobacterium* in suspension were studied for their effectiveness against benzopyrene. The result showed higher anti-mutagenic potential compared to bacteria-free suspension [74]. Among nine species of *Bifidobacterium*, *B. infantis BY12* and *B. lactis BI HN019* demonstrated higher binding ability with benzopyrene [75]. It was reported that the degree of anti-mutagenic effects of probiotics is related to the mutagen type and the phase of bacterial growth. *B. breve ATCC 15700* displayed a higher mutagenic activity against sodium azide, whereas no effect was observed in the exponential growth phase. Contrary to this result, *L. sakei 23K* demonstrated no anti-mutagenic properties in the stationary phase and a comparatively low percentage of anti-mutagenic properties in the exponential phase. However, *B. adolescentis ATCC 15703* expressed a higher degree of anti-mutagenicity against benzopyrene during the exponential phase [76]. Moreover, four strains of *Lactobacillus* in suspension showed higher anti-mutagenic activity against sodium azide as compared to the suspension without *Lactobacillus* [77].

It has been well documented that heavy metals (*e.g.*, cadmium, lead, *etc.*), as well as carcinogens (aflatoxin B1, & microcystin-LR) enter into the human body through contamination of the food chain [78]. In addition, the link between heavy metal intake and lung cancer has been established. In this scenario, probiotics play a crucial role in detoxifying heavy metals by binding to them, thereby reducing their intestinal absorption. As a result, heavy metal retention is reduced, and it gets eliminated through faeces [79]. For instance, the heavy metals' binding ability of *L. rhamnosus LC705*, *L. rhamnosus GG*, *B. breve Bbi99/E8*, and *Propionibacterium freudenreichiishermanii JS* were studied *in vitro*. These probiotics showed promising results in detoxifying heavy metals such as cadmium and lead, and toxin contaminants such as aflatoxin B1 (mycotoxin) and microcystin-LR (cynotoxin) [78].

4.3.2.2. Host Immune System Modulation

Modulating the host immune system with the use of appropriate probiotics is one of the most attractive and safe ways to prevent and treat lung cancers. As mentioned earlier, lung microbiota dysbiosis and the presence of specific bacterial strains mainly contribute to the development of a tumor and thereby lead to an immunosuppressive microenvironment. In this situation, various anti-inflammatory molecules, including PD-L1, CTLA-4, or TGF-β from M2 macrophages and Treg cells, lead to the inhibition of NK and T cell responses. As a consequence, tolerance and tumor immune evasion (immune dysregulation) occur. In this stage, immunotherapy treatments such as ICIs, modulation of lung microbiota with probiotics (bacterial aerosol spray) and/or selective treatment with antibiotics are the best options [39]. The criteria such as the ability of the probiotics to differentially regulate the formation of pro-inflammatory (*e.g.*, NK cells, IL17, & macrophages) and anti-inflammatory cytokines, and to create a balance between different types of T cell responses (*e.g.*, Th1, Th2, Th17, & Treg responses) provide benefits of probiotics therapy against lung cancers [15, 80]. The probiotics exert their anticancer activity by: (i) modulating the immunomodulatory characteristics of cancer cells *via* NK cells, macrophages, and T cells, and (ii) enhancing the formation of cytokines, anti-angiogenic and antioxidants factors, thereby resulting in the reduction of pro-carcinogenic enzymes and cancer-specific proteins [11] Fig. (**2**). NK cells produce IFN-γ cytokine (a major component in both innate and adaptive immunity), which in turn activates macrophages and neutrophils. Being a subset of CD4$^+$ T cell, Th17 cell generates IL-17 cytokine. Probiotics-based immunotherapy prevents the inhibition of NK cells, CD8$^+$ T cells, and Th17 cells by Treg cells and M2 macrophages. Probiotics also inhibit Th1, Th17, and M1 macrophages-based stimulation of tumor cell formation [39]. It is also reported that probiotics taken orally or intranasally lead to protective effects in airway mucosa with the activation of macrophages and/or NK cells [81, 82].

Lactic acid bacteria (LAB) are an important class of probiotics that can induce a cell-mediated immune response. In one study, administering mice with *L. pentosus* enhanced the activity of NK cells in the spleen. In addition, it also stimulated NK cells to produce IFN-γ through indirect action on IL-12 produced by CD11c$^+$ DCs after a Toll-like receptor (TLR) 2 and/or TLR4-based interaction between bacteria and DCs [83]. Another *Lactobacillus* species *L. reuteri* showed a significant enhancement (both in percentage and number) of CD4$^+$CD25$^+$FOXP3$^+$ T cells in the spleen [84]. In another study, *L. casei DN14001* and *Bifidobacterium lactis Bb12* were found to induce Treg cells [85].

4.3.2.3. Prevention and Management of Lung Cancer

It is stated earlier section that there are two major causes of lung cancer to occur, including (i) pathogens, and (ii) chronic lung diseases such as COPD and asthma. In the former case, major pathogens such as *Salmonella typhimurium, Pseudomonas aeruginosa,* and *Salmonella pneumoniae* are involved in the development of lung cancer. The probiotic strains of the genus, *Lactobacillus,* and *Bifidobacterium* were found to decrease a load of above-mentioned pathogens, not only in the intestine but also in the respiratory tract through the modulation of NK cells and macrophages [86]. The *L. rhamnosus CRL1501* strain showed the highest ability in decreasing the pathogen load by increasing cytokines' levels such as IFN-γ, IL-4, IL-6, and IL-10 in the bronchoalveolar lavage [87]. Patients with COPD and asthma expressively increase a higher risk of lung cancer [88, 89]. These chronic inflammatory diseases induce the production of reactive oxygen species (ROS) and/or nitrogen species (RNS) that may act as catalysts for the development of lung cancer in the patient. Therefore, probiotics with the above-mentioned genera prevent the development of lung cancer by controlling the inflammatory reactions in the airways [90].

Oral administration of probiotic strain, *L. paracasei L9*, was found to decrease allergic reactions in asthma, induced in a murine model. This was attributed to the balancing act of strain for Th1/Th2 responses, with Th1 as the dominant state [91]. In another study, six probiotic strains such as *L. plantarum NumRes8, L. rhamnosus NumRes6, B. breve M-16V, B. infantis NumRes251, B. animalis NumRes 252,* and *NumRes253* were tested against anti-allergic potential in ovalbumin (OVA) sensitized mice (BALB/c) model. Out of all, *B. breve M-16V* demonstrated the highest effectiveness in reducing acute allergic reactions by decreasing antibodies (IgE & IgG1) and interleukins (such as IL-4, IL-5, & IL-10) levels, along with the reduction in eosinophils count in bronchoalveolar lavage fluid [92].

4.4. Advances in Probiotic Therapy in Lung Cancer

Recombination of probiotic strains was found to exhibit promising results against lung cancer due to the higher activity of immune cells. For instance, recombination therapy involving sFlt-1 (FMS-like tyrosine kinase receptor) gene transferring system in *B. infantis* employed an electroporation technique for the treatment of the Lewis lung cancer in mice model [93]. The obtained results showed significant inhibition of tumor growth in mice, leading to the prolonged survival time [93]. The result was attributed to the expression of sFlt-1 at gene and protein levels that inhibited the vascular endothelial growth factor (VEGF) of endothelial cells in the human umbilical vein [93]. In another study, the same probiotic *B. infantis* was used for recombination, involving soluble kinase insert domain receptor (sKDR) for the treatment of induced Lewis lung cancer in mice model. Out of the two recombinant *B. infantis*, one with the plasmid pTRKH2-PsT/sKDR exhibited higher suppression of tumor growth as compared to another recombinant with pTRKH1-PsT plasmid. In addition, the necrosis rate of the tumor and subsequently prolonged survival time were also observed [94]. The study of various probiotics for the treatment of lung cancer, along with the mechanism of action, animal model or cell lines, and the obtained results are summarized in Table **1**.

4.5. Safety Aspects of Probiotics

Like drugs and drug delivery systems, probiotics are not completely free of side effects, even though a few of them such as *Lactobacillus* and *Bifidobacteria* are declared as GRAS. The occurrence of side effects is mainly due to the intake of probiotics related to the host susceptibility. However, the number and severity of the side effects are very rare compared to the synthetic drugs. The reported side effects due to probiotics usage include gastrointestinal distress, systemic infection, and antibiotic resistance. These safety concerns were reported to be strain-dependent. Gastrointestinal distress such as bloating is very occasionally observed in a patient administered with probiotics and it occurs in only immunocompromised patient groups, including geriatrics, newborn and pregnant women [95]. Another minor side effect of probiotic is a systemic infection with an occurrence of around 0.05-0.40% [96]. However, immunocompromised patients are more prone to invasive infections due to the intake of probiotics. Long-term usage of probiotics in combination with antibiotics is a possible reason for the development of antibiotic resistance and this resistance may be transferred to other bacteria as well. This resistance may lead to sepsis in children with short gut [97]. Moreover, there was a case of bacteraemia after the intake of *Bacillus clausii* [98]. Therefore, in the present context, safety aspects should be weighed against the risk factors generated due to the administration of probiotics.

Table. (1). Various studies of probiotics for the treatment of lung cancer.

Probiotic	Mechanism of Action	Animal Model/ Cell Lines	Results	References
L. casei	Direct Action	Mice and guinea pigs	Suppressed the regional and pulmonary lymph node metastasis	[60]
L. casei, L. plantarum, L. acidophilus, L. bulgaricus, Leuconostoc mesenterides, Streptococuss thermophilus and *B. bifdum*		Mouse	Showed antitumor effects in terms of increased body weight and mean survival time	[61]
L. lactis KC24		Lung carcinoma cell lines (SK-MES-1)	Inhibited the proliferation to a large extent (86.53%)	[62]
L. lactis NK34		SK-MES-1	Inhibited the proliferation	[63]
L. lactis NK 34 and *L. lactis KC24*		SK-MES-1	Exerted strong cytotoxic effect	[64]
L. acidophilus		Mice model	Enhanced the anticancer activity	[65]
L. casei CRL 431		BALB/c mice	Reduced the tumor growth and lung metastasis	[66]
B. breve, B. lactis, B. bifdum and *B. longum*		Antibiotic-treated (Abt) mice	Restrained the tumor progression	[68]
Co-administration of Bacillus subtilis and anticancer vaccine		Mice	Improved inhibition of metastasis by 2 to 2.5 times in combination therapy compared to mice treated with only vaccine	[69]
Enterococcus hirae and *Barnesiella intestinihominis* with anticancer drug		Lung and ovarian cancer patients	Improved efficacy of anticancer drug, leading to longer progression-free survival in advanced lung cancer	[70]

(Table 1) cont.....

Probiotic	Mechanism of Action	Animal Model/ Cell Lines	Results	References
Clostridium butyricum	Direct Action	Cancer patients	Reduced chemotherapy-induced diarrhoea and maintenance of homeostasis	[23]
Bacillus subtilis with cancer therapy		Cancer patients	Refined the intestinal microflora and eliminated the imbalance of gut microflora, resulting in decreased gastrointestinal complications	[71]
Lactobacillus, Bifidobacterium, and *Bacteroides*) with anticancer drugs		Cancer patients	Reduced the gut-related complications due to cancer therapy	[72]
B.longum, B. lactis and *B. breve*		Mouse	Reduced the tumor growth considerably	[73]
Various species of *Bifidobacterium*	Anti-mutagenic action	*Salmonella typhimurium* TA100	Showed higher anti-mutagenic potential against benzopyrene	[74]
B. infantis BY12 and *B. lactis BI HN019*		-----	Demonstrated higher binding ability with benzopyrene	[75]
B. breve ATCC 15700		-----	Displayed a higher mutagenic activity against sodium azide	[76]
B. adolescentis ATCC 15703		-----	Expressed a higher degree of anti-mutagenicity against benzopyrene.	[76]
L. casei, L. plantarum, and *L. brevis*		-----	Showed higher anti-mutagenic activity against sodium azide	[77]
L. rhamnosus LC705, L. rhamnosus GG, B. breve Bbi99/E8 and *Propionibacterium freudenreichiishermanii JS*	Heavy Metal and toxin neutralization	----	Detoxified heavy metals such as cadmium and lead, and toxin contaminants such as aflatoxin B1 and microcystin-LR	[78]

(Table 1) cont.....

Probiotic	Mechanism of Action	Animal Model/ Cell Lines	Results	References
L. pentosus S-PT84	Host immune system modulation	Mice	Enhanced the activity of NK cells in the spleen and also stimulated NK cells to produce IFN-γ	[83]
L. reuteri		Rat	Showed a significant enhancement (both in percentage and number) of CD4+, CD25+ and transcription factor (FOXP3+) T cells in the spleen	[84].
L. casei DN14001 and *B. lactis Bb12*		Rat	Induced the Treg cells	[85].
L. paracasei L9	Prevention and management of lung cancer	Murine	Decreased allergic reaction in asthma	[91]
L. plantarum NumRes8, L. rhamnosus NumRes6, B. breve M-16V, B. infantis NumRes251, B. animalis NumRes 252 and NumRes253		Mice (BALB/c) model	Reduced acute allergic reactions	[92]
sFlt-1 gene transferring system in *B. infantis*	Advances in probiotic therapy in lung cancer	Lewis lung cancer in mice model	Inhibited tumor growth and thereby, led to prolonged survival time	[93]
B. infantis was used for recombination involving sKDR		Lewis lung cancer in mice model	Suppressed the tumor growth, necrosis rate of tumor, and subsequently prolonged survival time	[94]

CONCLUDING REMARKS

In recent years, probiotics have gained huge medical attention owing to their positive impact not only on different cancers but also on different diseases. This has been proved through promising outcomes from different research on probiotics. Probiotics play a very crucial role in the prevention and treatment of lung cancer through the improvement of the immune system and/or anti-inflammatory responses. It seems to be better adjuvant to chemotherapy, radiotherapy, and/or surgery involving cancer with less chance of side effects. However, there are a few critical questions to be solved to make probiotic therapy more specific and reliable. Firstly, it is necessary to establish which strains of bacteria are solely responsible for the improvement or cure of a particular disease in a scientific manner. Secondly, it is very crucial to understand and determine the mechanism of action of a specific probiotic on lung cancer. Thirdly, a dosage regimen of probiotics is needed to be developed on a case-by-case basis. Finally, there is a necessity for validation of preclinical data through clinical trials for a better understanding of human health benefits exerted through probiotics' administration. To fulfill this, both short and long-term complementary human study, along with methodology standardization, is necessary for the recent future.

CONSENT FOR PUBLICATION

Not applicable.

CONFLICT OF INTEREST

The authors declare no conflict of interest, financial or otherwise.

ACKNOWLEDGEMENT

declared None.

REFERENCES

[1]   Siegel RL, Miller KD, Jemal A. Cancer statistics, 2019. CA Cancer J Clin 2019; 69(1): 7-34.
        [http://dx.doi.org/10.3322/caac.21551] [PMID: 30620402]

[2]   Bray F, Ferlay J, Soerjomataram I, Siegel RL, Torre LA, Jemal A. Global cancer statistics 2018: GLOBOCAN estimates of incidence and mortality worldwide for 36 cancers in 185 countries. CA Cancer J Clin 2018; 68(6): 394-424.
        [http://dx.doi.org/10.3322/caac.21492] [PMID: 30207593]

[3]   Guo H, Zhao L, Zhu J, *et al.* Microbes in lung cancer initiation, treatment, and outcome: Boon or bane? Semin Cancer Biol 2021.
        [PMID: 34029741]

[4]   Druesne-Pecollo N, Keita Y, Touvier M, *et al.* Alcohol drinking and second primary cancer risk in patients with upper aerodigestive tract cancers: a systematic review and meta-analysis of observational studies. Cancer Epidemiol Biomarkers Prev 2014; 23(2): 324-31.
        [http://dx.doi.org/10.1158/1055-9965.EPI-13-0779] [PMID: 24307268]

[5]   Divyashri G, Krishna Murthy TPK, Murahari M. Potential of Probiotics in the Management of Lung Cancer.Probiotic Research in Therapeutics. Singapore Pte Ltd., Springer Nature 2021; pp. 211-30.
        [http://dx.doi.org/10.1007/978-981-15-8214-1_10]

[6]   Vandeven N, Nghiem P. Pathogen-driven cancers and emerging immune therapeutic strategies. Cancer Immunol Res 2014; 2(1): 9-14.
        [http://dx.doi.org/10.1158/2326-6066.CIR-13-0179] [PMID: 24778160]

[7]   Alberg AJ, Brock MV, Ford JG, Samet JM, Spivack SD. Epidemiology of lung cancer: Diagnosis and management of lung cancer, 3rd ed: American College of Chest Physicians evidence-based clinical practice guidelines. Chest 2013; 143(5) (Suppl.): e1S-e29S.
        [http://dx.doi.org/10.1378/chest.12-2345] [PMID: 23649439]

[8]   Johnson DH, Schiller JH, Bunn PA Jr. Recent clinical advances in lung cancer management. J Clin Oncol 2014; 32(10): 973-82.
        [http://dx.doi.org/10.1200/JCO.2013.53.1228] [PMID: 24567433]

[9]   Wakelee H, Kelly K, Edelman MJ. 50 Years of progress in the systemic therapy of non-small cell lung cancer. In: American Society of Clinical Oncology educational book. American Society of Clinical Oncology Meeting, NIH Public Access, 2014; pp. 177.

[10]   Vivarelli S, Salemi R, Candido S, *et al.* Gut microbiota and cancer: from pathogenesis to therapy. Cancers (Basel) 2019; 11(1): 38.
[http://dx.doi.org/10.3390/cancers11010038] [PMID: 30609850]

[11]   Dasari S, Kathera C, Janardhan A, Praveen Kumar A, Viswanath B. Surfacing role of probiotics in cancer prophylaxis and therapy: A systematic review. Clin Nutr 2017; 36(6): 1465-72.
[http://dx.doi.org/10.1016/j.clnu.2016.11.017] [PMID: 27923508]

[12]   Joint FAO. WHO working group report on drafting guidelines for the evaluation of probiotics in food. 2002.

[13]   Hill C, Guarner F, Reid G, *et al.* The International Scientific Association for Probiotics and Prebiotics consensus statement on the scope and appropriate use of the term probiotic. Nat Rev Gastroenterol Hepatol 2014; 11(8): 506-14.
[http://dx.doi.org/10.1038/nrgastro.2014.66] [PMID: 24912386]

[14]   Varzakas T, Kandylis P, Dimitrellou D, Salamoura C, Zakynthinos G, Proestos C. Innovative and fortified food: probiotics, prebiotics, gmos, and superfood. 2018.
[http://dx.doi.org/10.1016/B978-0-08-101892-7.00006-7]

[15]   Legesse Bedada T, Feto TK, Awoke KS, Garedew AD, Yifat FT, Birri DJ. Probiotics for cancer alternative prevention and treatment. Biomed Pharmacother 2020; 129110409
[http://dx.doi.org/10.1016/j.biopha.2020.110409] [PMID: 32563987]

[16]   Bhat S, Bhat V, Hegde S, Palit M. Intelligent nutrition: Oral health promotion by probiotics. Archives of Medicine and Health Sciences 2013; 1(2): 140-4.
[http://dx.doi.org/10.4103/2321-4848.123027]

[17]   Rahbar Saadat Y, Yari Khosroushahi A, Pourghassem Gargari B. A comprehensive review of anticancer, immunomodulatory and health beneficial effects of the lactic acid bacteria exopolysaccharides. Carbohydr Polym 2019; 217: 79-89.
[http://dx.doi.org/10.1016/j.carbpol.2019.04.025] [PMID: 31079688]

[18]   WHO Report on Cancer: setting Priorities, Investing Wisely and Providing Care for All. Geneva: WHO 2020.

[19]   2018.Cancer: fact sheet https://www.who.int/news-room/fact-sheets/detail/cancer

[20]   Tian T, Olson S, Whitacre JM, Harding A. The origins of cancer robustness and evolvability. Integr Biol 2011; 3(1): 17-30.
[http://dx.doi.org/10.1039/C0IB00046A] [PMID: 20944865]

[21]   Hanahan D, Weinberg RA. Hallmarks of cancer: the next generation. Cell 2011; 144(5): 646-74.
[http://dx.doi.org/10.1016/j.cell.2011.02.013] [PMID: 21376230]

[22]   Chen W, Zheng R, Baade PD, *et al.* Cancer statistics in China, 2015. CA Cancer J Clin 2016; 66(2): 115-32.
[http://dx.doi.org/10.3322/caac.21338] [PMID: 26808342]

[23]   Tian Y, Li M, Song W, Jiang R, Li Y. Effects of probiotics on chemotherapy in patients with lung cancer. Oncol Lett 2019; 17(3): 2836-48.
[http://dx.doi.org/10.3892/ol.2019.9906] [PMID: 30854059]

[24]   Feng C, Feng M, Gao Y, *et al.* Clinicopathologic significance of intestinal-type molecules' expression and different EGFR gene status in pulmonary adenocarcinoma. Appl Immunohistochem Mol Morphol 2018. Ahead of print
[PMID: 29489510]

[25]   Toyoda Y, Nakayama T, Ioka A, Tsukuma H. Trends in lung cancer incidence by histological type in

Osaka, Japan. Jpn J Clin Oncol 2008; 38(8): 534-9.
[http://dx.doi.org/10.1093/jjco/hyn072] [PMID: 18689853]

[26]   Liu NN, Ma Q, Ge Y, *et al.* Microbiome dysbiosis in lung cancer: from composition to therapy. NPJ
Precis Oncol 2020; 4(1): 33.
[http://dx.doi.org/10.1038/s41698-020-00138-z] [PMID: 33303906]

[27]   Quigley EMM. Microbiota-brain-gut axis and neurodegenerative diseases. Curr Neurol Neurosci Rep
2017; 17(12): 94.
[http://dx.doi.org/10.1007/s11910-017-0802-6] [PMID: 29039142]

[28]   Zhang D, Li S, Wang N, Tan HY, Zhang Z, Feng Y. The cross-talk between gut microbiota and lungs
in common lung diseases. Front Microbiol 2020; 11: 301.
[http://dx.doi.org/10.3389/fmicb.2020.00301] [PMID: 32158441]

[29]   Zhang YJ, Li S, Gan RY, Zhou T, Xu DP, Li HB. Impacts of gut bacteria on human health and
diseases. Int J Mol Sci 2015; 16(12): 7493-519.
[http://dx.doi.org/10.3390/ijms16047493] [PMID: 25849657]

[30]   Wypych TP, Wickramasinghe LC, Marsland BJ. The influence of the microbiome on respiratory
health. Nat Immunol 2019; 20(10): 1279-90.
[http://dx.doi.org/10.1038/s41590-019-0451-9] [PMID: 31501577]

[31]   Dickson RP, Huffnagle GB. The lung microbiome: new principles forrespiratory bacteriology in health
and disease. PLoS Pathog 2015; 11(7)e1004923
[http://dx.doi.org/10.1371/journal.ppat.1004923] [PMID: 26158874]

[32]   Zhuang H, Cheng L, Wang Y, *et al.* Dysbiosis of the gut microbiome in lung cancer. Front Cell Infect
Microbiol 2019; 9: 112.
[http://dx.doi.org/10.3389/fcimb.2019.00112] [PMID: 31065547]

[33]   Ballesteros-Tato A, León B, Lund FE, Randall TD. Temporal changes in dendritic cell subsets, cross-
priming and costimulation *via* CD70 control CD8+ T cell responses to influenza. Nat Immunol 2010;
11(3): 216-24.
[http://dx.doi.org/10.1038/ni.1838] [PMID: 20098442]

[34]   Ho AWS, Prabhu N, Betts RJ, *et al.* Lung CD103+ dendritic cells efficiently transport influenza virus
to the lymph node and load viral antigen onto MHC class I for presentation to CD8 T cells. J Immunol
2011; 187(11): 6011-21.
[http://dx.doi.org/10.4049/jimmunol.1100987] [PMID: 22043017]

[35]   Ege MJ, Mayer M, Normand AC, *et al.* Exposure to environmental microorganisms and childhood
asthma. N Engl J Med 2011; 364(8): 701-9.
[http://dx.doi.org/10.1056/NEJMoa1007302] [PMID: 21345099]

[36]   Stein MM, Hrusch CL, Gozdz J, *et al.* Innate immunity and asthma risk in amish and hutterite farm
children. N Engl J Med 2016; 375(5): 411-21.
[http://dx.doi.org/10.1056/NEJMoa1508749] [PMID: 27518660]

[37]   Park CO, Kupper TS. The emerging role of resident memory T cells in protective immunity and
inflammatory disease. Nat Med 2015; 21(7): 688-97.
[http://dx.doi.org/10.1038/nm.3883] [PMID: 26121195]

[38]   Sathaliyawala T, Kubota M, Yudanin N, *et al.* Distribution and compartmentalization of human
circulating and tissue-resident memory T cell subsets. Immunity 2013; 38(1): 187-97.
[http://dx.doi.org/10.1016/j.immuni.2012.09.020] [PMID: 23260195]

[39]   Ramírez-Labrada AG, Isla D, Artal A, *et al.* The Influence of Lung Microbiota on Lung
Carcinogenesis, Immunity, and Immunotherapy. Trends Cancer 2020; 6(2): 86-97.
[http://dx.doi.org/10.1016/j.trecan.2019.12.007] [PMID: 32061309]

[40]   Nanno M, Shiohara T, Yamamoto H, Kawakami K, Ishikawa H. γδ T cells: firefighters or fire boosters
in the front lines of inflammatory responses. Immunol Rev 2007; 215(1): 103-13.

[http://dx.doi.org/10.1111/j.1600-065X.2006.00474.x] [PMID: 17291282]

[41]   Radicioni G, Cao R, Carpenter J, *et al.* The innate immune properties of airway mucosal surfaces are regulated by dynamic interactions between mucins and interacting proteins: the mucin interactome. Mucosal Immunol 2016; 9(6): 1442-54.
[http://dx.doi.org/10.1038/mi.2016.27] [PMID: 27072609]

[42]   Beck JM, Young VB, Huffnagle GB. The microbiome of the lung. Transl Res 2012; 160(4): 258-66.
[http://dx.doi.org/10.1016/j.trsl.2012.02.005] [PMID: 22683412]

[43]   Maddi A, Sabharwal A, Violante T, *et al.* The microbiome and lung cancer. J Thorac Dis 2019; 11(1): 280-91.
[http://dx.doi.org/10.21037/jtd.2018.12.88] [PMID: 30863606]

[44]   Sethi S. Bacterial infection and the pathogenesis of COPD. Chest 2000; 117(5) (Suppl. 1): 286S-91S.
[http://dx.doi.org/10.1378/chest.117.5_suppl_1.286S] [PMID: 10843957]

[45]   Martins D, Mendes F, Schmitt F. Microbiome: a supportive or a leading actor in lung cancer? Pathobiology 2021; 88(2): 198-207.
[http://dx.doi.org/10.1159/000511556] [PMID: 33352574]

[46]   WHO-Food and Agricultural Organization, Probiotics in Food: Health and Nutritional Properties and Guidelines for Evaluation, FAO Food and Nutritional Paper. FAO/WHO, Rome, 2006; No.8592-5-105513-0.

[47]   Adams CA. The probiotic paradox: live and dead cells are biological response modifiers. Nutr Res Rev 2010; 23(1): 37-46.
[http://dx.doi.org/10.1017/S0954422410000090] [PMID: 20403231]

[48]   Kandylis P, Pissaridi K, Bekatorou A, Kanellaki M, Koutinas AA. Dairy and non-dairy probiotic beverages. Curr Opin Food Sci 2016; 7: 58-63.
[http://dx.doi.org/10.1016/j.cofs.2015.11.012]

[49]   Sanders ME, Merenstein DJ, Ouwehand AC, *et al.* Probiotic use in at-risk populations. J Am Pharm Assoc (Wash DC) 2016; 56(6): 680-6.
[http://dx.doi.org/10.1016/j.japh.2016.07.001] [PMID: 27836128]

[50]   O'Toole PW, Marchesi JR, Hill C. Next-generation probiotics: the spectrum from probiotics to live biotherapeutics. Nat Microbiol 2017; 2(5): 17057.
[http://dx.doi.org/10.1038/nmicrobiol.2017.57] [PMID: 28440276]

[51]   Valdovinos MA, Montijo E, Abreu AT, *et al.* The Mexican consensus on probiotics in gastroenterology. Rev Gastroenterol Mex 2017; 82(2): 156-78.
[http://dx.doi.org/10.1016/j.rgmx.2016.08.004] [PMID: 28104319]

[52]   Kurakula M, Rao GSNK. Probiotics in lung cancer: an emerging field of multifarious potential and opportunities. 2021.
[http://dx.doi.org/10.1007/978-981-15-8214-1_7]

[53]   Georgiev K, Georgieva M. Antiproliferative effect of bulgarian spring water probiotics (laktera nature probiotic®) against human colon carcinoma cell line. World J Pharm Pharm Sci 2015; 4: 130-6.

[54]   Ricci A, Allende A, Bolton D, *et al.* Update of the list of QPS-recommended biological agents intentionally added to food or feed as notified to EFSA 5: suitability of taxonomic units notified to EFSA until September 2016. EFSA J 2017; 15(3)e04663
[PMID: 32625420]

[55]   Saber A, Alipour B, Faghfoori Z, Yari Khosroushahi A. Cellular and molecular effects of yeast probiotics on cancer. Crit Rev Microbiol 2017; 43(1): 96-115.
[http://dx.doi.org/10.1080/1040841X.2016.1179622] [PMID: 27561003]

[56]   WHO-Food and Agricultural Organization, Guidelines for the Evaluation of Probiotics in Food, FAO/WHO joint report., London, 2002.

[57]   Mattila-Sandholm T, Myllärinen P, Crittenden R, Mogensen G, Fondén R, Saarela M. Technological challenges for future probiotic foods. Int Dairy J 2002; 12(2-3): 173-82.
[http://dx.doi.org/10.1016/S0958-6946(01)00099-1]

[58]   Raman M, Ambalam P, Kondepudi KK, *et al.* Potential of probiotics, prebiotics and synbiotics for management of colorectal cancer. Gut Microbes 2013; 4(3): 181-92.
[http://dx.doi.org/10.4161/gmic.23919] [PMID: 23511582]

[59]   Plaza-Diaz J, Ruiz-Ojeda FJ, Gil-Campos M, Gil A. Mechanisms of action of probiotics. Adv Nutr 2019; 10 (Suppl. 1): S49-66.
[http://dx.doi.org/10.1093/advances/nmy063] [PMID: 30721959]

[60]   Matsuzaki T, Yokokura T, Azuma I. Anti-tumour activity of *Lactobacillus casei* on lewis lung carcinoma and line-10 hepatoma in syngeneic mice and guinea pigs. Cancer Immunol Immunother 1985; 20(1): 18-22.
[http://dx.doi.org/10.1007/BF00199768] [PMID: 3933816]

[61]   Kim HY, Bae HS, Baek YJ. *In vivo* antitumor effects of lactic acid bacteria on sarcoma 180 and mouse Lewis lung carcinoma. J Korean Cancer Assoc 1991; 23: 188-96.

[62]   Lee NK, Han KJ, Son SH, Eom SJ, Lee SK, Paik HD. Multifunctional effect of probiotic *Lactococcus lactis* KC24 isolated from kimchi. Lebensm Wiss Technol 2015; 64(2): 1036-41.
[http://dx.doi.org/10.1016/j.lwt.2015.07.019]

[63]   Han KJ, Lee NK, Park H, Paik HD. Anticancer and anti-inflammatory activity of probiotic *Lactococcus lactis* NK34. J Microbiol Biotechnol 2015; 25(10): 1697-701.
[http://dx.doi.org/10.4014/jmb.1503.03033] [PMID: 26165315]

[64]   Sharma A, Viswanath B, Park YS. Role of probiotics in the management of lung cancer and related diseases: An update. J Funct Foods 2018; 40: 625-33.
[http://dx.doi.org/10.1016/j.jff.2017.11.050]

[65]   Gui QF, Lu HF, Zhang CX, Xu ZR, Yang YH. Well-balanced commensal microbiota contributes to anti-cancer response in a lung cancer mouse model. Genet Mol Res 2015; 14(2): 5642-51.
[http://dx.doi.org/10.4238/2015.May.25.16] [PMID: 26125762]

[66]   Aragón F, Carino S, Perdigón G, de Moreno de LeBlanc A. Inhibition of growth and metastasis of breast cancer in mice by milk fermented with *Lactobacillus casei* CRL 431. J Immunother 2015; 38(5): 185-96.
[http://dx.doi.org/10.1097/CJI.0000000000000079] [PMID: 25962107]

[67]   Zamberi NR, Abu N, Mohamed NE, *et al.* The antimetastatic and antiangiogenesis effects of kefir water on murine breast cancer cells. Integr Cancer Ther 2016; 15(4): NP53-66.
[http://dx.doi.org/10.1177/1534735416642862] [PMID: 27230756]

[68]   Cheng M, Qian L, Shen G, *et al.* Microbiota modulate tumoral immune surveillance in lung through a γδT17 immune cell-dependent mechanism. Cancer Res 2014; 74(15): 4030-41.
[http://dx.doi.org/10.1158/0008-5472.CAN-13-2462] [PMID: 24947042]

[69]   Tanasienko OA, Cheremshenko NL, Titova GP, *et al.* Elevation of the efficacy of antitumor vaccine prepared on the base of lectines from *B. subtilis* B-7025 upon its combined application with probiotics *in vivo*. Exp Oncol 2005; 27(4): 336-8.
[PMID: 16404358]

[70]   Daillère R, Vétizou M, Waldschmitt N, *et al. Enterococcushirae* and *Barnesiellaintestinihominis* facilitate cyclophosphamide-induced therapeutic immunomodulatory effects. Immunity 2016; 45(4): 931-43.
[http://dx.doi.org/10.1016/j.immuni.2016.09.009] [PMID: 27717798]

[71]   Serkova M, Urtenova MA, Tkachenko EI, *et al.* On the possibilities of correction of changes of the gastrointestinal tract microbiota in patients with lung cancer treated receiving chemotherapy. Eksperimental'naiaiklinicheskaiagastroenterologiia1/4. Exp Clin Gastroenterol 2013; 11: 15-20.

[72]   Serkova MIu, Urtenova MA, Tkachenko EI, *et al.* [On the possibilities of correction of changes of the gastrointestinal tract microbiota in patients with lung cancer treated receiving chemotherapy]. Eksp Klin Gastroenterol 2013; 11(11): 15-20.
[PMID: 24933973]

[73]   Sivan A, Corrales L, Hubert N, *et al.* Commensal *Bifidobacterium* promotes antitumor immunity and facilitates anti–PD-L1 efficacy. Science 2015; 350(6264): 1084-9.
[http://dx.doi.org/10.1126/science.aac4255] [PMID: 26541606]

[74]   Pei-Ren L, Roch-Chuiyu , Cheng-Chun C, Ya-Hui T. Antimutagenic activity of several probiotic *bifidobacteria* against Benzo[a]pyrene. J Biosci Bioeng 2002; 94(2): 148-53.
[http://dx.doi.org/10.1016/S1389-1723(02)80135-9]

[75]   Shoukat S, Aslam MZ, Rehman A, Zhang B. Screening of *Bifidobacterium* strains to bind with Benzo[a]pyrene under food stress factors and the mechanism of the process. J Food Process Preserv 2019; 43(7): 101-9.
[http://dx.doi.org/10.1111/jfpp.13956]

[76]   Chalova VI, Lingbeck JM, Kwon YM, Ricke SC. Extracellular antimutagenic activities of selected probiotic *Bifidobacterium* and *Lactobacillus* spp. as a function of growth phase. J Environ Sci Health B 2008; 43(2): 193-8.
[http://dx.doi.org/10.1080/03601230701795262] [PMID: 18246512]

[77]   Abbas Ahmadi M, Tajabadi Ebrahimi M, Mehrabian S, Tafvizi F, Bahrami H, Dameshghian M. Antimutagenic and anticancer effects of lactic acid bacteria isolated from Tarhana through Ames test and phylogenetic analysis by 16S rDNA. Nutr Cancer 2014; 66(8): 1406-13.
[http://dx.doi.org/10.1080/01635581.2014.956254] [PMID: 25330454]

[78]   Halttunen T, Collado MC, El-Nezami H, Meriluoto J, Salminen S. Combining strains of lactic acid bacteria may reduce their toxin and heavy metal removal efficiency from aqueous solution. Lett Appl Microbiol 2008; 46(2): 160-5.
[http://dx.doi.org/10.1111/j.1472-765X.2007.02276.x] [PMID: 18028332]

[79]   Gayathri D, Rashmi BS. Anti-cancer properties of probiotics: a natural strategy for cancer prevention. EC Nutr 2016; 5: 1191-202.

[80]   Kausar H, Jeyabalan J, Aqil F, *et al.* Berry anthocyanidins synergistically suppress growth and invasive potential of human non-small-cell lung cancer cells. Cancer Lett 2012; 325(1): 54-62.
[http://dx.doi.org/10.1016/j.canlet.2012.05.029] [PMID: 22659736]

[81]   Choi SS, Kim Y, Han KS, You S, Oh S, Kim SH. Effects of *Lactobacillus* strains on cancer cell proliferation and oxidative stress *in vitro*. Lett Appl Microbiol 2006; 42(5): 452-8.
[http://dx.doi.org/10.1111/j.1472-765X.2006.01913.x] [PMID: 16620202]

[82]   Kim JE, Kim JY, Lee KW, Lee HJ. Cancer chemopreventive effects of lactic acid bacteria. J Microbiol Biotechnol 2007; 17(8): 1227-35.
[PMID: 18051589]

[83]   Koizumi S, Wakita D, Sato T, *et al.* Essential role of Toll-like receptors for dendritic cell and NK1.1+ cell-dependent activation of type 1 immunity by *Lactobacillus pentosus* strain S-PT84. Immunol Lett 2008; 120(1-2): 14-9.
[http://dx.doi.org/10.1016/j.imlet.2008.06.003] [PMID: 18620001]

[84]   Rowland IR, Bearne CA, Fischer R, Pool-Zobel BL. The effect of lactulose on DNA damage induced by DMH in the colon of human flora-associated rats. Nutr Cancer 1996; 26(1): 37-47.
[http://dx.doi.org/10.1080/01635589609514461] [PMID: 8844720]

[85]   Gavresea F, Vagianos C, Korontzi M, *et al.* Beneficial effect of synbiotics on experimental colon cancer in rats. Turk J Gastroenterol 2018; 29(4): 494-501.
[http://dx.doi.org/10.5152/tjg.2018.17469] [PMID: 30249566]

[86]   Hardy H, Harris J, Lyon E, Beal J, Foey A. Probiotics, prebiotics and immunomodulation of gut

mucosal defences: homeostasis and immunopathology. Nutrients 2013; 5(6): 1869-912.
[http://dx.doi.org/10.3390/nu5061869] [PMID: 23760057]

[87]   Salva S, Villena J, Alvarez S. Immunomodulatory activity of *Lactobacillus rhamnosus* strains isolated from goat milk: Impact on intestinal and respiratory infections. Int J Food Microbiol 2010; 141(1-2): 82-9.
[http://dx.doi.org/10.1016/j.ijfoodmicro.2010.03.013] [PMID: 20395002]

[88]   Qu YL, Liu J, Zhang LX, *et al.* Asthma and the risk of lung cancer: a meta-analysis. Oncotarget 2017; 8(7): 11614-20.
[http://dx.doi.org/10.18632/oncotarget.14595] [PMID: 28086224]

[89]   Houghton AM. Mechanistic links between COPD and lung cancer. Nat Rev Cancer 2013; 13(4): 233-45.
[http://dx.doi.org/10.1038/nrc3477] [PMID: 23467302]

[90]   Mortaz E, Adcock IM, Folkerts G, Barnes PJ, Paul Vos A, Garssen J. Probiotics in the management of lung diseases. Mediators Inflamm 2013; 2013: 1-10.
[http://dx.doi.org/10.1155/2013/751068] [PMID: 23737654]

[91]   Wang X, Hui Y, Zhao L, Hao Y, Guo H, Ren F. Oral administration of *Lactobacillus paracasei* L9 attenuates PM2.5-induced enhancement of airway hyperresponsiveness and allergic airway response in murine model of asthma. PLoS One 2017; 12(2)e0171721
[http://dx.doi.org/10.1371/journal.pone.0171721] [PMID: 28199353]

[92]   Hougee S, Vriesema AJM, Wijering SC, *et al.* Oral treatment with probiotics reduces allergic symptoms in ovalbumin-sensitized mice: a bacterial strain comparative study. Int Arch Allergy Immunol 2010; 151(2): 107-17.
[http://dx.doi.org/10.1159/000236000] [PMID: 19752564]

[93]   Zhu H, Li Z, Mao S, *et al.* Antitumor effect of sFlt-1 gene therapy system mediated by *Bifidobacterium Infantis* on Lewis lung cancer in mice. Cancer Gene Ther 2011; 18(12): 884-96.
[http://dx.doi.org/10.1038/cgt.2011.57] [PMID: 21921942]

[94]   Li ZJ, Zhu H, Ma BY, *et al.* Inhibitory effect of *Bifidobacterium infantis*-mediated sKDR prokaryotic expression system on angiogenesis and growth of Lewis lung cancer in mice. BMC Cancer 2012; 12(1): 155.
[http://dx.doi.org/10.1186/1471-2407-12-155] [PMID: 22536942]

[95]   Szajewska H, Horvath A, Piwowarczyk A. Meta-analysis: the effects of *Saccharomyces boulardii* supplementation on *Helicobacter pylori* eradication rates and side effects during treatment. Aliment Pharmacol Ther 2010; 32(9): 1069-79.
[http://dx.doi.org/10.1111/j.1365-2036.2010.04457.x] [PMID: 21039671]

[96]   Martín-Muñoz MF, Fortuni M, Caminoa M, Belver T, Quirce S, Caballero T. Anaphylactic reaction to probiotics. Cow's milk and hen's egg allergens in probiotic compounds. Pediatr Allergy Immunol 2012; 23(8): 778-84.
[http://dx.doi.org/10.1111/j.1399-3038.2012.01338.x] [PMID: 22957765]

[97]   Rautio M, Jousimies-Somer H, Kauma H, *et al.* Liver abscess due to a *Lactobacillus rhamnosus* strain indistinguishable from *L. rhamnosus* strain GG. Clin Infect Dis 1999; 28(5): 1159-60.
[http://dx.doi.org/10.1086/514766] [PMID: 10452653]

[98]   Gargar JD, Divinagracia RM. When good things go bad: a case series of bacteremia from probiotics. Chest 2019; 155(4): 92A.
[http://dx.doi.org/10.1016/j.chest.2019.02.091]

CHAPTER 11

Probiotics-based Anticancer Immunity in Head and Neck Cancer

Shanth Kumar Sushma[1], Shivaraju Amrutha[1] and **Alwarappan Sankaranarayanan[1,*]**

[1] *Department of Life Sciences, Sri Sathya Sai University for Human Excellence Kamalapur, Navanihal, Kalaburagi, Karnataka State, India*

Abstract: Every day we are used to hearing about cancer and its effects. Head and neck cancer is one of the types of cancer which is leading to mortality. Treatment of cancer is crucial to lead a happy and healthy life. Till today several medical strategies, such as radiotherapy, chemotherapy, *etc.*, have come forward to eradicate cancer, but along with these approaches, probiotics are also taking part to dissolve this problem. In simple words, probiotics are microorganisms that are present in fermented foods like yogurt, cheese, creams, fermented milk, *etc.*, which, when administered to the host, provide health benefits. Some familiar probiotics are *Lactobacillus bulgaricus*, *L. casei* and *Streptococcus thermophilus,* which are involved in cancer treatment. Much evidence has proven its health benefits. This chapter focuses on how probiotics act on cancer cells with an introduction to head and neck cancer, thereby triggering our interest to probe into further research on treating cancer using probiotics.

Keywords: Chemotherapy, DNA damage, Head and neck cancer, *Lactobacillus bulgaricusL. casei*, Radiotherapy, Probiotics, , *Streptococcus thermophilus.*

1. INTRODUCTION

Cancer has become more prominent in every nook and corner of the world. "Head and neck cancer" includes distinct kinds of tumors which metastasise in or around the mouth, nose, and throat [1]. Comparatively, men are 2-3 times more affected by head and neck cancer than women. Among all cancers, head and neck cancer is the 6th prominent cancer, accounting for 500,000 cases every year [2]. The use of alcohol, cigarettes and human papillomavirus (HPV) infection is thought to be the leading causes of head and neck cancer.

---
[*] **Corresponding authors Alwarappan Sankaranarayanan:** Department of Life Sciences, Sri Sathya Sai University for Human Excellence, Kamalapur, Navanihal, Kalaburagi, Karnataka State, India; E-mail: drsankarkamal@gmail.com

Mitesh Kumar Dwivedi, Alwarappan Sankaranarayanan & Sanjay Tiwari (Eds.)
All rights reserved-© 2023 Bentham Science Publishers

The most prevalent type of head and neck cancer is squamous cell carcinoma (SCC) [3]. The SCC begins in the squamous cells, which are thin, flattened cells that cover the outermost layer of the skin. Squamous cells are found in the lungs, mucous membranes, digestive tract, and urinary tract, in addition to the skin. SCC of the skin is known as cutaneous squamous cell carcinoma (cSCC). This transpires due to the mutation in squamous cell's DNA, resulting in unregulated cell division [4]. People under the age of 40 or above are more prone to this cancer. When it comes to the matter of cure, all types of head and neck cancers are curable, if they are found early. However, after a certain stage, they can be treatable but not curable. The life expectancy for the head and neck cancer patients is between 1-5 years after diagnosis, through the common cancer treatments, which include surgery, chemotherapy, radiotherapy, immunotherapy, targeted therapy, *etc.* However, the recent strategy, which uses probiotics, has gained more attention than the other cancer treatments, which use live bacteria delivered through food and capsules.

Probiotics are live bacteria that give health advantages, when supplemented through yoghurt, milk, cheese, creams, *etc.*, according to the world health organization (WHO) [5]. The most prevalent probiotics present in meals are lactic acid-producing bacteria. Probiotics have long been known to have a wide range of health advantages in both humans and livestock. They aid in the protection of the host against hazardous bacteria as well as the immune system's strengthening. Probiotics have also been shown to aid in metabolic issues and digestion problems. Although the exact methods by which probiotic bacteria provide health advantages are uncertain, they could include competitive exclusion of enteric pathogens, production of antimicrobial metabolites, neutralization of dietary carcinogens and activation of the immune system [6]. The current chapter discusses the types of head and neck cancer, the role of probiotics in cancer treatment, the mode of delivery and the challenges in using probiotics to treat head and neck cancer.

2. TYPES OF HEAD AND NECK CANCER

Head and neck malignancies are a major concern in our nation, accounting for around one-third of all cancer cases [7]. Head and neck cancer includes different types of cancer which are widely spread with common risk factors, namely, alcohol, tobacco and HPV infection [8]. In certain parts of India and Southeast Asia, the practice of blending tobacco with betel nuts has been related to head and neck squamous cell carcinoma (HNSCC). More than 200 million individuals are thought to padlock in this practice around the world, coming to a 2.8-times higher hazard of creating HNSCC, and this increments to more than 10 times when smoking is additionally practiced [9]. Tobacco products have been around for millennia, but only in the last 60-70 years, we have gained a better knowledge of their harmful consequences (Table. **1**). This new knowledge has paved the way for educational and regulatory initiatives targeted at lowering cigarette consumption. Many carcinogens are thought to damage DNA structure by forming DNA adducts, which is thought to be a frequent mutagenesis route. Moreover, oxidative-induced lesions and damages occur, in protein cross-linked by carcinogens [10]. The different types of head and neck cancer are presented in Table. **1**.

Table. (1). Different types of head and neck cancer, their symptoms and associated genes.

Type of Cancer	Area Affected	Gene Involved	Symptoms	Reference
Oropharyngeal cancer	Oropharynx	TP53	Sore throat, trouble in swallowing, ear pain, & lump in the back of mouth or throat	[11] [12]
Hypopharyngeal cancer	Hypopharynx (bottom part of the throat)	p16	Change in voice, hoarseness, & trouble in breathing	[13] [14]
Laryngeal cancer	Larynx	p16	Hoarseness, & pain while swallowing	[15] [16]
Lip and Oral cavity cancer	Any part of the mouth	TP53	Chronic sore throat, swelling of lips, gums, cheek, & patches in the mouth, & bleeding in the mouth	[12] [17]
Nasopharyngeal cancer	Nasopharynx (upper part of the throat)	MST1R	Lump in the neck, blood in saliva, nasal congestion, headache, & frequent ear infections	[18] [19]
Paranasal sinus and Nasal cavity cancer	Any of the sinuses	-	Nasal discharge, & bleeding from the nose	[20]
Salivary gland cancer	Any of the salivary gland	AR	Difficulty in opening mouth, weak facial muscles on one side of face, persistent pain in salivary gland, & rapid tumour growth	[21] [22] [23]
Squamous cell neck cancer	Outermost surface of the skin	P53	Firm red nodule, ulcer, scaly patch inside the mouth, & itching	[24] [25]
Soft tissue sarcoma	Soft tissues	PTCH1	Noticeable lump, & pain	[26] [27]
Thyroid cancer	Thyroid cells	RAS, BRAF	Lump in the neck, change in voice, difficulty in swallowing, & pain in the throat.	[28] [29]

[**Abbreviations**: TP53, tumour suppressor gene; MST1R, macrophage stimulating 1 receptor; AR, androgen receptor; PTCH1, protein patched homolog; RAS, Rat sarcoma virus; BRAF, B-Raf proto-oncogene serine / threonine-protein kinase]

3. HISTORICAL PERSPECTIVE OF CANCER TREATMENTS

Chemotheraphy, radiotheraphy, and targeted drug therapy have taken a role in treating the cancer. Since the day cancer evolved, the history of head and neck cancer advanced and underwent many adjustments on the flip of the century. Starting from the historical instances, there have been texts on the way to deal with and study patients. Two of the oldest medical manuscripts that discussed the management of cancer patients are the Edwin Smith and Ebers Papyrus. The term "cancer" was coined by Hippocrates. Hippocrates clarified cancer treatments and skin cancer in his doctrine [30]. Hippocrates and Galen were credited with identifying cancer as a disease caused by an imbalance of the four primary bodily humours: phlegm, yellow, blood, and black bile. Hippocrates hypothesised that when there is a larger amount of black bile secretion, it initiates cancer [31]. For superficial tumor types, cancer therapy was primarily centred on the adoption of a healthy diet, cautery, and radical surgical techniques [32]. There was a lot of fresh information on how to treat such oral cancer in the 17th century, compared with 16th century. Cancer of the tongue was treated with cauterization, which was later substituted using surgical tools in the 18th century. The 19th century saw tremendous advances in surgical, diagnostic, and anaesthetic procedures, as well as a better knowledge of causes of the disease. One cancer treatment technique that gained popularity is Modified Radical Neck Dissection (MRND) [30]. When there is evidence of more widespread lymph node metastasis, this sort of neck dissection is undertaken. In the case of neck dissection, in 1885, Botlin elucidated the benefits of removing glands of the neck in the treatment of head and neck cancer. These fearless, and careful endeavours to destroy the disease were, to a great extent, with serious patient grimness and mortality. The standards of sedation were destitute and there were no facilities for blood transfusion or anti-toxins. Also, the enormous areas of tissue that were taken out, brought about huge injuries that were habitually unfit to be shut agreeably [9].

Initially, the two scientists, namely Rontgen and Becquerel looked into using X-rays for diagnostic purposes, but subsequently discovered that they were harmful to cells, hinting that they may be used to treat cancer [33]. In 1920, Claudius Regaud proved that radiation fractionation could be used to treat a variety of human tumors while reducing the treatment's side effects [34]. Despite these accomplishments, prior to World War II, medicinal and interventional therapies treating tumors were primarily radical methods aimed at eradicating the illness completely before it could spread and cause metastasis throughout the body. As a result, in patients with advanced tumor pathology or when the surgical act failed, surgical therapy, which is frequently the only therapeutic alternative despite its devastating potential, was useless [35]. In the mid-nineteenth century, the introduction of chemotherapy and subsequent advancements in modern medical tumor therapy marked a watershed movement in cancer treatment. Further, the discovery and production of novel chemicals laid the groundwork for the development of effective therapeutic approaches in patients with advanced solid tumors of various types or haematological drug regimens, either alone or in combination with surgery and radiotherapy [33].

Shortly after World War II, new therapeutic strategies for the treatment of malignancies were found, focusing on the use of chemicals that mirrored the structure of normal metabolite, interrupting the enzyme chains required for purine synthesis and thus suppressing cell development. The most frequent anti-metabolites are folate analogues (methotrexate & aminopterin), and pyrimidine analogues (fluorouracil, capecitabine, & gemcitabine), purine analogues (mercaptopurine) [36]. Following that, the finding of gene alterations responsible for neoplastic transformation led to advances in DNA structure and the development of new molecular methods for DNA analysis [37].

In addition, novel anti-tumor therapy techniques utilising new biotechnology pharmaceuticals have been created in the previous 20 years. These tactics have considerably improved the efficacy of cancer therapies as well as cancer patient's survival rates. Monoclonal antibodies (mAbs) and novel immunotherapeutic medicines have enabled the development of new individualised therapeutic regimens (personalised medicine) with extremely high effectiveness and little toxicity for cancer patients [38] (Fig. **1**).

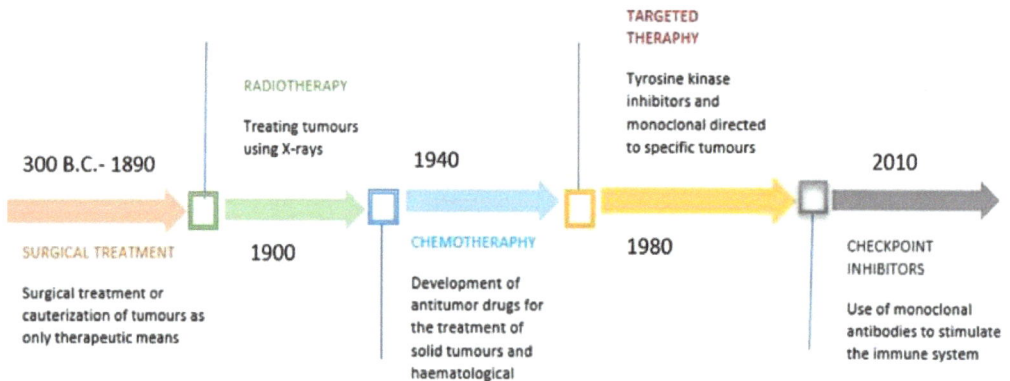

Fig. (1). Schematic representation of different types of cancer treatments (from the year 1890-2010)

Finally, several research institutions have been producing therapeutic anticancer vaccines based on the unique features of the tumour in order to boost the immune system's anticancer action and identify how cancer cells die. Vaccination induces an increase in immunological response in this technique, resulting in their eradication. However, due to the heterogeneity that distinguishes each tumor, the development of these vaccines is difficult [39]. The type of treatment primarily depends on the location of tumor, phase of the tumor, victim's age and his other wellbeing conditions. The essential treatment of cancer is performed by specialists.

4. GUT MICROBIOTA DYSBIOSIS IN HEAD AND NECK CANCER

Head and neck squamous cell carcinoma (HNSCC) has occupied the sixth position among the common cancer-affected the human population worldwide [40]. HNSCC is mainly originated from the epithelial cells of laryngeal, oropharynx, mouth and lips. Alcohol, obesity, smoking, tobacco chewing and inflammation modify the microbiota in diverse anatomic sites [41].

In head and neck cancer, bacterial infection mediated especially the oral pathogens *Porphyromonas gingivalis* and *F. nucleatum* evidenced to promote the tumor development in mice [42]. Further the microbiome enriched with *Fusobacterium, Leptotrichia, Selenomonas* and *Treponema* in oral HNSCC, as per the report [43]. The gut microbiota alter the metabolic phenotype and influence the innate immunity which leads to various disorders including malignancy. The inflammation in oral cavity called 'peridontitis' is linked to various cancers including oesophageal and oropharyngeal [44]. Various molecular databases including the Microbial Kyoto Encyclopedia of Genes and Genomes (KEGG) pathway and protein network mechanisms has played a pivotal in understanding the development of HNSCC [43]. As per the recent report the dysbiosis in oral microbiota promotes the oral HNSCC development [45].

5. ROLE OF PROBIOTICS IN TREATMENT OF HEAD AND NECK CANCER

Cancer, the deadly malignant tumor and the leading cause of disease and death, has no appropriate cure till now [1]. However, current clinical management uses the standard drug as treatment. Nevertheless, stability, long-term safety of these synthetic and various chemotherapeutic agents is uncertain. In addition, these cytotoxic medicines are related to severe facet side effects that are sometimes worse than the malignancy of cancer itself (that affect cell division, cause nausea, damage to mouth and pharynx mucosa, and fatigue). These drugs impair quality of life or contribute to the event of drug resistance and do not seem to be cheap for many patients. Therefore, probiotics have attracted much attention due to their ability to modulate cancer cell proliferation and apoptosis, which has been studied both *in vitro* and *in vivo*. The potential application of these properties in novel therapies could be an alternative to more invasive treatments such as chemotherapy and radiotherapy [2]. These are used as drugs or dietary supplements to help in maintaining the health-promoting microbial balance in the digestive tract of humans and other hosts [1]. Probiotics are relatively cheaper and readily available to cancer patients without any prescription restrictions [3]. Due to their unique properties, probiotics can reduce the risk and severity of chemotherapy, surgery, and radiation-related toxicity associated with radiation therapy, thus reducing the side effects associated with cancer treatment. Other unique properties of probiotics are that they slow down tumorigenesis and inhibit the proliferation of cancer cells [3]. The effects of different probiotics on animal models of cancer are shown in Table. **2**.

Table. (2). General effects of probiotics on tumour-bearing or tumour-induced animal models *in vivo*.

Probiotic Strain	Model	Induction	Result	References
Lactobacillus acidophilus, *Lactobacillus casei* *Lactobacillus lactis biovar diacetylactis* DRC-1	Rat	DMH	↓TI; ↓TV; ↓ TM	[46]
*Bifidobacterium lactis*KCTC 5727	SPF C57BL rat	DLD-1 cells injection	↓ TI; ↓ TV	[47]
Bacillus polyfermenticus	CD-1 mice	TNBS	↓ TI; ↓ TV	[48]
Lactobacillus rhamnosus GG MTCC #1408 *Lactobacillus acidophilus* NCDC #1	SD rats	TNBS	↓ TI; ↓ TM	[49]
Lactobacillus plantarum	BALB/c mice	AOM, DSS	↓TI, cell cycle arrest Induction of apoptosis.	[50]
Lactobacillus plantarum	BALB/c mice	CT26 cells injection	↓TV, Induction of necrosis.	[51]
Lactobacillus plantarum (AdF10) *Lactobacillus rhamnosus* GG	SD rats	DMH 4 weeks	↓TI; ↓TV; ↓ TM	[52]
Lactobacillus salivarius Ren	F344 rats	DMH 10 weeks	↓ TI	[53]
Lactobacillus acidophilus *Bifidobacteria bifidum* *Bifidobacteria infantum*	SD rats	antibiotics DMH	↓ TI; ↓ TV	[54]
Lactobacillus rhamnosus GG CGMCC 1.2134	SD rats	DMH 10 weeks	↓ TI; ↓ TV; ↓ TM, and induction of apoptosis.	[55]

(Table 2) cont.....

Probiotic Strain	Model	Induction	Result	References
Pediococcus pentosaceus GS4	Swiss albino mice	-	↓ TP and induction of apoptosis	[56]
Lactobacillus casei BL23	C57BL/6 mice	-	↓ TI	[57]

[**Abbreviations:** ↓, Decrease; TI, tumour incidence; TV, tumour volume; TM, tumour multiplicity; TP, tumour progression; AOM, azoxymethane; DMH, 1,2 dimethylhydrazine dihydrochloride; DSS, dextran sulphate sodium; TNBS, trinitrobenzene sulfonic acid; SD rat, Sprague-Dawley rat]

Probiotics are mainly classified into microorganisms or strains of microorganisms and lactic and non-lactic yeasts. *Lactococcus, Bifidobacterium, Lactobacillus,* and *Enterococcus* are common bacterial probiotics. In addition, *Bacteroidales, Bacillus* spp, *Escherichia coli, Enterococci* and *Weissella* spp, *Clostridiales, Saccharomyces cerevisiae var. debaryomyces, Hanseniaspora,* and *Metschni-kowia boulardii, Candida, Kluyveromyces, Pichia,* are accepted as potential probiotic bacteria and yeasts [3]. The main mechanisms of action of probiotics for antitumor and anti-mutagenic activity include: binding, degradation and inhibition of the effector by probiotics; interference with carcinogens and converting toxic and reactive carcinogens into non-toxic compounds and their removal; lowering the pH in the gut due to short-chain fatty acids (SCFAs) formed during the breakdown of indigestible carbohydrates; modulation and enhancing host immunity through the secretion of anti-inflammatory molecules [3]. In a systematic retrospective study, currently administered probiotic strains (mainly *Bifidobacterium & Lactobacillus*) with specific dosage (additional daily dose not to exceed 5.0×10^{10} CFU/day, mean 2.0×10^9 CFU/day) showed no serious side effects. The results suggest that it is safe to use these probiotics in immunocompromised patients [58].

Thyroid carcinoma is the most common endocrine malignancy of the head and neck. It has also been established that probiotics modulation of the gut microbiome has a valuable approach in the management of thyroid cancer [59]. In addition, oral mucositis is a common and severe side effect in head and neck cancer patients who are treated with radiation and chemotherapy [15]. It interferes with normal eating and oral hygiene activities. When probiotic pills containing *L. brevis* CD2 (Table. **3**) were given to adult patients during and after the acute phases of the cancer treatment, both the frequency and severity of mucositis decreased significantly compared to the placebo group in a randomized double-blind research [15]. *Bifidobacterium breve* lw01 probiotic exerted anticancer effect on head and neck cancer cells by releasing exopolysaccharides (EPSs), thereby controlling the cell cycle arrest and cell death (Table. **3**) [3]. The *Lactobacillus brevis* helps in preventing radiation mucositis in people with head and neck cancer. Researchers conducted a parallel, randomized, double-blind, placebo-controlled study on 46 patients who had undergone radiation therapy for head and neck malignancies [16]. Patients were assigned standard treatment with *Bacillus clausii* UBBC07 or standard treatment with placebo [16]. *B. clausii* UBBC07 was administered as an oral suspension with 2 billion spores twice a day for 30 days or until all radiation fractions were completed. The study showed that the treatment effectively reduced oral mucosal inflammation through restoration of disturbed microflora, anti-inflammatory effects and enhanced immunity [16]. Xia *et al.* [13] found that administering the patients with a probiotic cocktail containing *L. plantarum* MH-301,10^9 CFU, *B. animalis* subsp. *Lactis* LPL-RH, 10^9 CFU, *L. rhamnosus* LGG-18,10^9 CFU, and *L. acidophilus* 10^9 CFU for 7 weeks (one capsule, 2 times a day) from the first day of chemoradiotherapy, significantly reduced the severity of oral mucositis. According to Chattopadhyay *et al.* [13], oral glutamine (OG) delayed the beginning of oral mucositis (20 days for the test group and 11.6 days for the control). In the probiotic-treated group, the onset was 10 days, while in the placebo-controlled group, it was 8 days.

Table. (3). Effects of different probiotics and their metabolites on head and neck cancer.

Probiotics	Type of Cancer	Mode of Metabolites Supplement	Effect	Reference
Lactobacillus brevis CD2	Head and neck cancer	as pills	Changed gut microbiota composition after 2 months of MD plus probiotics	[59]
Lactobacillus lactis	Nasopharyngeal carcinoma	-	Enhanced the immune response of patients and reduced the severity of oral mucositis through modification of gut microbiota	[60]
Streptococcus salivarius M18	Head and neck cancer	-	Probiotic intervention changed oral health and the composition of the plaque and saliva bacterial communities	[61]
Bifidobacterium. breve lw01	Head and neck cancer	EPA (Exopolysaccharide)	Regulated cell cycle arrest and cell apoptosis promotion	[62]
Saccharomyces boulardii	Oropharyngeal cancer T3 N2 MO	Amphotericin B 60mg/day for 4 weeks	Decreased the fever and after 6 months, partial remission of the tumor with no signs of residual infection	[63]

(Table 3) cont.....

Probiotics	Type of Cancer	Mode of Metabolites Supplement	Effect	Reference
Acetobacter syzygii, Lactobacillus acidophilus	Squamous cell carcinoma of the oral cavity	Pronase and lipase	Metabolites of *A. syzygii* induced apoptosis	[64]

Furthermore, butyrate is generated by *Firmicutes* species *(Ruminococcaceae, Lachnospiraceae, & Clostridiaceae)* and is the most studied of SCFAs and have been shown to decrease proliferation and increase apoptosis in cancer cells *in vitro* [12]. Nissle's (1917) experiment with *E. coli* bacteria in mice revealed that large numbers of bacterial cells congregate in tumors, suggesting that probiotic bacteria could be a tumor-targeted delivery system that could be used in immunocompromised patients.

Periodontal pathogens such as *Fusobacterium periodonticum, Filifactor alocis, Bulleidia extraextructa, Eubacterium infirmum, Gemella morbillorum, Streptococcus constellatus,* and *Streptococcus intermedius,* promote oral epithelial cell neoplasm progression, development, and metastasis; these have been reversed by bacteriocin or nisin treatment which acts as an antitumor agent [14]. Bacteriocin/nisin is produced by bound probiotics such as *Bifidobacterium* and *Lactobacillus, Lactococcus, Streptococcus, etc* [15]. Squamous cell carcinoma treated with increasing concentrations of nisin ZP enhanced apoptosis and decreased cell proliferation, clonogenic capacity, and sphere formation [16]. To analyze the *in vivo* relevance of the *in vitro* findings, a mouse model of the oral floor simulating human OSCC was used. Mice that received Nisin ZP (800 mg/kg b.w. daily) had a significant reduction in the tumor volume and suppressed the pathogen-induced tumorigenesis without affecting the mice [17].

Squamous cell malignant neoplastic disease of the mouth includes 94% of all malignancies. Probiotic microorganisms *Acidobacter syzygii* and *Lactobacillus acidophilus,* exerted an anti-proliferative impact by secretion of metabolites pronase and lipase (Table. **3**). The administration of these secretions was dose-dependent. Therefore, the LC50 concentration of each metabolite secretion was tested on each cancer cell *(Acidobacter syzygii:* 60 µg/mL and *Lactobacillus acidophilus*: 10 µg/mL) and normal cells *(Acidobacter syzygii:* 10 µg/mL and *Lactobacillus acidophilus*: 80 µg/mL). The results showed that the metabolites caused high toxicity in cancer cells, whereas there was no significant effect on the normal cells [18].

Cancer patients are at increased risk of infection due to immunodeficiency and damage to the epithelium of the oral and gastrointestinal tract (GIT) as well as damage to the epithelium of the GIT from chemotherapy or radiation therapy. A patient with oropharyngeal epithelial malignancy received an extensive regimen before surgery and after chemotherapy; and underwent a lengthy and strenuous surgery. One week after the surgery, the jejunal screen was removed. The PEG nasogastric tube collection began three days after surgery. However, the patient had a fever above 40°C, and exhibited increased white blood cell (WBC) count and CRP. Therefore, each oral and PEG intake were stopped, and a couple of completely different sorts of probiotic (powder form of Biofermin-R, fine granules of *Lactobacillus* and myaBM, *Clostridium*) were introduced to raise the normal intestinal flora. The patient's fever and different inflammatory reactions decreased to normal ranges. One week after, the oral intake of probiotics was started, and the patient had no fever or inflammation, with a stable scenario [19].

6. MODE OF DELIVERY OF PROBIOTICS

Probiotic delivery systems are nutritional products widely used to replenish the natural gut flora. The effectiveness of these delivery systems varies considerably in producing beneficial effects on patient health. Probiotic delivery systems can be classified into conventional pharmaceutical formulations and unique commercial food products (Fig. **2**) [65]. Pharmaceutical formulations for probiotic use currently include, among others, granules, capsules and tablets (pills). Different ways of encapsulation are explored by the researchers, along with the trade for encapsulation of various ingredients of interest (Fig. **3**) [66].

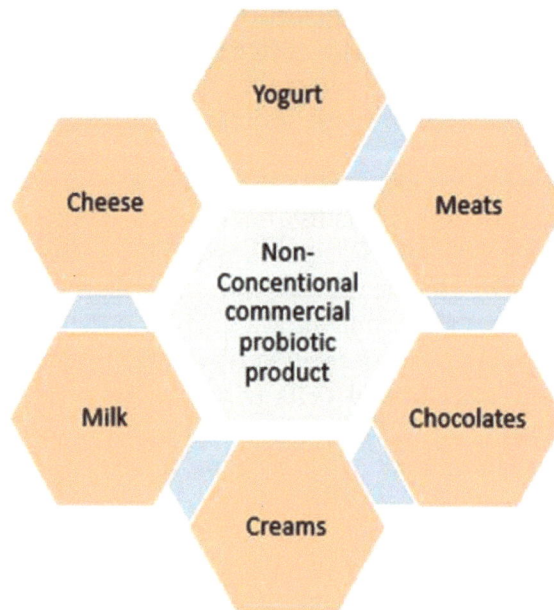

Fig. (2). Non-commercial products of probiotics.

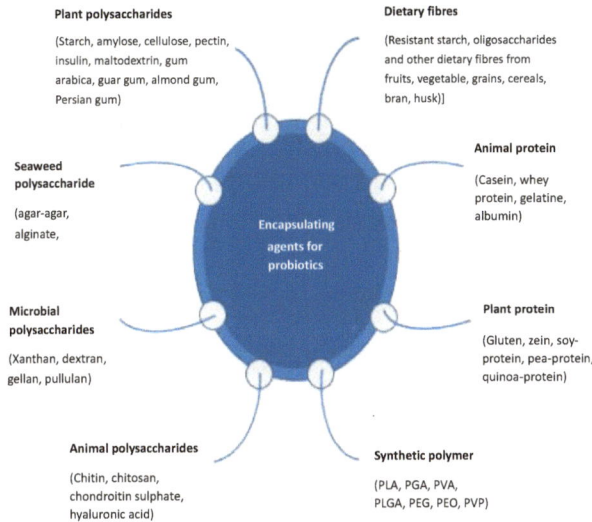

Fig. (3). Different types of agents used for encapsulating probiotics.

7. FUTURE PERSPECTIVE

As radiotherapy and chemotherapy had high and long-term side effects, especially mucositis in oropharynx, the probiotics-based treatment has a high prospective in treating cancer, especially head and neck cancer. The researchers are initiated a various dimensions to treat the head and neck cancer including probiotics and immunotherapy methods. A growing research interest indicated that microbiota plays a significant role in the development and curability of cancer. The probiotic organisms modulate immune and inflammatory responses in cancer and can serve as potential cancer therapeutics. For example, the administration of *L. plantarum* and *L. casei* inhibited cell proliferation and apoptosis [67, 68]. Especially, *L. brevis* CD2 worked well against the adverse effects in patients with head and neck squamous cell carcinoma. Probiotics can also be used as a vector for drug delivery or gene therapy in the field of cancer treatment. Further, the engineered probiotic bacteria can be delivered at the tumor site by exploiting the affinity of anaerobic strains for anaerobic tumor microenvironment. Hence, the probiotics as prominent tool play a pivotal role in the treatment of cancer, especially head and neck cancer.

CONCLUSION

The consumption of probiotics mediated through food and supplement, is a feasible and the cheapest way to prevent the cancer onset, and progression and mitigate the side effects generated through the current anticancer treatment such as chemo- and radiotherapy. Probiotic such as *Lactobacillus casei* has shown decreased carcinogenesis, increased cytotoxic T lymphocytes as well as decreased oropharyngeal mucositis in head and neck cancer patients. Moreover, *L. brevis* CD2 decreased the incidence and severity of oral mucositis in head and neck cancer patients. Collectively, microbiota manipulation, especially probiotics, can prevent the cancer onset, improve clinical efficacy and mitigate the adverse effect of anticancer therapies.

CONSENT FOR PUBLICATION

Not applicable.

CONFLICT OF INTEREST

The authors declare no conflict of interest, financial or otherwise.

ACKNOWLEDGEMENTS

The authors are grateful to the management and authorities of Sri Sathya Sai University for Human Excellence, for their encouragement and support for the publication of this chapter.

REFERENCES

[1]   Argiris A, Karamouzis MV, Raben D, Ferris RL. Head and neck cancer. Lancet 2008; 371(9625): 1695-709.
        [http://dx.doi.org/10.1016/S0140-6736(08)60728-X] [PMID: 18486742]

[2]   St John MAR, Abemayor E, Wong DTW. Recent new approaches to the treatment of head and neck cancer. Anticancer Drugs 2006; 17(4): 365-75.
        [http://dx.doi.org/10.1097/01.cad.0000198913.75571.13] [PMID: 16549993]

[3]   Mody MD, Rocco JW, Yom SS, Haddad RI, Saba NF. Head and neck cancer. Lancet 2021; 398(10318): 2289-99.
        [http://dx.doi.org/10.1016/S0140-6736(21)01550-6] [PMID: 34562395]

[4]   Squamous Cell Carcinoma: Pictures, Symptoms, and More. https://www.healthline.com/health/squamous-cell-skin-cancer (accessed Apr. 25, 2022).

[5]   Kechagia M, Basoulis D, Konstantopoulou S, *et al.* Health benefits of probiotics: a review. ISRN Nutr 2013; 2013: 1-7.
        [http://dx.doi.org/10.5402/2013/481651] [PMID: 24959545]

[6]   Zielińska D, Kołożyn-Krajewska D. Food-Origin Lactic Acid Bacteria May Exhibit Probiotic Properties: Review. BioMed Res Int 2018; 2018: 1-15.
        [http://dx.doi.org/10.1155/2018/5063185] [PMID: 30402482]

[7]   Shah SB, Sharma S, D'Cruz AK. Head and neck oncology: The Indian scenario. South Asian J Cancer 2016; 5(3): 104-5.
        [http://dx.doi.org/10.4103/2278-330X.187572] [PMID: 27606291]

[8]   B. R, M. S, G. A, and P. Tk, Role of tobacco in the development of head and neck squamous cell carcinoma in an eastern Indian population, Asian Pac. J. Cancer Prev. APJCP, vol. 9, no. 3, 2008,

Accessed: 25, 2022. [Online]. Available: https://pubmed.ncbi.nlm.nih.gov/18990006/

[9] Chin D, Boyle GM, Porceddu S, Theile DR, Parsons PG, Coman WB. Head and neck cancer: past, present and future. Expert Rev Anticancer Ther 2006; 6(7): 1111-8.
[http://dx.doi.org/10.1586/14737140.6.7.1111] [PMID: 16831082]

[10] Jethwa AR, Khariwala SS. Tobacco-related carcinogenesis in head and neck cancer. Cancer Metastasis Rev 2017; 36(3): 411-23.
[http://dx.doi.org/10.1007/s10555-017-9689-6] [PMID: 28801840]

[11] Jamal Z, Anjum F. Oropharyngeal Squamous Cell Carcinoma.StatPearls. Treasure Island, FL: StatPearls Publishing 2022. [Online] http://www.ncbi.nlm.nih.gov/books/NBK563268/

[12] Usman S, Jamal A, Teh M-T, Waseem A. Major Molecular Signaling Pathways in Oral Cancer Associated With Therapeutic Resistance 2021. https://www.frontiersin.org/article/10.3389/froh.2020.603160
[http://dx.doi.org/10.3389/froh.2020.603160]

[13] Sanders O, Pathak S. Hypopharyngeal Cancer.StatPearls. Treasure Island, FL: StatPearls Publishing 2022. [Online] http://www.ncbi.nlm.nih.gov/books/NBK567720/

[14] Wendt M, Romanitan M, Näsman A, *et al.* Presence of human papillomaviruses and p16 expression in hypopharyngeal cancer. Head Neck 2014; 36(1): 107-12.
[http://dx.doi.org/10.1002/hed.23394] [PMID: 23737140]

[15] Koroulakis A, Agarwal M. Laryngeal Cancer.StatPearls. Treasure Island, FL: StatPearls Publishing 2022. [Online] http://www.ncbi.nlm.nih.gov/books/NBK526076/

[16] What Causes Laryngeal Cancer? https://www.webmd.com/cancer/laryngeal-cancer-causes (accessed Apr. 25, 2022).

[17] Oral Cancer: Symptoms, Causes, Treatments, and More. https://www.webmd.com/oral-health/guide/oral-cancer (accessed Apr. 25, 2022).

[18] Wu L, Li C, Pan L. Nasopharyngeal carcinoma: A review of current updates. Exp Ther Med 2018; 15(4): 3687-92.
[http://dx.doi.org/10.3892/etm.2018.5878] [PMID: 29556258]

[19] Yu G, Hsu WL, Coghill AE, *et al.* Whole-Exome Sequencing of Nasopharyngeal Carcinoma Families Reveals Novel Variants Potentially Involved in Nasopharyngeal Carcinoma. Sci Rep 2019; 9(1): 9916.
[http://dx.doi.org/10.1038/s41598-019-46137-4] [PMID: 31289279]

[20] Boulton CH. Equine nasal cavity and paranasal sinus disease: A review of 85 cases. J Equine Vet Sci 1985; 5(5): 268-75.
[http://dx.doi.org/10.1016/S0737-0806(85)80062-9]

[21] To VSH, Chan JYW, Tsang RKY, Wei WI. Review of salivary gland neoplasms. ISRN Otolaryngol 2012; 2012: 1-6.
[http://dx.doi.org/10.5402/2012/872982] [PMID: 23724273]

[22] Williams L, Thompson LDR, Seethala RR, *et al.* Salivary duct carcinoma: the predominance of apocrine morphology, prevalence of histologic variants, and androgen receptor expression. Am J Surg Pathol 2015; 39(5): 705-13.
[http://dx.doi.org/10.1097/PAS.0000000000000413] [PMID: 25871467]

[23] Dalin M, Watson P, Ho A, Morris L. Androgen Receptor Signaling in Salivary Gland Cancer. Cancers (Basel) 2017; 9(12): 17.
[http://dx.doi.org/10.3390/cancers9020017] [PMID: 28208703]

[24] Amri K. Squamous Cell Carcinoma: Causes, Symptoms & Treatment | USA Health Articles 2021. https://usahealtharticles.com/squamous-cell-carcinoma/

[25] Sugerman PB, Joseph BK, Savage NW. The role of oncogenes, tumour suppressor genes and growth factors in oral squamous cell carcinoma: a case of apoptosis *versus* proliferation. Oral Dis 1995; 1(3):

172-88.
[http://dx.doi.org/10.1111/j.1601-0825.1995.tb00181.x] [PMID: 8705824]

[26]   Rougraff BT, Lawrence J, Davis K. Length of symptoms before referral: prognostic variable for high-grade soft tissue sarcoma? Clin Orthop Relat Res 2012; 470(3): 706-11.
[http://dx.doi.org/10.1007/s11999-011-2192-4] [PMID: 22183474]

[27]   Ping XL, Ratner D, Zhang H, *et al.* PTCH mutations in squamous cell carcinoma of the skin. J Invest Dermatol 2001; 116(4): 614-6.
[http://dx.doi.org/10.1046/j.1523-1747.2001.01301.x] [PMID: 11286632]

[28]   Nguyen QT, Lee EJ, Huang MG, Park YI, Khullar A, Plodkowski RA. Diagnosis and treatment of patients with thyroid cancer. Am Health Drug Benefits 2015; 8(1): 30-40.
[PMID: 25964831]

[29]   Kopczyńska E, Junik R, Tyrakowski T. [BRAF gene mutation in thyroid cancer]. Pol Merkuriusz Lek 2006; 20(116): 210-3.
[PMID: 16708643]

[30]   Woźniak A, Szyfter K, Szyfter W, Florek E. [Head and neck cancer--history]. Przegl Lek 2012; 69(10): 1079-83.
[PMID: 23421095]

[31]   Tsoucalas G, Sgantzos M. Hippocrates (ca 460-370 BC) on nasal cancer p. 4.

[32]   Faguet GB. A brief history of cancer: Age-old milestones underlying our current knowledge database. Int J Cancer 2015; 136(9): 2022-36.
[http://dx.doi.org/10.1002/ijc.29134] [PMID: 25113657]

[33]   Arruebo M, Vilaboa N, Sáez-Gutierrez B, *et al.* Assessment of the evolution of cancer treatment therapies. Cancers (Basel) 2011; 3(3): 3279-330.
[http://dx.doi.org/10.3390/cancers3033279] [PMID: 24212956]

[34]   Moulder JE, Seymour C. Radiation fractionation: the search for isoeffect relationships and mechanisms. Int J Radiat Biol 2018; 94(8): 743-51.
[http://dx.doi.org/10.1080/09553002.2017.1376764] [PMID: 28967281]

[35]   Hajdu SI. A note from history: Landmarks in history of cancer, part 1. Cancer 2011; 117(5): 1097-102.
[http://dx.doi.org/10.1002/cncr.25553] [PMID: 20960499]

[36]   Tiwari M. Antimetabolites: Established cancer therapy. J Cancer Res Ther 2012; 8(4): 510-9.
[http://dx.doi.org/10.4103/0973-1482.106526] [PMID: 23361267]

[37]   Krause DS, Van Etten RA. Tyrosine kinases as targets for cancer therapy N. Engl. J. Med., 14;353 (2): 172-87.
[http://dx.doi.org/10.1056/NEJMra044389]

[38]   Scott AM, Allison JP, Wolchok JD. Monoclonal antibodies in cancer therapy 2012.

[39]   Falzone L, Salomone S, Libra M. Evolution of Cancer Pharmacological Treatments at the Turn of the Third Millennium. Front Pharmacol 2018; 9: 1300.
[http://dx.doi.org/10.3389/fphar.2018.01300] [PMID: 30483135]

[40]   Ferlay J, Colombet M, Soerjomataram I, *et al.* Estimating the global cancer incidence and mortality in 2018: GLOBOCAN sources and methods. Int J Cancer 2019; 144(8): 1941-53.
[http://dx.doi.org/10.1002/ijc.31937] [PMID: 30350310]

[41]   Chen J. J.C. Domingue CL Sears 2018. Microbiota Dysbiosis in select Human cancers: Evidence of Association and Casualty.PMD 28822617. Semin Immunol
[http://dx.doi.org/10.1016/j.smim.2017.08.001] [PMID: 28822617]

[42]   Gallimidi AB, Fischman S, Revach B, *et al.* Periodontal pathogens *Porphyromonas gingivalis* and *Fusobacterium nucleatum* promote tumor progression in an oral-specific chemical carcinogenesis model. Oncotarget 2015; 6(26): 22613-23.

[http://dx.doi.org/10.18632/oncotarget.4209] [PMID: 26158901]

[43]   Kim YK, Kwon EJ, Yu Y, *et al.* Microbial and molecular differences according to the location of head and neck cancers. Cancer Cell Int 2022; 22(1): 135.
[http://dx.doi.org/10.1186/s12935-022-02554-6] [PMID: 35346218]

[44]   Irfan M, Delgado RZR, Frias-Lopez J. The oral microbiome and cancer. Front Immunol 2020; 11591088
[http://dx.doi.org/10.3389/fimmu.2020.591088] [PMID: 33193429]

[45]   Frank DN, Qiu Y, Cao Y, *et al.* A dysbiotic microbiome promotes head and neck squamous cell carcinoma. Oncogene 2022; 41(9): 1269-80.
[http://dx.doi.org/10.1038/s41388-021-02137-1] [PMID: 35087236]

[46]   Kumar A, Singh NK, Sinha PR. Inhibition of 1,2-dimethylhydrazine induced colon genotoxicity in rats by the administration of probiotic curd. Mol Biol Rep 2010; 37(3): 1373-6.
[http://dx.doi.org/10.1007/s11033-009-9519-1] [PMID: 19330535]

[47]   Kim SW, Kim HM, Yang KM, *et al. Bifidobacterium lactis* inhibits NF-κB in intestinal epithelial cells and prevents acute colitis and colitis-associated colon cancer in mice. Inflamm Bowel Dis 2010; 16(9): 1514-25.
[http://dx.doi.org/10.1002/ibd.21262] [PMID: 20310012]

[48]   Altonsy MO, Andrews SC, Tuohy KM. Differential induction of apoptosis in human colonic carcinoma cells (Caco-2) by *Atopobium*, and commensal, probiotic and enteropathogenic bacteria: Mediation by the mitochondrial pathway. Int J Food Microbiol 2010; 137(2-3): 190-203.
[http://dx.doi.org/10.1016/j.ijfoodmicro.2009.11.015] [PMID: 20036023]

[49]   Verma A, Shukla G. Synbiotic (*Lactobacillus rhamnosus+Lactobacillus acidophilus*+inulin) attenuates oxidative stress and colonic damage in 1,2 dimethylhydrazine dihydrochloride-induced colon carcinogenesis in Sprague–Dawley rats. Eur J Cancer Prev 2014; 23(6): 550-9.
[http://dx.doi.org/10.1097/CEJ.0000000000000054] [PMID: 25025584]

[50]   Lee HA, Kim H, Lee KW, Park KY. Dead Nano-Sized *Lactobacillus plantarum* Inhibits Azoxymethane/Dextran Sulfate Sodium-Induced Colon Cancer in Balb/c Mice. J Med Food 2015; 18(12): 1400-5.
[http://dx.doi.org/10.1089/jmf.2015.3577] [PMID: 26595186]

[51]   Hu J, Wang C, Ye L, *et al.* Anti-tumour immune effect of oral administration of *Lactobacillus plantarum* to CT26 tumour-bearing mice. J Biosci 2015; 40(2): 269-79.
[http://dx.doi.org/10.1007/s12038-015-9518-4] [PMID: 25963256]

[52]   Walia S, Kamal R, Kanwar SS, Dhawan DK. Cyclooxygenase as a target in chemoprevention by probiotics during 1,2-dimethylhydrazine induced colon carcinogenesis in rats. Nutr Cancer 2015; 67(4): 603-11.
[http://dx.doi.org/10.1080/01635581.2015.1011788] [PMID: 25811420]

[53]   Zhang M, Fan X, Fang B, Zhu C, Zhu J, Ren F. Effects of *Lactobacillus salivarius* Ren on cancer prevention and intestinal microbiota in 1, 2-dimethylhydrazine-induced rat model. J Microbiol 2015; 53(6): 398-405.
[http://dx.doi.org/10.1007/s12275-015-5046-z] [PMID: 26025172]

[54]   Kuugbee ED, Shang X, Gamallat Y, *et al.* Structural Change in Microbiota by a Probiotic Cocktail Enhances the Gut Barrier and Reduces Cancer *via* TLR2 Signaling in a Rat Model of Colon Cancer. Dig Dis Sci 2016; 61(10): 2908-20.
[http://dx.doi.org/10.1007/s10620-016-4238-7] [PMID: 27384052]

[55]   Gamallat Y, Meyiah A, Kuugbee ED, *et al. Lactobacillus rhamnosus* induced epithelial cell apoptosis, ameliorates inflammation and prevents colon cancer development in an animal model. Biomed Pharmacother 2016; 83: 536-41.
[http://dx.doi.org/10.1016/j.biopha.2016.07.001] [PMID: 27447122]

[56]   Dubey V, Ghosh AR, Bishayee K, Kuda-Bukhsh AR. Bishayee and A.R. Kuda-Bukhsh, Appraisal of the anti-cancer potential of probiotic Pediococcus pentosaceus GS4 against colon cancer: invitro and invivo approaches 23, 2016
[http://dx.doi.org/10.1016/j.jff.2016.02.032]

[57]   Górska A, Przystupski D, Niemczura MJ, Kulbacka J. Probiotic Bacteria: A Promising Tool in Cancer Prevention and Therapy. Curr Microbiol 2019; 76(8): 939-49.
[http://dx.doi.org/10.1007/s00284-019-01679-8] [PMID: 30949803]

[58]   Lu K, Dong S, Wu X, Jin R, Chen H. Probiotics in Cancer 2021. https://www.frontiersin.org/article/10.3389/fonc.2021.638148
[http://dx.doi.org/10.3389/fonc.2021.638148]

[59]   Pellegrini M, Ippolito M, Monge T, *et al.* Gut microbiota composition after diet and probiotics in overweight breast cancer survivors: a randomized open-label pilot intervention trial. Nutrition 2020; 74110749
[http://dx.doi.org/10.1016/j.nut.2020.110749] [PMID: 32234652]

[60]   Jiang C, Wang H, Xia C, *et al.* A randomized, double-blind, placebo-controlled trial of probiotics to reduce the severity of oral mucositis induced by chemoradiotherapy for patients with nasopharyngeal carcinoma. Cancer 2019; 125(7): 1081-90.
[http://dx.doi.org/10.1002/cncr.31907] [PMID: 30521105]

[61]   Rakita A, Nikolić N, Mildner M, Matiasek J, Elbe-Bürger A. Re-epithelialization and immune cell behaviour in an *ex vivo* human skin model. Sci Rep 2020; 10(1): 1.
[http://dx.doi.org/10.1038/s41598-019-56847-4] [PMID: 31913322]

[62]   Wang L, Wang Y, Li Q, *et al.* Exopolysaccharide, Isolated From a Novel Strain *Bifidobacterium breve* lw01 Possess an Anticancer Effect on Head and Neck Cancer – Genetic and Biochemical Evidences 2019. https://www.frontiersin.org/article/10.3389/fmicb.2019.01044
[http://dx.doi.org/10.3389/fmicb.2019.01044]

[63]   Lu K, Dong S, Wu X, Jin R, Chen H. Probiotics in Cancer. Front Oncol 2021; 11638148
[http://dx.doi.org/10.3389/fonc.2021.638148] [PMID: 33791223]

[64]   Wan Mohd Kamaluddin WNF, Rismayuddin NAR, Ismail AF, *et al.* Probiotic inhibits oral carcinogenesis: A systematic review and meta-analysis. Arch Oral Biol 2020; 118104855
[http://dx.doi.org/10.1016/j.archoralbio.2020.104855] [PMID: 32801092]

[65]   Boyle RJ, Robins-Browne RM, Tang MLK. Probiotic use in clinical practice: what are the risks? Am J Clin Nutr 2006; 83(6): 1256-64.
[http://dx.doi.org/10.1093/ajcn/83.6.1256] [PMID: 16762934]

[66]   Yoha KS, Nida S, Dutta S, Moses JA, Anandharamakrishnan C. Targeted Delivery of Probiotics: Perspectives on Research and Commercialization. Probiotics Antimicrob Proteins 2022; 14(1): 15-48.
[http://dx.doi.org/10.1007/s12602-021-09791-7] [PMID: 33904011]

[67]   Jiang C, Wang H, Xia C, *et al.* A randomized, double-blind, placebo-controlled trial of probiotics to reduce the severity of oral mucositis induced by chemoradiotherapy for patients with nasopharyngeal carcinoma. Cancer 2019; 125(7): 1081-90.
[http://dx.doi.org/10.1002/cncr.31907] [PMID: 30521105]

[68]   De Sanctis V, Belgioia L, Cante D, *et al. Lactobacillus brevis* CD2 for Prevention of Oral Mucositis in Patients With Head and Neck Tumors: A Multicentric Randomized Study. Anticancer Res 2019; 39(4): 1935-42.
[http://dx.doi.org/10.21873/anticanres.13303] [PMID: 30952736]

SUBJECT INDEX

A

Acids 50, 75, 79, 80, 81, 120, 123, 126, 127, 190, 200, 217, 238
  butyric 123, 126
  conjugated linoleic 50, 80
  deoxyribonucleic 238
  gastric 120
  lipoic 75
  lipoteichoic 75, 81, 190, 217
  nucleic 127
  organic 200
Actinic keratosis (AK) 72, 74, 76
Actinomycetes 2
Action 18, 24, 25, 151, 242, 266
  antitumor 24, 25
  immune system's anticancer 266
  inflammatory 18
  inhibitory 151
  mucociliary 242
Activation 6, 47, 48, 49, 52, 53, 55, 80, 81, 121, 131, 132, 217, 250
  macrophage 53, 250
Activity 48, 53, 54, 81, 84, 94, 95, 97, 99, 103, 104, 105, 106, 110, 131, 133, 152, 155, 196, 197, 220, 242, 244, 246
  antagonistic 97, 244
  anti-inflammatory 95, 110
  antimicrobial 94, 95
  antioxidant 246
  anti-proliferative 84, 104, 110, 152
  anti-tumor 99, 131, 220
  carcinogenic 244
  glucosidase 48
  immunomodulatory 95, 155
  respiratory 242
Agents 3, 20, 81, 144, 215, 216, 267, 271, 273
  anti-cervical cancer 216
  antimicrobial 3
  antioxidant 81
  antitumor 271
  chemotherapeutic 267

Allergic reactions 250
Antiapoptotic proteins 17
Antibiotic therapy 56
Antigen-presenting cells (APCs) 47, 122, 131, 214
Anti-inflammatory 6, 47, 80, 81, 82, 99, 148, 195, 216, 249, 270
  cytokines 6, 80, 81, 148, 195, 216, 249
  effects 47, 82, 99, 270
Anti-mutagenic 53, 94, 95, 244, 248, 253, 269
  action 248, 253
  activity 244, 269
  effects 248
  properties 53, 94, 95, 248
Anti-proliferative 17, 47, 80, 218, 220
  effects 17, 80, 218, 220
  properties 47
Antitumor 16, 23, 42, 55, 190, 192, 197
  effects 23, 42, 197
  immunity 16, 55, 190, 192
Apoptosis 6, 50, 52, 53, 54, 80, 81, 103, 104, 124, 126, 127, 129, 130, 131, 151, 152, 154, 216, 218, 220, 238, 268
  cellular 80, 81
  epithelial cell 238
  gastric cell 6
  of adenocarcinoma cells 124, 127
  of cancerous cells 129
  regulating 130
  related proteins 126
Apoptotic responses 102, 103, 129
Arginine deiminase activity 82

B

Bacillus 125, 127, 128, 150, 247, 252, 253
  clausii 252
  licheniformis 125, 127
  mesentericus 128, 150
  subtilis 247, 252, 253
Bacterial 53, 74, 194,
  carcinogenesis 53

www.ingramcontent.com/pod-product-compliance
Lightning Source LLC
Chambersburg PA
CBHW050813220326
41598CB00006B/197